Diagnostic and Interventional Imaging in Various Diseases

Diagnostic and Interventional Imaging in Various Diseases

Guest Editors

Romica Cergan
Adrian Costache
Mihai Dumitru

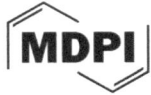

Basel • Beijing • Wuhan • Barcelona • Belgrade • Novi Sad • Cluj • Manchester

Guest Editors

Romica Cergan	Adrian Costache	Mihai Dumitru
Carol Davila University of Medicine and Pharmacy	Carol Davila University of Medicine and Pharmacy	Carol Davila University of Medicine and Pharmacy
Bucharest	Bucharest	Bucharest
Romania	Romania	Romania

Editorial Office
MDPI AG
Grosspeteranlage 5
4052 Basel, Switzerland

This is a reprint of the Special Issue, published open access by the journal *Medicina* (ISSN 1648-9144), freely accessible at: https://www.mdpi.com/journal/medicina/special_issues/1N0C43UEIB.

For citation purposes, cite each article independently as indicated on the article page online and as indicated below:

Lastname, A.A.; Lastname, B.B. Article Title. *Journal Name* **Year**, *Volume Number*, Page Range.

ISBN 978-3-7258-2729-9 (Hbk)
ISBN 978-3-7258-2730-5 (PDF)
https://doi.org/10.3390/books978-3-7258-2730-5

© 2024 by the authors. Articles in this book are Open Access and distributed under the Creative Commons Attribution (CC BY) license. The book as a whole is distributed by MDPI under the terms and conditions of the Creative Commons Attribution-NonCommercial-NoDerivs (CC BY-NC-ND) license (https://creativecommons.org/licenses/by-nc-nd/4.0/).

Contents

About the Editors vii

Preface ix

Romica Cergan, Mihai Dumitru and Adrian Costache
Diagnostic and Interventional Imaging in Various Diseases
Reprinted from: *Medicina* **2024**, *60*, 1810, https://doi.org/10.3390/medicina60111810 1

Alexandra Floriana Nemes, Adrian Ioan Toma, Vlad Dima, Sorina Crenguta Serboiu, Andreea Ioana Necula, Roxana Stoiciu, et al.
Use of Lung Ultrasound in Reducing Radiation Exposure in Neonates with Respiratory Distress: A Quality Management Project
Reprinted from: *Medicina* **2024**, *60*, 308, https://doi.org/10.3390/medicina60020308 4

Valentina Opancina, Nebojsa Zdravkovic, Slobodan Jankovic, Dragan Masulovic, Elisa Ciceri, Bojan Jaksic, et al.
Predictors of Intrahospital Mortality in Aneurysmal Subarachnoid Hemorrhage after Endovascular Embolization
Reprinted from: *Medicina* **2024**, *60*, 1134, https://doi.org/10.3390/medicina60071134 18

Jasmin J. Nukovic, Valentina Opancina, Elisa Ciceri, Mario Muto, Nebojsa Zdravkovic, Ahmet Altin, et al.
Neuroimaging Modalities Used for Ischemic Stroke Diagnosis and Monitoring
Reprinted from: *Medicina* **2023**, *59*, 1908, https://doi.org/10.3390/medicina59111908 30

Eugen Horatiu Stefanescu, Nicolae Constantin Balica, Sorin Bogdan Motoi, Laura Grigorita, Madalina Georgescu and Gheorghe Iovanescu
High-Resolution Computed Tomography in Middle Ear Cholesteatoma: How Much Do We Need It?
Reprinted from: *Medicina* **2023**, *59*, 1712, https://doi.org/10.3390/medicina59101712 45

Muhammad Qasim Javed, Swati Srivastava, Badi Baen Rashed Alotaibi, Usman Anwer Bhatti, Ayman M. Abulhamael and Syed Rashid Habib
A Cone Beam Computed Tomography-Based Investigation of the Frequency and Pattern of Radix Entomolaris in the Saudi Arabian Population
Reprinted from: *Medicina* **2023**, *59*, 2025, https://doi.org/10.3390/medicina59112025 55

Josefa Alarcón Apablaza, Gonzalo Muñoz, Carlos Arriagada, Cristina Bucchi, Telma S. Masuko and Ramón Fuentes
Odontoma Recurrence. The Importance of Radiographic Controls: Case Report with a 7-Year Follow-Up
Reprinted from: *Medicina* **2024**, *60*, 1248, https://doi.org/10.3390/medicina60081248 66

Crenguța Sorina Șerboiu, Cătălin Aliuș, Adrian Dumitru, Dana Țăpoi, Mariana Costache, Adriana Elena Nica, et al.
Gallbladder Pancreatic Heterotopia—The Importance of Diagnostic Imaging in Managing Intraoperative Findings
Reprinted from: *Medicina* **2023**, *59*, 1407, https://doi.org/10.3390/medicina59081407 77

Ramona-Andreea Rizescu, Iulia Alecsandra Sălcianu, Alexandru Șerbănoiu, Radu Tudor Ion, Lucian Mihai Florescu, Ioana-Andreea Gheonea, et al.
Can MRI Accurately Diagnose and Stage Endometrial Adenocarcinoma?
Reprinted from: *Medicina* **2024**, *60*, 512, https://doi.org/10.3390/medicina60030512 90

Beatrice Anghel, Crenguta Serboiu, Andreea Marinescu, Iulian-Alexandru Taciuc, Florin Bobirca and Anca Daniela Stanescu
Recent Advances and Adaptive Strategies in Image Guidance for Cervical Cancer Radiotherapy
Reprinted from: *Medicina* **2023**, *59*, 1735, https://doi.org/10.3390/medicina59101735 . . . . **100**

Alexandru Șerbănoiu, Rareș Nechifor, Andreea Nicoleta Marinescu, Gheorghe Iana, Ana Magdalena Bratu, Iulia Alecsandra Sălcianu, et al.
Prostatic Artery Origin Variability: Five Steps to Improve Identification during Percutaneous Embolization
Reprinted from: *Medicina* **2023**, *59*, 2122, https://doi.org/10.3390/medicina59122122 . . . . **120**

Isabela Ioana Loghin, Andrei Vâță, Ioana Florina Mihai, George Silvaș, Șerban Alin Rusu, Cătălina Mihaela Luca and Carmen Mihaela Dorobăț
Profile of Newly Diagnosed Patients with HIV Infection in North-Eastern Romania
Reprinted from: *Medicina* **2023**, *59*, 440, https://doi.org/10.3390/medicina59030440 . . . . **131**

About the Editors

Romica Cergan

Romica Cergan is an Associate Professor of Anatomy at Carol Davila University of Medicine and Pharmacy, Bucharest, Romania. He also holds the position of Head of the Radiology Department at Foisor Clinical Hospital in Bucharest. His research activity is illustrated by 38 articles published in journals indexed in Web of Science with a high impact factor and his Hirsch Index of 12. His focus is on CT and MRI use for complex pathologies, mainly orthopedic cases in the last few years. Knowing the anatomy enables the clinician to conduct a proper management of the pathology.

Adrian Costache

Adrian Costache is a Professor of Pathology at Carol Davila University of Medicine and Pharmacy, Bucharest, Romania. He also holds the position of Coordinator of the Ultrasound Teaching Unit at Cantacuzino Clinical Hospital in Bucharest. His research activity is illustrated by 35 articles published in journals indexed in Web of Science with a high impact factor and his Hirsch Index of 11. His focus is on ultrasonography used for complex pathologies and ultrasound-guided procedures. Currently, he has five PhD students under coordination with research in the fields of artificial intelligence, ultrasound-guided procedures, molecular diagnostics, and head and neck pathology.

Mihai Dumitru

Mihai Dumitru is a Senior Lecturer (full tenure track) of Otorhinolaryngology at Carol Davila University of Medicine and Pharmacy, Bucharest, Romania. He also holds the position of Consultant ENT Surgeon at Bucharest University Emergency Hospital. His research activity is illustrated by 45 articles published in journals indexed in Web of Science with a high impact factor and his Hirsch Index of 11. His focus is on head and neck oncology, ultrasonography in otorhinolaryngology, and artificial intelligence. Moreover, he has strong interdisciplinary activity with fellow allergologists, ophthalmologists, and pathologists.

Preface

The following Special Issue, entitled **Diagnostic and Interventional Imaging in Various Diseases**, presents current up-to-date applications of imaging modalities for solving complex pathologies. The modern approach to medicine is a team effort and there is an increasing tendency toward personalized medicine. This research will gain the attention of fellow specialists in various fields of activity: imaging, pathology, surgery, neurology, neurosurgery, otorhinolaryngology, dentistry, gynecology, urology, and radiotherapy. We would like to thank the contributing authors who hail from all over the world: Italy, Serbia, Romania, Saudi Arabia, Pakistan, Turkey, Slovenia, Mexico, Chile, and Brazil.

Romica Cergan, Adrian Costache, and Mihai Dumitru
Guest Editors

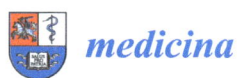

Editorial

Diagnostic and Interventional Imaging in Various Diseases

Romica Cergan [1], Mihai Dumitru [2,*] and Adrian Costache [3]

[1] Anatomy Department, Carol Davila University of Medicine and Pharmacy, 050474 Bucharest, Romania; r.cergan@gmail.com
[2] ENT Department, Carol Davila University of Medicine and Pharmacy, 050474 Bucharest, Romania
[3] Pathology Department, Carol Davila University of Medicine and Pharmacy, 050474 Bucharest, Romania; adriancostacheeco@yahoo.com
* Correspondence: orldumitrumihai@yahoo.com

Citation: Cergan, R.; Dumitru, M.; Costache, A. Diagnostic and Interventional Imaging in Various Diseases. *Medicina* **2024**, *60*, 1810. https://doi.org/10.3390/medicina60111810

Received: 29 October 2024
Accepted: 1 November 2024
Published: 4 November 2024

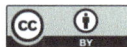

Copyright: © 2024 by the authors. Published by MDPI on behalf of the Lithuanian University of Health Sciences. Licensee MDPI, Basel, Switzerland. This article is an open access article distributed under the terms and conditions of the Creative Commons Attribution (CC BY) license (https://creativecommons.org/licenses/by/4.0/).

Diagnostic and interventional imaging is a cornerstone in the management of cases in various medical and surgical domains, such as neonatology, neurology, neurosurgery, otorhinolaryngology, dentistry, gynecology and urology.

Neonatal sonography is one of the newest instruments available in the diagnostic imaging newborns. The main advantage of performing lung sonography is that this imaging modality does not expose the newborn to radiation and permits serial imaging with the dynamic visualization of the progression or resolution of the pulmonary pathology. A recent study revealed that implementing lung sonography on a large scale diminished the dose of radiation by 30% per ventilated newborn [1]. It is therefore evident that sonography is the stethoscope of the future.

One domain that relies heavily on diagnostic and interventional imaging modalities is neuroimaging. Almost all improvements in the outcome and survival of neurology and neurosurgery patients in the last decade have been due to the extended availability of interventional neuroradiology procedures. However, when facing aneurysmal subarachnoid hemorrhage (ASAH), 19.7% of patients continue to die during hospitalization despite the use of endovascular interventions [2]. Moreover, ischemic stroke cases benefit from the use of a combination of contrast CT scans and MRI scans, which requires close cooperation between the neurologist and imaging specialist [3]. These data show that further improvements in both the pre-hospital and on-arrival management of patients with ASAH or ischemic stroke are required in order to reduce mortality rates further.

The viscerocranium is the anatomical region with the highest density of landmarks per voxel. The successful management of such cases relies on diagnostic imaging. Otorhinolaryngology and head and neck surgeons require numerous imaging modalities such as CT of the mastoid bone and cone beam CT of the sinuses. There is a good-to-excellent correlation between the findings of temporal bone high-resolution CT scans (HRCT) at the level of the mastoid bone and intraoperative lesions, particularly in tegmen tympani erosion, sigmoid plate dehiscence, malleus erosion, and scutum erosion [4]. The successful management of these cases at the level of the viscerocranium requires a multidisciplinary team of ear, nose and throat (ENT) surgeons, and dentists. Endodontic treatment should be conducted with careful cone beam CT imaging in order to prevent complications in cases with radix entomolaris [5]. Faster imaging equipment and targeted imaging protocols are necessary for the long-term follow up of such cases [6].

Emergency imaging requires trained diagnostic imaging specialists to be integrated into teams with general surgeons and pathologists. Without a complete imaging protocol, there are many anatomical variants that could result in the occurrence of complications and incidents during laparoscopic surgery [7].

Another task requiring extensive diagnostic procedures is the staging of oncological diseases. MRI is increasingly considered the gold standard for the presurgical staging of soft tissue tumors. Endometrial carcinoma can be detected on T2-weighted images taken after intravenous gadolinium chelates bolus caused by variations in vascularity; these images can be compared to the myometrium in order to differentiate it from the fluid filling the endometrial cavity. These real-life data show that the contrast of these tumors was assessed as low in 30 cases (67%), intermediate in 3 cases (7%) and heterogenous in 12 cases (26%) [8]. The further development of MRI protocols should focus on diminishing interobserver variability.

Imaging is highly important during the performance of radiation therapy. Novel techniques related to cervical cancer focus on adaptative strategies that reduce the radiation field and exposure of the patient [9].

Novel interventional radiology techniques have been implemented in order to undertake the minimally invasive management of pelvic pathology. An in-depth knowledge of the variability in the periprostatic vascular plexus is necessary in order to achieve the selective embolization of the prostatic parenchyma and prevent complications [10]. These procedures should be included in all core curricula of interventional radiology training.

Recent surge of infectious diseases in the aftermath of COVID-19 pandemics increased the number of imaging tests required for serial management of pathology progression. Imaging studies are needed for long term long term follow up of HIV, hepatitis and tuberculosis cases [11].

In conclusion, diagnostic and interventional imaging is the cornerstone to completing and correcting the management of complex pathologies. Medicine is now entering a new era of technology in which artificial intelligence (AI)-powered diagnostic tools will enhance the management of workflow in already crowded radiology departments.

Author Contributions: Conceptualization, R.C.; methodology, M.D.; software, A.C.; validation, R.C.; formal analysis, A.C.; investigation, M.D.; resources, A.C.; data curation, R.C.; writing—original draft preparation, M.D.; writing—review and editing, R.C.; visualization, M.D.; supervision, A.C.; project administration, R.C.; funding acquisition, A.C. All authors have read and agreed to the published version of the manuscript.

Funding: This research received no external funding.

Conflicts of Interest: The authors declare no conflict of interest.

References

1. Nemes, A.F.; Toma, A.I.; Dima, V.; Serboiu, S.C.; Necula, A.I.; Stoiciu, R.; Ulmeanu, A.I.; Marinescu, A.; Ulmeanu, C. Use of Lung Ultrasound in Reducing Radiation Exposure in Neonates with Respiratory Distress: A Quality Management Project. *Medicina* **2024**, *60*, 308. [CrossRef] [PubMed]
2. Opancina, V.; Zdravkovic, N.; Jankovic, S.; Masulovic, D.; Ciceri, E.; Jaksic, B.; Nukovic, J.J.; Nukovic, J.A.; Adamovic, M.; Opancina, M.; et al. Predictors of Intrahospital Mortality in Aneurysmal Subarachnoid Hemorrhage after Endovascular Embolization. *Medicina* **2024**, *60*, 1134. [CrossRef] [PubMed]
3. Nukovic, J.J.; Opancina, V.; Ciceri, E.; Muto, M.; Zdravkovic, N.; Altin, A.; Altaysoy, P.; Kastelic, R.; Velazquez Mendivil, D.M.; Nukovic, J.A.; et al. Neuroimaging Modalities Used for Ischemic Stroke Diagnosis and Monitoring. *Medicina* **2023**, *59*, 1908. [CrossRef] [PubMed]
4. Stefanescu, E.H.; Balica, N.C.; Motoi, S.B.; Grigorita, L.; Georgescu, M.; Iovanescu, G. High-Resolution Computed Tomography in Middle Ear Cholesteatoma: How Much Do We Need It? *Medicina* **2023**, *59*, 1712. [CrossRef] [PubMed]
5. Javed, M.Q.; Srivastava, S.; Alotaibi, B.B.R.; Bhatti, U.A.; Abulhamael, A.M.; Habib, S.R. A Cone Beam Computed Tomography-Based Investigation of the Frequency and Pattern of Radix Entomolaris in the Saudi Arabian Population. *Medicina* **2023**, *59*, 2025. [CrossRef] [PubMed]
6. Alarcón Apablaza, J.; Muñoz, G.; Arriagada, C.; Bucchi, C.; Masuko, T.S.; Fuentes, R. Odontoma Recurrence. The Importance of Radiographic Controls: Case Report with a 7-Year Follow-Up. *Medicina* **2024**, *60*, 1248. [CrossRef] [PubMed]
7. Șerboiu, C.S.; Aliuș, C.; Dumitru, A.; Țăpoi, D.; Costache, M.; Nica, A.E.; Alexandra-Ana, M.; Antoniac, I.; Grădinaru, S. Gallbladder Pancreatic Heterotopia—The Importance of Diagnostic Imaging in Managing Intraoperative Findings. *Medicina* **2023**, *59*, 1407. [CrossRef] [PubMed]
8. Rizescu, R.-A.; Sălcianu, I.A.; Șerbănoiu, A.; Ion, R.T.; Florescu, L.M.; Gheonea, I.-A.; Iana, G.; Bratu, A.M. Can MRI Accurately Diagnose and Stage Endometrial Adenocarcinoma? *Medicina* **2024**, *60*, 512. [CrossRef] [PubMed]
9. Anghel, B.; Serboiu, C.; Marinescu, A.; Taciuc, I.-A.; Bobirca, F.; Stanescu, A.D. Recent Advances and Adaptive Strategies in Image Guidance for Cervical Cancer Radiotherapy. *Medicina* **2023**, *59*, 1735. [CrossRef] [PubMed]

10. Șerbănoiu, A.; Nechifor, R.; Marinescu, A.N.; Iana, G.; Bratu, A.M.; Sălcianu, I.A.; Ion, R.T.; Filipoiu, F.M. Prostatic Artery Origin Variability: Five Steps to Improve Identification during Percutaneous Embolization. *Medicina* **2023**, *59*, 2122. [CrossRef] [PubMed]
11. Loghin, I.I.; Vâță, A.; Mihai, I.F.; Silvaș, G.; Rusu, Ș.A.; Luca, C.M.; Dorobăț, C.M. Profile of Newly Diagnosed Patients with HIV Infection in North-Eastern Romania. *Medicina* **2023**, *59*, 440. [CrossRef] [PubMed]

Disclaimer/Publisher's Note: The statements, opinions and data contained in all publications are solely those of the individual author(s) and contributor(s) and not of MDPI and/or the editor(s). MDPI and/or the editor(s) disclaim responsibility for any injury to people or property resulting from any ideas, methods, instructions or products referred to in the content.

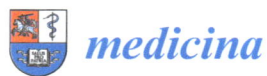 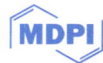

Article

Use of Lung Ultrasound in Reducing Radiation Exposure in Neonates with Respiratory Distress: A Quality Management Project

Alexandra Floriana Nemes [1,2,3], Adrian Ioan Toma [2,3,*], Vlad Dima [4,*], Sorina Crenguta Serboiu [1,5], Andreea Ioana Necula [2], Roxana Stoiciu [2], Alexandru Ioan Ulmeanu [1,6], Andreea Marinescu [1] and Coriolan Ulmeanu [1,6]

[1] Faculty of Medicine. Doctoral School, Carol Davila University of Medicine and Pharmacy, 050474 Bucharest, Romania
[2] Department of Neonatology, Life Memorial Hospital, 010719 Bucharest, Romania;
[3] Faculty of Medicine, Titu Maiorescu University, 040441 Bucharest, Romania
[4] Department of Neonatology, Filantropia Hospital, 011132 Bucharest, Romania
[5] Department of Radiology, University Emergency Hospital Bucharest, 050098 Bucharest, Romania
[6] Department of Toxicology, Grigore Alexandrescu Children's Hospital, 011743 Bucharest, Romania
* Correspondence: adrian.toma@prof.utm.ro (A.I.T.); vlad.dima@spitalulfilantropia.ro (V.D.)

Abstract: *Background and Objectives:* Our quality management project aims to decrease by 20% the number of neonates with respiratory distress undergoing chest radiographs as part of their diagnosis and monitoring. *Materials and Methods:* This quality management project was developed at Life Memorial Hospital, Bucharest, between 2021 and 2023. Overall, 125 patients were included in the study. The project consisted of a training phase, then an implementation phase, and the final results were measured one year after the end of the implementation phase. The imaging protocol consisted of the performance of lung ultrasounds in all the patients on CPAP (continuous positive airway pressure) or mechanical ventilation (first ultrasound at about 90 min after delivery) and the performance of chest radiographs after endotracheal intubation in any case of deterioration of the status of the patient or if such a decision was taken by the clinician. The baseline characteristics of the population were noted and compared between years 2021, 2022, and 2023. The primary outcome measures were represented by the number of X-rays performed in ventilated patients per year (including the patients on CPAP, SIMV (synchronized intermittent mandatory ventilation), IPPV (intermittent positive pressure ventilation), HFOV (high-frequency oscillatory ventilation), the number of X-rays performed per patient on CPAP/year, the number of chest X-rays performed per mechanically ventilated patient/year and the mean radiation dose/patient/year. There was no randomization of the patients for the intervention. The results were compared between the year before the project was introduced and the 2 years across which the project was implemented. *Results:* The frequency of cases in which no chest X-ray was performed was significantly higher in 2023 compared to 2022 (58.1% vs. 35.8%; $p = 0.03$) or 2021 (58.1% vs. 34.5%; $p = 0.05$) (a decrease of 22.3% in 2023 compared with 2022 and of 23.6% in 2023 compared with 2021). The frequency of cases with one chest X-ray was significantly lower in 2023 compared to 2022 (16.3% vs. 35.8%; $p = 0.032$) or 2021 (16.3% vs. 44.8%; $p = 0.008$). The mean radiation dose decreased from 5.89 Gy $\times$ cm^2 in 2021 to 3.76 Gy $\times$ cm^2 in 2023 (36% reduction). However, there was an increase in the number of ventilated patients with more than one X-ray (11 in 2023 versus 6 in 2021). We also noted a slight annual increase in the mean number of X-rays per patient receiving CPAP followed by mechanical ventilation (from 1.80 in 2021 to 2.33 in 2022 and then 2.50 in 2023), and there was a similar trend in the patients that received only mechanical ventilation without a statistically significant difference in these cases. *Conclusions:* The quality management project accomplished its goal by obtaining a statistically significant increase in the number of ventilated patients in which chest radiographs were not performed and also resulted in a more than 30% decrease in the radiation dose per ventilated patient. This task was accomplished mainly by increasing the number of patients on CPAP and the use only of lung ultrasound in the patients on CPAP and simple cases.

Citation: Nemes, A.F.; Toma, A.I.; Dima, V.; Serboiu, S.C.; Necula, A.I.; Stoiciu, R.; Ulmeanu, A.I.; Marinescu, A.; Ulmeanu, C. Use of Lung Ultrasound in Reducing Radiation Exposure in Neonates with Respiratory Distress: A Quality Management Project. *Medicina* **2024**, *60*, 308. https://doi.org/10.3390/medicina60020308

Academic Editor: Marina Aiello

Received: 17 January 2024
Revised: 4 February 2024
Accepted: 8 February 2024
Published: 10 February 2024

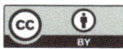

Copyright: © 2024 by the authors. Licensee MDPI, Basel, Switzerland. This article is an open access article distributed under the terms and conditions of the Creative Commons Attribution (CC BY) license (https://creativecommons.org/licenses/by/4.0/).

Keywords: lung ultrasound; chest radiographs; neonatal intensive care unit

1. Introduction

Respiratory distress in neonates within the initial 24 h following birth is among the most prevalent neonatal conditions with the main cause of neonatal intensive care unit (NICU) admissions [1,2].

Neonatal respiratory distress (RD) arises from pulmonary immaturity and a deficit in surfactant, leading to inadequate respiratory function shortly after birth. In cases where RD worsens, the administration of surfactant is indicated based on the following criteria: (1) if FiO_2 exceeds more than 0.3 on CPAP pressure at or above 6 cm H_2O or (2) if lung ultrasound is suggestive of surfactant deficiency. Early surfactant administration is currently recommended, even before radiographic confirmation, based on findings from observational studies [3,4].

The diagnosis and management of neonatal lung disorders heavily rely on radiographs, and using the right radiographic approach is crucial for both patient safety and accurate diagnosis. It is important to utilize the ALARA (as low as reasonably achievable) principle when using ionizing radiation in medical imaging to minimize radiation exposure to the greatest extent possible [5,6]. In an NICU, it has been documented that estimated radiation exposure is low, ranging from 24 to 32 μGy per chest X-ray [6].

Even though a chest X-ray is usually sufficient to diagnose TTN (transient tachypnea of the newborn), RDS (respiratory distress syndrome) or congenital pneumonia, it has been shown from emerging studies that lung ultrasound has greater reliability and usefulness in various forms of respiratory distress [7–9].

Lung ultrasound (LU) has demonstrated its reliability in identifying infants who will need admission to the Neonatal Intensive Care Unit (NICU) due to transient neonatal tachypnea or respiratory distress syndrome as well as to predict the need for surfactant administration [10,11].

Transient Tachypnea of the Newborn (TTN) is the most common form of respiratory distress in newborns. The pathophysiological substrate is represented by the lack of absorption of fetal lung fluid, thus producing intra-alveolar exudate and interstitial edema. From an ultrasound point of view, type A lines (>3 per field) are present with the appearance of interstitial edema and in the lower lung fields a "white lung" appearance with confluent B-type lines—a pattern named a double lung point [12–14].

The main sonographic features of respiratory distress syndrome (RDS) involve the presence of numerous compact B-lines, leading to a "white lung" appearance, which is accompanied by a thickened and irregular pleural line. Multiple subpleural lung consolidations appear as small hypoechoic regions. It is worth noting that these patterns do not show immediate improvement even after the administration of surfactant [15,16].

Congenital pneumonia represents a frequent pathology of the newborn with a variety of sonographic findings, such as the absence of pleural line, subpleural consolidation with air bronchogram and interstitial syndrome [17].

Our quality management project has the aim to decrease by 20% the number of neonates with respiratory distress in which the chest radiograph is used in the diagnosis and monitoring of the evolution of the patient, after a period of implementation of 1 year, measured 1 year after the end of the implementation phase, compared with the year preceding the beginning of the project, by using lung ultrasound in the diagnosis and monitoring of the patients and by having clear criteria for the use of chest radiographs. By this approach, the aim is to decrease the radiation exposure of these fragile patients without affecting the diagnosis and the management of the cases.

2. Materials and Methods
2.1. Sample and Variables Analyzed

This quality management project was accomplished at Life Memorial Hospital, Bucharest. Data collection was conducted in the period between January 2021 and December 2023. A study sample of 125 patients was chosen for this research. In 2021, 29 patients were included, followed by 53 patients in 2022, and 43 patients in 2023.

The hospital's Ethics Committee approved the quality management project before data collection.

We considered 2021 as the year of baseline (that will serve for comparison) and started to apply the method of lung ultrasound throughout 2022 and 2023 (see below for the description of the quality management program.

The inclusion criteria were admission to the Neonatal Intensive Care Unit (NICU), presence of respiratory distress, and record of treatment involving either CPAP or mechanical ventilation.

The following exclusion criteria were used: individuals with a congenital diaphragmatic hernia, necrotizing enterocolitis, or other malformations that necessitated the utilization of X-ray radiation regardless of their admission to the Neonatal Intensive Care Unit (NICU).

The clinical records of the included cases were analyzed. There were a couple of baseline variables that would be compared between the groups (years of study) to assess if the pathologies and the severity of the cases were comparable and to exclude sampling biases [18]: gestational age gender, type of delivery, treatment administered in the delivery room, type of respiratory ventilation support in the Neonatal Intensive Care Unit (NICU), pulmonary pathology, doses of administered surfactant (if any), and the presence of congenital infections

The primary outcome measures were represented by the number of ventilated patients that received X-rays each year (including the patients on CPAP, SIMV, IPPV, and HFOV), the number of X-rays performed per patient on CPAP/year, the number of chest X-rays performed per mechanically ventilated patient/year and the mean radiation dose/patient/year. The years 2021, 2022, and 2023 were compared. As the number of patients each year could not be equal, we decided to use for comparison the percent of patients receiving X-rays from the total number of patients receiving respiratory support.

As stated from the beginning, this has not been a randomized trial but rather a quality management project. We implemented a set of measures in order to decrease the number of patients. Accordingly, we compared the year 2021 when lung ultrasound was not a standard of care and 2022 and 2023 when the project has been implemented. All the ventilated (or CPAP) patients were included in the project. So, we did not have a calculated sample, but we had all the patients born during the 3-year period that needed any form of mechanical ventilation.

2.2. Quality Management Project Design

The resources utilized for the project were human resources and material resources.

The human resources were represented by the physicians of the neonatology unit—6 doctors—certified in neonatology; two of them were also certified in ultrasound with courses in lung ultrasound.

The neonatal unit has a functioning ultrasound machine (see below the specifications) that is available 24/7. The radiology service is also available 24/7 with qualified personnel who can perform and interpret the ultrasounds.

The first phase of the project has been a training phase with two components
- All the doctors of the units have been trained in the use and interpretation of lung ultrasound.
- A protocol for the performance of the imaging procedures has been established (Table 1)—also with training the staff for its use.

Table 1. Imaging procedures protocol in patients with respiratory distress.

Lung ultrasound
- Performed in all the patients 60–90 min after delivery
- Performed as needed in the case of ventilated patients or patients on CPAP *
Indications for chest radiographs (X-rays)
- After intubation, check the status of the patient and the position of the ET tube
- At any deterioration of the clinical status of a ventilated patient
- For confirming the diagnosis of a pneumothorax
- As decided by the clinicians' clinical judgement **

* Lung ultrasound performed by the bedside clinician. In case of doubt, the images were sent electronically to the expert for a second opinion. ** The attending physician had the freedom to decide to perform a chest X-ray in any case of a patient with respiratory distress not mentioned above, based on their clinical judgement, but had to state the reason in the patient's record.

An implementation phase followed, beginning on 1 January 2022. During this phase, the patients were managed according to the new imaging protocol.

The indications for mechanical ventilation or surfactant administration were established according to the national [19] and European guidelines [4]—in case of different indications, the national guidelines have priority.

To ensure unity of practice, weekly reviews of the records of the patients with respiratory distress, lung ultrasounds and chest X-rays were performed with the staff and experts.

On 1 January 2023, we considered the transition period finished, and we followed the accomplishments of the objectives of the program.

2.3. Lung Ultrasound Criteria/Findings

Lung ultrasound examination was performed in all patients included in the study, using the linear probe of 8–10 MHz frequency in anterior and lateral fields, with a scanning depth of 4–5 cm adjusted to the infant's birth weight and gestational age. The device used was a GE Vivid S60 (Manufacturer, General Electric HealthCare, Waukesha, West Milwaukee and Madison, WI, USA). To maintain the safety of the examination, the mechanical index (MI) and thermal index (TI) were maintained below 1.0.

Ultrasound images of normal lung semiology (A lines, B lines, normal lung appearance) are presented in Figure 1a,b. Typical images of ultrasound findings in lung diseases in patients in our study are shown in Figures 2–4.

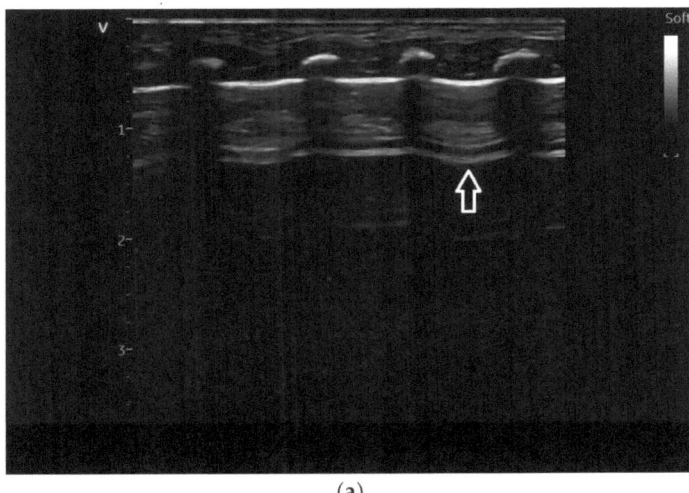

(a)

Figure 1. *Cont.*

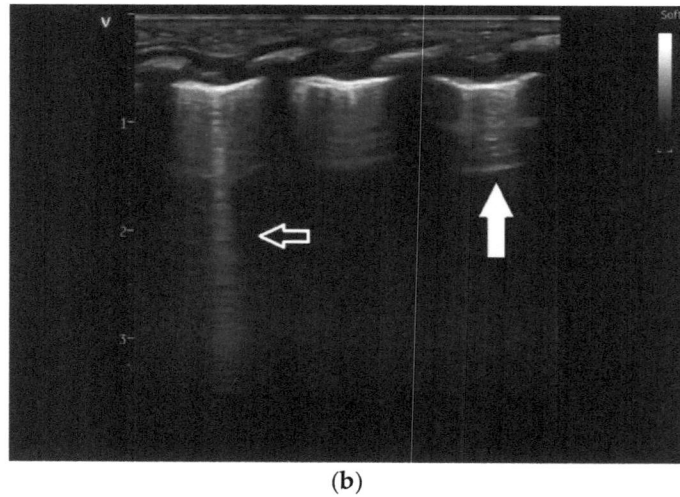

Figure 1. (a) Lung ultrasound. Normal image: A line—arrow—horizontal line parallel to the pleural line; (b) lung ultrasound. Normal image: A line—horizontal line parallel to the pleural line—reflection of the parietal pleura—white arrow—B line—white contour arrow—vertical line, with the origin at the visceral pleura, like a laser beam.

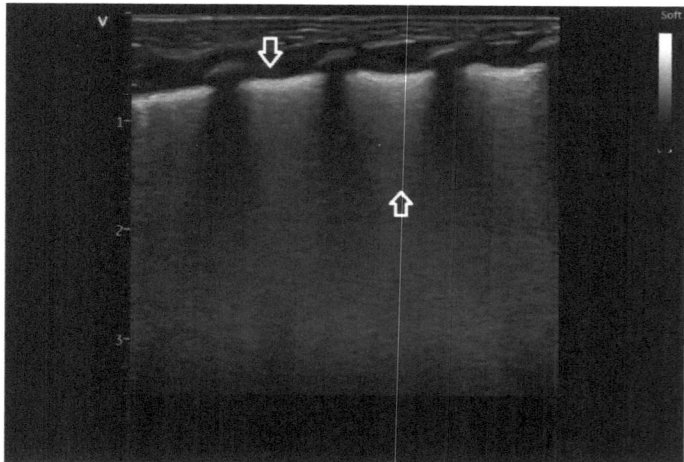

Figure 2. Lung ultrasound appearance of respiratory distress syndrome due to surfactant deficiency—white lung image, coalescent B-type lines occupying all lung fields—vertical arrow up; thickened pleural line–vertical downward arrow. Compare with Figure 1—normal lung.

2.4. Statistics

Patient data were gathered and stored in a centralized, anonymized database. All analyses and graphical representations were performed using SPSS Statistics software (version 18.0 IBM Corporation; Armonk, NY, USA). The analysis of the correlation between the number of pulmonary X-rays and lung pathologies was performed using the one-way ANOVA test. The statistical significance for the test was chosen to be $p < 0.05$ [20].

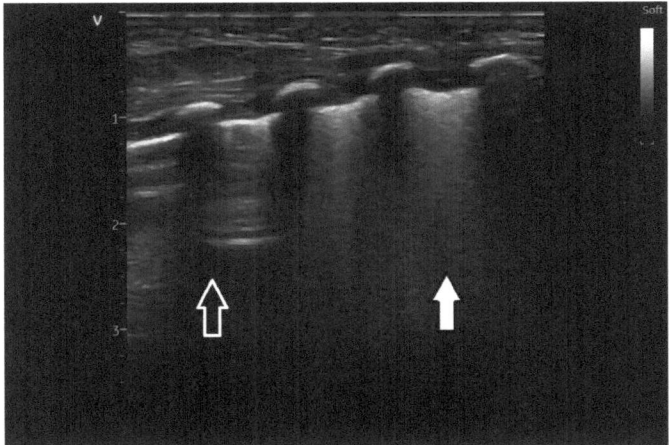

Figure 3. Lung ultrasound pattern in transient tachypnea of the newborn—double lung point—type A and type B lines visible in the upper lung fields—arrow with white outline; white lung appearance in the lower lung fields—white arrow. Compare with Figure 1—normal lung and Figure 2—lung ultrasound appearance in respiratory distress syndrome.

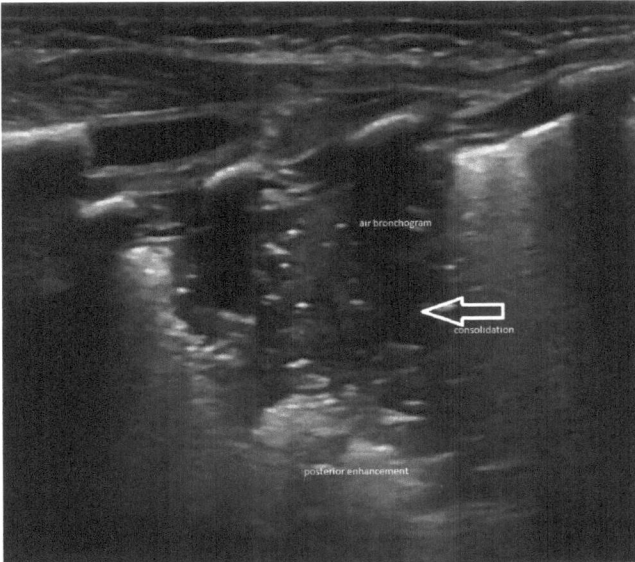

Figure 4. Lung ultrasound appearance in congenital pneumonia. Consolidation—arrow, air bronchogram—white spots and posterior enhancement with anfractuous appearance—shred sign.

3. Results

Overall, 125 patients were included in the quality management protocol from Life Memorial Hospital. The mean gestational age was 34.92 weeks (standard deviation ± 2.12) and the median was 35 weeks. In 2023, the average gestation age was significantly higher compared to that recorded in 2022 (36.14 vs. 34.92; $p = 0.009$) (Table 2).

Table 2. Descriptive data of gestational age and birth weight (g) compared by study years.

Parameters	Year of Study			One-Way ANOVA Test
	2021	2022 *	2023 **	
	Gestational age			
mean ± SD	35.55 ± 1.80	34.92 ± 2.12 [d]	36.14 ± 11.87 [d,b]	
median	35	35	36	0.012
limits	32–39	30–39	30–39	
	Birth weight			
mean ± SD	2680 ± 562.56	2504 ± 621.79 [d]	2803 ± 535.10 [d,c]	
median	2670	2420	2890	0.043
limits	1230–3500	1410–7592	1500–3670	

One-way ANOVA test post hoc Tukey HSD * 2022 vs. 2021; ** 2023 vs. 2021 and 2023 vs. 2022. [b] $p < 0.01$; [c] $p < 0.05$; [d] $p > 0.05$.

In 2023, the average birth weight was significantly higher compared to that recorded in 2022 (2803 vs. 2504; $p = 0.035$) (Table 2).

3.1. Correlations by Year of Study

The characteristics of each group per year regarding the pulmonary X-ray use, applied treatment and associated pathologies can be found in Table 3.

Table 3. Comparative clinical data by year of study.

Parameters	Year of Study						Chi-Square Test Likelihood Ratio
	2021 ($n = 29$)	2022 ($n = 53$)	p Value for Chi2 Test 2022 vs. 2021	2023 ($n = 43$)	p Value for Chi2 Test 2023 vs. 2021	p Value for Chi2 Test 2023 vs. 2022	
Male	24 (82.8%)	30 (56.6%)	0.018	22 (51.2%)	0.007	0.597	0.013
CPAP	18 (62.1%)	44 (83.0%)	0.036	35 (81.4%)	0.070	0.837	0.087
VM	16 (55.2%)	18 (34.0%)	0.064	14 (32.6%)	0.058	0.885	0.110
CPAP followed by VM	5 (17.2%)	9 (17.0%)	0.976	6 (14.0%)	0.706	0.686	0.901
Pulmonary Rx	19 (65.5%)	33 (62.3%)	0.771	18 (41.9%)	0.050	0.048	0.067
Associated pathologies							
SDR	21 (72.4%)	44 (83.0%)	0.260	31 (72.1%)	0.976	0.200	0.359
TTN	5 (17.2%)	8 (15.1%)	0.800	7 (16.3%)	0.915	0.874	0.967
Congenital pneumonia	3 (10.3%)	1 (1.9%)	0.091	0 (0%)	0.032	0.368	0.045
Meconium aspiration	0 (0%)	1 (1.9%)	0.459	1 (2.3%)	0.412	0.882	0.580
Pneumothorax	1 (3.4%)	0 (0%)	0.176	5 (11.6%)	0.221	0.011	0.014

There was a significant decrease in the proportion of males from 2021 (82.8%) to 2022 (56.6%) and 2023 (51.2%). The changes from 2021 to both 2022 and 2023 are statistically significant, indicating a notable shift in the gender distribution over the years.

There was a significant increase in the use of CPAP from 2021 (62.1%) to 2022 (83.0%). However, the slight decrease in 2023 (81.4%) was not significantly different from 2022, suggesting a stable and continuous administration of CPAP.

No statistical differences were noted in the administration of MV (mechanical ventilation) from 2021 to 2023, while in the group of patients treated with CPAP followed by MV, the percentages remained relatively stable across the three years with no significant changes. This suggests a consistent approach in using CPAP followed by ventilation mode for patients with CPAP failure over the study period.

Regarding pulmonary X-rays, the considerable decrease in the use of chest radiographs from 2021 to 2023 could be due to advancements in preventive measures, such as the implementation of lung ultrasound protocol, improvements in early treatment protocols, or changes in the prevalence of pulmonary-related conditions.

The stability in the rates of RDS and TTN suggests that there has not been a significant change in their prevalence or the effectiveness of preventive measures.

Moreover, the significant increase in 2023 of pneumothorax warrants attention. It could suggest changes in clinical practices, an increase in predisposing factors, or variations in reporting or diagnostic criteria. The frequency of cases in which no pulmonary X-rays were performed was significantly higher in 2023 compared to 2022 (58.1% vs. 35.8%; $p = 0.03$) or 2021 (58.1% vs. 34.5%; $p = 0.05$). The frequency of cases with pulmonary X-rays was significantly lower in 2023 compared to 2022 (16.3% vs. 35.8%; $p = 0.032$) or 2021 (16.3% vs. 44.8%; $p = 0.008$) (Table 4).

Table 4. Descriptive data of comparative pulmonary Rx number by study years.

Lung Rx Number	2021 ($n = 29$)	2022 * ($n = 53$)	2023 ** ($n = 43$)	Chi-Square Test Likelihood Ratio
0	10 (34.5%)	19 (35.8%) [d]	25 (58.1%) [c,c]	
1	13 (44.8%)	19 (35.8%) [d]	7 (16.3%) [b,c]	
2	4 (13.8%)	8 (15.1%) [d]	5 (11.6%) [d,d]	0.146
3	2 (6.9%)	3 (5.7%) [d]	5 (11.6%) [d,d]	
≥4	0 (0.0%)	4 (7.6%) [d]	1 (2.3%) [d,d]	

Chi2 test * 2022 vs. 2021; ** 2023 vs. 2021 and 2023 vs. 2022. [b] $p < 0.01$; [c] $p < 0.05$; [d] $p > 0.05$.

3.2. Correlations between X-rays and Categories of Treatment Applied to Patients

The basic characteristics and the pathology encountered were analyzed separately for the subgroups of patients treated with CPAP (Table 5), CPAP followed by MV (Table 6) and MV (Table 7).

Table 5. Number of X-rays/patient CPAP. $p = 0.208$.

	N	Mean	Std. Deviation	Std. Error	95% Confidence Interval for Mean		Minimum	Maximum
					Lower Bound	Upper Bound		
2021	18	0.67	0.907	0.214	0.22	1.12	0	3
2022	44	1.02	1.320	0.199	0.62	1.42	0	6
2023	35	0.57	1.065	0.180	0.21	0.94	0	4
Total	97	0.79	1.172	0.119	0.56	1.03	0	6

Table 6. Number of X-rays/patient CPAP followed by MV. $p = 0.688$.

	N	Mean	Std. Deviation	Std. Error	95% Confidence Interval for Mean		Minimum	Maximum
					Lower Bound	Upper Bound		
2021	5	1.80	0.837	0.374	0.76	2.84	1	3
2022	9	2.33	1.732	0.577	1.00	3.66	1	6
2023	6	2.50	1.049	0.428	1.40	3.60	1	4
Total	20	2.25	1.333	0.298	1.63	2.87	1	6

The mean number of X-rays per CPAP patient was lowest in 2023 (0.57) and highest in 2022 (1.02). However, the overall p-value of 0.208 suggests that these differences across the years are not statistically significant.

The wide range of standard deviations each year indicates variability in the number of X-rays per patient.

Table 7. Number of X-rays/ventilated patient. $p = 0.155$.

	N	Mean	Std. Deviation	Std. Error	95% Confidence Interval for Mean		Minimum	Maximum
					Lower Bound	Upper Bound		
2021	16	1.50	0.730	0.183	1.11	1.89	1	3
2022	18	2.11	1.410	0.332	1.41	2.81	1	6
2023	14	2.21	0.975	0.261	1.65	2.78	1	4
Total	48	1.94	1.119	0.161	1.61	2.26	1	6

The total analysis over the three years shows a mean of 0.79 X-rays per patient, with a 95% confidence interval ranging from 0.56 to 1.03, reflecting the average tendency across the study period.

The absence of statistically significant differences year over year suggests that the variation in the number of X-rays per CPAP patient may be attributed to the learning curve of decreasing the use of chest X-rays. These results can be useful for understanding the typical radiographic imaging needs of CPAP patients and for assessing the consistency of X-ray usage in CPAP treatment over the specified period.

The slight annual increase in the mean number of X-rays (from 1.80 in 2021 to 2.33 in 2022, and then 2.50 in 2023) could indicate a trend toward more frequent use of X-rays in managing patients who require both CPAP and VM.

The high standard deviations, especially in 2022 and 2023, point to significant variability in the number of X-rays per patient. This variability might reflect differences in individual patient conditions, the complexity of cases, or varied clinical judgments about the necessity for X-ray imaging.

The total analysis over the three years shows a mean of 2.25 X-rays per patient, with a 95% confidence interval ranging from 1.63 to 2.87, indicating a general trend toward a higher number of X-rays for patients undergoing CPAP followed by VM compared to CPAP alone.

There is a noticeable increase in the mean number of X-rays per ventilated patient from 2021 (1.50) to 2022 (2.11) and 2023 (2.21). This suggests a potential upward trend in the use of X-rays in ventilated patients over these years.

The wide range of standard deviations indicates high variability in the number of X-rays per patient each year, suggesting individualized care and differences in patient conditions or treatment protocols.

The analysis over the three years shows a mean of 1.94 X-rays per patient, indicating an overall tendency toward nearly two X-rays per ventilated patient on average.

Regarding the radiation dose received per year, we used a mean dose of $9\ Gy \times cm^2$ and analyzed the following data presented in Table 8.

Table 8. Radiation dose per year.

Parameter	2021	2022	2023
N	29	53	43
Pulmonary X-ray	19	33	18
Radiation dose (mean = $9\ Gy \times cm^2$)	171	297	162
Radiation dose/ventilated patient (including CPAP)	5.89	5.6	3.76

Considering 2022 as the comparison year, 2021 had a 57.57% rate of radiation dose/patient, while 2023 had a reduction of 54.54% after using lung ultrasound concomitantly with pulmonary X-rays. There has been a reduction in the mean radiation dose per patient from $5.89\ Gy \times cm^2$ in 2021 to $3.76\ Gy \times cm^2$ in 2023 (a 36% reduction).

The number of cases increased significantly from 2021 to 2022, and then decreased in 2023, but it remained higher than in 2021. This might reflect changes in the number of patients undergoing pulmonary X-rays or changes in lung ultrasound practices.

4. Discussion

Our quality management project accomplished its goal, i.e., to decrease the number of neonates that received respiratory support (mechanical ventilation or CPAP) in which chest X-rays were performed by more than 20% compared with the year before the implementation of the project.

As such a project, randomization and isolation of the intervention in order to assess its efficacy were not entirely possible. As a consequence, we cannot state certainly that this reduction has been related solely to the use of ultrasound. Instead, we noticed an increase in the use of CPAP in the patients in the need for respiratory support between 2021 and 2022 and, since we performed less chest X-rays in the patients on CPAP, this could have been a contributing factor. Another confounding factor could have been the difference in gestational age between 2022 and 2023 (but not between 2021 and 2023), but the main difference in the percent of patients receiving chest X-rays has been between 2021 and 2023 (in which case, no significant difference in the gestational ages was noticed). Another factor could have been the incidence of the different respiratory conditions (pneumonia, transient tachypnea of the newborn, respiratory distress syndrome), but in these cases there was no noted difference between the years. In conclusion, we consider that the main factor that could be related to a reduction in the percent of X-rays performed, together with the more widespread use of lung ultrasound, could be the more frequent use of CPAP as the only respiratory support technique.

We consider the strong points of the study to be the implementation of a lung ultrasound teaching program for all the doctors in the NICU and the study design as a quality management protocol. During the first year (2022), there was a learning curve in the use of both LU and chest X-rays with a decrease in pulmonary radiographs in 2022 and 2023. We showed that it is possible, through teaching and the judicious use of lung ultrasound, to decrease the number of patients that were exposed to X-rays, especially in the case of patients on CPAP.

Our choice for lung ultrasound has been supported by the ease of using the method and a good diagnostic value for the neonatal lung pathology [21,22]. Lung ultrasound (LUS) presents distinct signs linked to respiratory distress, which can be better identified by observing the lung tissue in real time and conducting multiple ultrasounds across the lung fields in various planes [21]. It is important to note that ultrasound is known for being influenced by the operator's skill, which can introduce potential errors. However, adhering to a standardized approach can reduce operator variability and enhance diagnostic precision [22].

While there have been concerns about excessive radiation exposure in NICU radiographic examinations, the research reviewed consistently found that the radiation levels in most individual radiographic procedures are minimal in modern NICUs [23,24]. Nonetheless, it remains crucial to adhere to the ALARA ("as low as reasonably achievable") principle, because NICU patients are exceptionally susceptible to the long-term cumulative effects of radiation exposure throughout their lives [25–27]. A study from Gao that analyzed 1381 patients admitted to the NICU over three years showed that lung ultrasound is completely reliable for diagnosis and lung disease differential diagnosis and could potentially replace pulmonary X-ray use [9].

Previously published papers have shown that neonatologists can attain a high level of proficiency in lung ultrasound following training programs of 2 days or more (either on site or combined with e-learning) [28]. As a result, the use of pulmonary X-rays has decreased, and more focus has been put on preventive management therapies as well as ultrasound-guided surfactant therapy [28,29].

Considering the potential risks associated with ultrasound examinations, it is important to recognize that while ultrasound is generally considered less harmful than other imaging techniques like radiology or CT scans, it still carries real biological risks that should be considered [12,15,30]. Ultrasound examinations can induce thermal effects, such as overheating and mechanical effects, particularly cavitation, on living tissues. If these effects surpass specific thresholds, they have the potential to harm living tissues [12,25,30].

We are aware also of certain weak points and limitations of the project. Two of them are represented by the monocentric design of the study and the fact that there has not been a uniform approach to the indications for X-rays, allowing freedom for the clinician in the decision to perform this procedure. This approach could also be considered a strong point, because we left the clinicians' choice in order to establish the diagnosis modality for the patient, trying to decrease the risk of under-diagnosing certain pathologies and harming the patient by not performing an X-ray when needed. It is our belief, though, that positive results (decreasing the use of X-rays) could be obtained better by education than by constraint and regulations and that results obtained this way will be more durable and safer for the patients. The monocentric character of the project lead to a smaller number of patients included. We consider though that the lessons learned in this project (see below) could provide us with more experience for a multicentric approach with the same goal.

Another limitation could be considered the fact that the patients included were not of small gestational ages (not less than 30 weeks GA). This could be also an issue for a future research or quality management project.

A notable issue in our quality management project surfaced when, despite a reduction in the overall number of X-rays, there was a rising trend in the number of X-rays administered per mechanically ventilated patient. The fact that we did not obtain the expected results in the case of the mechanically ventilated patients suggested the topic of a future direction of quality management research project, in which, by education and support for the staff, we will aim for a decrease in the use of chest radiographs in this category of patients. Looking ahead, our objective is to explore in greater detail the factors underlying the increased frequency of X-rays for individual patients, which is likely linked to inherent variations. We aim to deepen our understanding and refine the number of X-rays conducted. Our future strategy involves standardizing the utilization of X-rays and implementing the pulmonary X-ray protocol. This shift ensures that decisions regarding X-ray procedures are no longer solely reliant on physician opinions.

An Italian panel from 10 centers has shown that their guidelines outline specific criteria aimed at maintaining a superior level of neonatal care within NICUs. These criteria encompass various aspects such as protocols for procedures, facility requirements, recommended equipment, quality control measures, radiation protection protocols for both infants and staff and communication regarding radiation-related risks. This approach aims to establish a standardized framework for managing exposures in NICUs while still allowing for adaptability and flexibility as needed [31].

Another limitation could have been that we did not use other imaging modalities to compare the results with LU. Other imaging modalities are used more and more in the diagnosis and appreciation of prognosis of lung diseases in the neonate [32–35]. Of these, lung MRI, both fetal and neonatal, is worth mentioning.

Regarding fetal MRI, it is tempting to try to use this for establishing the prognosis in the lung conditions in the newborn. However, in a review published this year, the studies using fetal MRI for prognosis were used in most of the cases in patients with congenital diaphragmatic hernia and in a small number of patients with congenital lung malformations [30]. The indication for fetal MRI, as also mentioned in this paper, is pulmonary hypoplasia [30], so this is not the case in the premature infants with respiratory distress that do not have hypoplastic lungs (like the patients with diaphragmatic hernia) but rather lungs deficient in the production of surfactant (RDS) or with delayed absorption of lung fluid (TTN) or meconium aspiration or pneumonia. The same review concludes that for the moment, the prognostic value depends on the volumetric assessment and that the prediction of postnatal respiratory outcome could be feasible if emerging techniques could be employed and validated in pathological lungs [32]. This could be, though, a future direction of study.

Also, a future direction of study could be the use of neonatal lung MRI, now a very promising imaging technique, especially with ultrafast sequences and short exposure times and the availability of newer portable techniques [33–35]. Feasibility studies have shown the possibility of using this method in the NICU [33].

There are, although, several points to be discussed regarding neonatal lung MRI:

- The studies show good correlations between MRI patterns and chronic conditions like bronchopulmonary dysplasia [33–35] but do not mention the use of the method in the acute setting like respiratory distress syndrome and transient tachypnea of the newborn.
- The cost of an MRI in the NICU is far greater than the cost of a MRI, and this is not a technique to be used yet in all the neonates.
- The aim of our project has been to decrease the use of the X-rays by using simple diagnostic and assessment methods, like clinical examination, history, blood gases and ultrasound, and MRI is obviously not a simple technique to be used in all the settings.
- Although MRI is a promising and very accurate technique for the assessment of neonatal lungs, it is not yet passed into usual clinical practice, and it is not mentioned in the RDS guidelines like X-rays and ultrasound. Accordingly, since our goal has been to provide a model to be simple and replicated in all the units, we did not include lung MRI in our assessment protocol.

We would though consider in the future the use of MRI in a smaller group of patients, as the other studies did, in order to demonstrate the value of this technique.

5. Conclusions

The quality management project accomplished its goal by resulting in a statistically significant increase in the number of ventilated patients in which chest radiographs were not performed and also resulted in a more than 30% decrease in the radiation dose per ventilated patient. This task was accomplished mainly by increasing the number of patients on CPAP and the use only of lung ultrasound in the patients on CPAP and in simple cases.

As we did not perform a study with a control group, we cannot say for certain that this reduction was the result of only the use of lung ultrasound. Instead, we could consider that a bundle of care has been applied, consisting of the increased use of CPAP, increased use of lung ultrasound and more awareness to the indications of the X-rays.

The detection of more frequent use of chest radiographs in the case of more severe cases suggested to our group that the next quality management goal in the appropriate use of chest radiographs will be the introduction of more restrictive criteria and the improvement of the skills of the staff in using the lung ultrasound not only in the monitoring of the premature infants with respiratory distress syndrome or transient tachypnea of the newborn but also in the monitoring of all the categories of ventilated neonates.

Author Contributions: Conceptualization, A.I.T. and A.F.N. methodology, A.I.T., C.U. and V.D.; formal analysis, A.I.U., A.F.N. and A.I.N.; investigation, A.I.N., R.S., A.M. and S.C.S.; data curation, A.I.N.; writing—original draft preparation, A.F.N.; writing—review and editing, V.D.; visualization, A.F.N.; supervision, C.U.; project administration, A.I.U. All authors have read and agreed to the published version of the manuscript.

Funding: This research received no external funding.

Institutional Review Board Statement: The study was conducted in accordance with the Declaration of Helsinki and approved by the Institutional Ethics Committee of Life Memorial Hospital, Bucharest. No 21/28.12.2020.

Informed Consent Statement: Informed consent was obtained from all subjects involved in the study.

Data Availability Statement: The database of the study can be accessed upon request at the address adrian.toma@prof.utm.ro.

Acknowledgments: The authors would like to thank Francesco Raimondi and Almudena Alonso Ojembarrena for the mentorship and inspiration in performing research in the field of lung ultrasound.

Conflicts of Interest: The authors declare no conflicts of interest.

Abbreviations

ANOVA	analysis of variance
CPAP	continuous positive airway pressure
ET tube	endotracheal tube
Gy	Gray
HFOV	High-frequency oscillatory ventilation
H_2O	water
IPPV	intermittent positive pressure ventilation
LU	lung ultrasound
MHz	megahertz
N	number
NICU	neonatal intensive care unit
NY	New York
RD	respiratory distress
RDS	respiratory distress syndrome
SIMV	synchronized intermittent mandatory ventilation
TTN	transient tachypnea of the newborn
WI	Wisconsin
Vs	versus
X-rays	radiograph

References

1. Rachuri, H.; Oleti, T.P.; Murki, S.; Subramanian, S.; Nethagani, J. Diagnostic Performance of Point of Care Ultrasonography in Identifying the Etiology of Respiratory Distress in Neonates. *Indian J. Pediatr.* **2017**, *84*, 267–270. [CrossRef]
2. Liu, J.; Chen, X.X.; Li, X.W.; Chen, S.W.; Wang, Y.; Fu, W. Lung ultrasonography to diagnose transient tachypnea of the newborn. *Chest* **2016**, *149*, 1269–1275. [CrossRef]
3. Ammirabile, A.; Buonsenso, D.; Di Mauro, A. Lung Ultrasound in Pediatrics and Neonatology: An Update. *Healthcare* **2021**, *9*, 1015. [CrossRef]
4. Sweet, D.G.; Carnielli, V.P.; Greisen, G.; Hallman, M.; Klebermass-Schrehof, K.; Ozek, E.; Pas, A.T.; Plavka, R.; Roehr, C.C.; Saugstad, O.D.; et al. European Consensus Guidelines on the Management of Respiratory Distress Syndrome: 2022 Update. *Neonatology* **2023**, *120*, 3–23. [CrossRef]
5. Don, S.; Whiting, B.R.; Rutz, L.J.; Apgar, B.K. New exposure indicators for digital radiography simplified for radiologists and technologists. *Am. J. Roentgenol.* **2012**, *199*, 1337–1341. [CrossRef]
6. Makri, T.; Yakoumakis, E.; Papadopoulou, D.; Gialousis, G.; Theodoropoulos, V.; Sandilos, P.; Georgiou, E. Radiation risk assessment in neonatal radiographic examinations of the chest and abdomen: A clinical and Monte Carlo dosimetry study. *Phys. Med. Biol.* **2006**, *51*, 5023–5033. [CrossRef]
7. Raimondi, F.; Yousef, N.; Rodriguez Fanjul, J.; De Luca, D.; Corsini, I.; Shankar-Aguilera, S.; Dani, C.; Di Guardo, V.; Lama, S.; Mosca, F.; et al. A multicenter lung ultrasound study on transient tachypnea of the neonate. *Neonatology* **2019**, *115*, 263–268. [CrossRef] [PubMed]
8. Raimondi, F.; Migliaro, F.; Corsini, I.; Meneghin, F.; Dolce, P.; Pierri, L.; Perri, A.; Aversa, S.; Nobile, S.; Lama, S.; et al. Lung Ultrasound Score Progress in Neonatal Respiratory Distress Syndrome. *Pediatrics* **2021**, *147*, e2020030528. [CrossRef] [PubMed]
9. Gao, Y.-Q.; Qiu, R.-X.; Liu, J.; Zhang, L.; Ren, X.-L.; Qin, S.-J. Lung ultrasound completely replaced chest X-ray for diagnosing neonatal lung diseases: A 3-year clinical practice report from a neonatal intensive care unit in China. *J. Matern.-Fetal Neonatal Med.* **2020**, *35*, 3565–3572. [CrossRef] [PubMed]
10. Poerio, A.; Galletti, S.; Baldazzi, M.; Martini, S.; Rollo, A.; Spinedi, S.; Raimondi, F.; Zompatori, M.; Corvaglia, L.; Aceti, A. Lung ultrasound features predict admission to the neonatal intensive care unit in infants with transient neonatal tachypnoea or respiratory distress syndrome born by caesarean section. *Eur. J. Pediatr.* **2020**, *180*, 869–876. [CrossRef] [PubMed]
11. Raimondi, F.; Migliaro, F.; Corsini, I.; Meneghin, F.; Pierri, L.; Salomè, S.; Perri, A.; Aversa, S.; Nobile, S.; Lama, S.; et al. Neonatal Lung Ultrasound and Surfactant Administration. *Chest* **2021**, *160*, 2178–2186. [CrossRef] [PubMed]
12. Riccabona, M. (Ed.) *Pediatric Ultrasound: Requisites and Applications*, 2nd ed.; Springer: Berlin/Heidelberg, Germany, 2020.

13. Liu, J.; Wang, Y.; Fu, W.; Yang, C.S.; Huang, J.J. The 'Double Lung Point': An Ultrasound Sign Diagnostic of Transient Tachypnea of the New-born. *Medicine* 2014, *91*, e197–e202. [CrossRef] [PubMed]
14. Corsini, I.; Parri, N.; Gozzini, E.; Coviello, C.; Leonardi, V.; Poggi, C.; Giacalone, M.; Bianconi, T.; Tofani, L.; Raimondi, F.; et al. Lung Ultrasound for the Differential Diagnosis of Respiratory Distress in Neonates. *Neonatology* 2018, *115*, 77–84. [CrossRef] [PubMed]
15. Volpicelli, G.; Elbarbary, M.; Blaivas, M.; Lichtenstein, D.A.; Mathis, G.; Kirkpatrick, A.W.; Melniker, L.; Gargani, L.; Noble, V.E.; Via, G.; et al. International evidence-based recommendations for point of care lung ultrasound. *Intensive Care Med.* 2012, *38*, 577–591. [CrossRef] [PubMed]
16. Vergine, M.; Copetti, R.; Brusa, G.; Cattarossi, L. Lung Ultrasound Accuracy in Respiratory Distress Syndrome and Transient Tachypnea of the Newborn. *Neonatology* 2014, *106*, 87–93. [CrossRef] [PubMed]
17. Liu, J.; Ma, H.-R.; Fu, W. Lung Ultrasound to Diagnose Pneumonia in Neonates with Fungal Infection. *Diagnostics* 2022, *12*, 1776. [CrossRef] [PubMed]
18. Higgins, J.P.T.; Altman, D.G.; Sterne, J.A.C. Chapter 8: Assessing risk of bias in included studies. In *Cochrane Handbook for Systematic Reviews of Interventions Version 5.2.0 (Updated June 2017)*; Higgins, J.P.T., Churchill, R., Chandler, J., Cumpston, M.S., Eds.; Cochrane: Hoboken, NJ, USA, 2017.
19. Ognean, L. (Ed.) *Managementul Sindromului de Detresă Respiratorie Prin Deficit de Surfactant*; Asociația de Neonatologie din România: Bucharest, Romania, 2023.
20. Boiculese, L.V.; Dascalu, C. *Informatica Medicala*; Editura Venus: Bucuresti, Romania, 2001.
21. Raimondi, F.; Migliaro, F.; Sodano, A.; Ferrara, T.; Lama, S.; Vallone, G.; Capasso, L. Use of neonatal chest ultrasound to predict noninvasive ventilation failure. *Pediatrics* 2014, *134*, e1089–e1094. [CrossRef]
22. Lichtenstein, D.A.; Mauriat, P. Lung ultrasound in the critically ill neonate. *Curr. Pediatr. Rev.* 2012, *8*, 217–223. [CrossRef]
23. Gislason-Lee, A.J. Patient X-ray Exposure and ALARA in the Neonatal Intensive Care Unit: Global Patterns. *Pediatr. Neonatol.* 2021, *62*, 3–10. [CrossRef]
24. Gilley, R.; David, L.R.; Leamy, B.; Moloney, D.; Moore, N.; England, A.; Waldron, M.; Maher, M.; McEntee, M.F. Establishing weight-based diagnostic reference lev-els for neonatal chest X-rays. *Radiography* 2023, *29*, 812–817. [CrossRef]
25. Armpilia, C.I.; Fife, I.A.J.; Croasdale, P.L. Radiation dose quantities and risk in neonates in a special care baby unit. *Br. J. Radiol.* 2002, *75*, 590–595. [CrossRef]
26. Donadieu, J.; Zeghnoun, A.; Roudier, C.; Maccia, C.; Pirard, P.; André, C.; Adamsbaum, C.; Kalifa, G.; Legmann, P.; Jarreau, P.-H. Cumulative effective doses delivered by radiographs to preterm infants in a neonatal intensive care unit. *Pediatrics* 2006, *117*, 882–888. [CrossRef] [PubMed]
27. Yu, C.-C. Radiation Safety in the Neonatal Intensive Care Unit: Too Little or Too Much Concern? *Pediatr. Neonatol.* 2010, *51*, 311–319. [CrossRef] [PubMed]
28. Rodriguez-Fanjul, J.; Benet, N.; de Lliria, C.R.G.; Porta, R.; Guinovart, G.; Bobillo-Pérez, S. Lung Ultrasound Protocol Decreases Radiation in Newborn Population without Side Effects: A Quality Improvement Project. *Med. Intensiv. (Engl. Ed.)* 2023, *47*, 16–22. [CrossRef]
29. Raschetti, R.; Yousef, N.; Vigo, G.; Marseglia, G.; Centorrino, R.; Ben-Ammar, R.; Shankar-Aguilera, S.; De Luca, D. Ecography-guided surfactant therapy to improve timeliness of surfactant replacement: A quality improvement project. *J. Pediatr.* 2019, *212*, 137–143. [CrossRef] [PubMed]
30. Kurepa, D.; Zaghloul, N.; Watkins, L.; Liu, J. Neonatal lung ultrasound exam guidelines. *J. Perinatol.* 2018, *38*, 11–22. [CrossRef] [PubMed]
31. del Vecchio, A.; Salerno, S.; Barbagallo, M.; Chirico, G.; Campoleoni, M.; Cannatà, V.; Genovese, E.; Granata, C.; Magistrelli, A.; Tomà, P. Italian Inter-Society Expert Panel Position on Radiological Exposure in Neonatal Intensive Care Units. *Ital. J. Pediatr.* 2020, *46*, 159. [CrossRef] [PubMed]
32. Whitby, E.; Gaunt, T. Fetal lung MRI and features predicting post-natal outcome: A scoping review of the current literature. *Br. J. Radiol.* 2023, *96*, 20220344. [CrossRef]
33. Hahn, A.D.; Higano, N.S.; Walkup, L.L.; Thomen, R.P.; Cao, X.; Merhar, S.L.; Tkach, J.A.; Woods, J.C.; Fain, S.B. Pulmonary MRI of neonates in the intensive care unit using 3D ultrashort echo time and a small footprint MRI system. *J. Magn. Reson. Imaging* 2017, *45*, 463–471. [CrossRef]
34. Higano, N.S.; Spielberg, D.R.; Reck, R.J.; Schapiro, A.H.; Walkup, L.L.; Hahn, A.D.; Tkach, J.A.; Kingma, P.S.; Merhar, S.L.; Fain, S.B.; et al. Neonatal Pulmonary Magnetic Resonance Imaging of Bronchopulmonary Dysplasia Predicts Short-Term Clinical Outcomes. *Am. J. Resp. Crit. Care Med.* 2018, *198*, 1302–1311. [CrossRef]
35. Hysinger, E.B.; Higano, N.S.; Critser, P.J.; Woods, J.C. Imaging in Neonatal Respiratory Disease. *Paediatr. Respir. Rev.* 2022, *43*, 44–52. [CrossRef] [PubMed]

Disclaimer/Publisher's Note: The statements, opinions and data contained in all publications are solely those of the individual author(s) and contributor(s) and not of MDPI and/or the editor(s). MDPI and/or the editor(s) disclaim responsibility for any injury to people or property resulting from any ideas, methods, instructions or products referred to in the content.

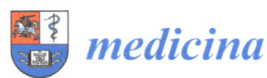

Article

Predictors of Intrahospital Mortality in Aneurysmal Subarachnoid Hemorrhage after Endovascular Embolization

Valentina Opancina [1,2,3,*,†], **Nebojsa Zdravkovic** [4,†], **Slobodan Jankovic** [2,5], **Dragan Masulovic** [6], **Elisa Ciceri** [3], **Bojan Jaksic** [7], **Jasmin J. Nukovic** [8,9], **Jusuf A. Nukovic** [8,9], **Miljan Adamovic** [10,11], **Miljan Opancina** [10,12], **Nikola Prodanovic** [2,13], **Merisa Nukovic** [8], **Tijana Prodanovic** [2,14] and **Fabio Doniselli** [15]

1. Department of Radiology, Faculty of Medical Sciences, University of Kragujevac, 34000 Kragujevac, Serbia
2. University Clinical Center Kragujevac, 34000 Kragujevac, Serbia
3. Diagnostic Imaging and Interventional Neuroradiology Unit, Department of Neurosurgery, Fondazione IRCCS Istituto Neurologico Carlo Besta, 20133 Milan, Italy
4. Department of Medical Statistics and Informatics, Faculty of Medical Sciences, University of Kragujevac, 34000 Kragujevac, Serbia
5. Department of Pharmacology and Toxicology, Faculty of Medical Sciences, University of Kragujevac, 34000 Kragujevac, Serbia
6. Department of Radiology, Medical Faculty, University of Belgrade, 11120 Belgrade, Serbia
7. Faculty of Medicine, University of Kosovska Mitrovica, 11000 Belgrade, Serbia
8. Department of Radiology, General Hospital Novi Pazar, 36300 Novi Pazar, Serbia
9. Faculty of Pharmacy and Health Travnik, University of Travnik, 72270 Travnik, Bosnia and Herzegovina
10. Faculty of Medical Sciences, University of Kragujevac, 34000 Kragujevac, Serbia
11. Pharmacy Institution "Zdravlje Lek", Prvomajska 100, 11000 Belgrade, Serbia
12. Faculty of Medicine, Military Medical Academy, University of Defense, 11000 Belgrade, Serbia
13. Department of Surgery, Faculty of Medical Sciences, University of Kragujevac, 34000 Kragujevac, Serbia
14. Department of Pediatrics, Faculty of Medical Sciences, University of Kragujevac, 34000 Kragujevac, Serbia
15. Department of Neuroradiology, Fondazione IRCCS Istituto Neurologico Carlo Besta, 20133 Milan, Italy
* Correspondence: valentina.opancina@gmail.com
† These authors contributed equally to this work.

Abstract: *Background and Objectives*: Aneurysmal subarachnoid hemorrhage (ASAH) is defined as bleeding in the subarachnoid space caused by the rupture of a cerebral aneurysm. About 11% of people who develop ASAH die before receiving medical treatment, and 40% of patients die within four weeks of being admitted to hospital. There are limited data on single-center experiences analyzing intrahospital mortality in ASAH patients treated with an endovascular approach. Given that, we wanted to share our experience and explore the risk factors that influence intrahospital mortality in patients with ruptured intracranial aneurysms treated with endovascular coil embolization. *Materials and Methods*: Our study was designed as a clinical, observational, retrospective cross-sectional study. It was performed at the Department for Radiology, University Clinical Center Kragujevac in Kragujevac, Serbia. The study inclusion criteria were ≥18 years, admitted within 24 h of symptoms onset, acute SAH diagnosed on CT, aneurysm on DSA, and treated by endovascular coil embolization from January 2014 to December 2018 at our institution. *Results*: A total of 66 patients were included in the study—48 (72.7%) women and 18 (27.3%) men, and 19.7% of the patients died during hospitalization. After adjustment, the following factors were associated with in-hospital mortality: a delayed ischemic neurological deficit, the presence of blood in the fourth cerebral ventricle, and an elevated urea value after endovascular intervention, increasing the chances of mortality by 16.3, 12, and 12.6 times. *Conclusions*: Delayed cerebral ischemia and intraventricular hemorrhage on initial head CT scan are strong predictors of intrahospital mortality in ASAH patients. Also, it is important to monitor kidney function and urea levels in ASAH patients, considering that elevated urea values after endovascular aneurysm embolization have been shown to be a significant risk factor for intrahospital mortality.

Keywords: intracranial aneurysm; subarachnoid hemorrhage; endovascular embolization; risk factors; mortality

Citation: Opancina, V.; Zdravkovic, N.; Jankovic, S.; Masulovic, D.; Ciceri, E.; Jaksic, B.; Nukovic, J.J.; Nukovic, J.A.; Adamovic, M.; Opancina, M.; et al. Predictors of Intrahospital Mortality in Aneurysmal Subarachnoid Hemorrhage after Endovascular Embolization. *Medicina* **2024**, *60*, 1134. https://doi.org/10.3390/medicina60071134

Academic Editors: Iosif Marincu, Romica Cergan, Adrian Costache and Mihai Dumitru

Received: 5 June 2024
Revised: 28 June 2024
Accepted: 10 July 2024
Published: 15 July 2024

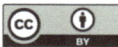

Copyright: © 2024 by the authors. Licensee MDPI, Basel, Switzerland. This article is an open access article distributed under the terms and conditions of the Creative Commons Attribution (CC BY) license (https://creativecommons.org/licenses/by/4.0/).

1. Introduction

Aneurysmal subarachnoid hemorrhage (ASAH) is defined as "bleeding in the subarachnoid space caused by the rupture of a cerebral aneurysm" [1–3]. Epidemiological ASAH data suggest that 9 out of 100,000 people in the US and almost 600,000 people worldwide experience it annually [4]. About 11% of people who develop ASAH die before receiving medical treatment, and 40% of patients end up dying within four weeks of being admitted to the hospital [5]. ASAH has a great impact on morbidity, so up to 30% of surviving patients show some degree of disability [5].

After providing emergency medical assistance, selecting an adequate diagnostic modality, and establishing a diagnosis, the next step is the treatment of brain injury caused by the aneurysm bleeding [6]. This is achieved by excluding the source of the bleeding from the circulation, whereby the speed of response in terms of the treatment reduces the mortality of these patients [7]. More precisely, if the exclusion of the cerebral aneurysm from the circulation is performed on the second day after the subarachnoid hemorrhage, the outcome of such patients is better than if it is done later [8]. An aneurysm that caused an ASAH can be treated with an open surgical method by placing a metal clip whose role is to occlude the neck of the aneurysm [9]. However, the treatment option is decided with interdisciplinary consent. Endovascular embolization (EE) is a minimally invasive method and involves "performing the procedure using a catheter under fluoroscopic guidance from the entry point in the artery (usually the femoral artery in the groin) to the parent artery where the aneurysm is" [10]. Two randomized trials that compared endovascular treatment with a surgical approach in cerebral aneurysms after their rupture, the International Subarachnoid Aneurysm Trial (ISAT) and the Barrow Ruptured Aneurysm Trial, came to the conclusion that the patients treated with the endovascular method had better functional outcomes in the first year after treatment. It should be noted that the authors also stated that the complete occlusion rate after endovascular treatment was only about 50% in the long term and frequent retreatment may be required [10–14]. Significant morbidity or mortality take place in 8% to 23% of patients with rebleeding [15]. The most important period is the first six hours after the initial bleeding, as up to 90% of rebleeding occurs in that time frame [16,17]. Also, the risk groups of patients for this complication include those who have a more severe form of ASAH and a large aneurysm, as well as those who wait for aneurysm embolization for a long time [18].

Still, data on intrahospital mortality for treated ruptured intracranial aneurysms vary from 8.3% to 66.7% [19]. A recent study explored mortality risk factors in ASAH patients with subarachnoid hemorrhage hospitalized in an Intensive Care Unit (ICU) and revealed mortality of 40% and the following predictors: aspiration pneumonia, septic shock, a CT-diagnosed midline shift, inter-hospital transfer, and hypernatremia (all during the first 72 h in the ICU). It was also stated that endovascular or surgical treatment performed within the first 72 h was a good prognostic factor [20]. There are limited data on single-center experiences analyzing intrahospital mortality in ASAH patients treated with an endovascular approach. Given that, we wanted to share our experience and explore the risk factors that influence intrahospital mortality in patients with ruptured intracranial aneurysms treated with endovascular coil embolization.

2. Materials and Methods

Our study was designed as a clinical, observational, retrospective cross-sectional study. It was performed at the Department for Radiology, University Clinical Center Kragujevac in Kragujevac, Serbia. The study was approved by the Institutional Ethics Board and conducted according to the principles of the Helsinki Declaration.

The study inclusion criteria were ≥18-year-old patients, admitted within 24 h of symptoms onset, a first-time intracranial aneurysm rupture diagnosed by CT and digital subtraction angiography, and treated with endovascular coil embolization (EE) from January 2014 to December 2018 at our institution. We excluded patients who had been treated with EE previously due to an aneurysm rupture, who had CT scans with artefacts, incomplete medical documentation, hepatorenal dysfunction, or malignant disease, and pregnant women. The interventional procedure was performed by two neuroradiologists with expertise in the field, and the CT scans were assessed by three experienced neuroradiologists at our institution. Most of the procedures were done within 72 h from the ictus. The indication and timing of the treatment were decided by a decision of a multidisciplinary board, including neurosurgeons, neurologists, neuroradiologists, and an interventional radiologist.

An ASAH was diagnosed on CT upon admission with the presence of blood in the subarachnoid space, while an aneurysm was diagnosed on DSA. Laboratory results that were taken in account were divided into three groups, depending on the day of the endovascular procedure: 24 to 48 h before the procedure, on the day when the endovascular procedure was performed, and 24 to 48 h after the procedure.

Our study explored the following variables from the patient files: socio-demographic data; the clinical picture prior to admission; scales: the Hunt and Hesse scale (HHS) and the Glasgow Coma Scale (GCS), both performed on admission [21], and the Fisher scale (FS) performed using the initial head CT scan [22]; the findings of the initial CT scan; a lumbar puncture and/or ventriculoperitoneal shunt; the application of mechanical ventilation after EE; the aneurysm features seen on DSA; the characteristics of the interventional procedure; hospitalization length, the time frame from admission to the hospital to the interventional procedure, and the duration of symptoms prior to admission; and laboratory analysis, which included the blood count, coagulation tests, and biochemistry analysis.

Statistics

We used SPSS version 23 software (SPSS Inc., Chicago, IL, USA) to analyze the study data [22]. Descriptive statistics were used initially. In order to describe continuous variables, the mean and standard deviation (if there was normal distribution) or the median and interquartile range (if there was not normal distribution) were used. We displayed categorical variables using rates and percentages. In order to test the normality of the data distribution, the Kolmogorov–Smirnov test was performed. The Mann–Whitney test was used for continuous variables and contingency tables were used for categorical variables when the significance of differences in the study groups was explored. The influence of study variables on death outcome was checked by univariate logistic regression and later on with multivariate logistic regression with the use of a backward conditional method. The Hosmer–Lemeshow, Cox–Snell, and Nagelkerke tests were used to explore the quality of the multivariate logistic regression model.

3. Results

After applying the inclusion and exclusion criteria of the study, the study included and analyzed a total of 66 ASAH patients. Of these, 48 (72.7%) were women and 18 (27.3%) were men. The youngest patient was 30 years old and the oldest 80 years old, while the mean age of the patients was 54 years. All patients were treated with endovascular aneurysm embolization, of whom 33 developed cerebral vasospasm, 14 patients developed hydrocephalus, and 42 developed brain edema. Thirteen patients (19.7%) died during hospitalization.

Table 1 presents the main characteristics of the study population. The variables explored in the laboratory analysis of the study population are presented in Table 2.

Table 1. Characteristics of study population.

Risk Factors	Patients Alive (n = 53)	Death Outcome (n = 13)	p Value
Age (Mean ± SD, Median [IQR])	52.43 ± 9.964, 54 [17]	60.38 ± 12.725, 56 [21]	0.054
Age category (20–40/40–60/>60 years)	8/31/14 (15.1%/58.5%/26.4%)	1/6/6 (7.7%/46.2%/46.2%)	0.360
Gender (male/female, %/%)	13/40 (24.5%/75.5%)	5/8 (38.5%/61.5%)	0.312
Caffeine usage (no/yes)	23/30 (43.4%/56.6%)	5/8 (38.5%/61.5%)	0.747
Smoking (no/yes)	29/24 (54.7%/45.3%)	7/6 (53.8%/46.2%)	0.955
DM as comorbidity (no/yes)	51/2 (96.2%/3.8%)	12/1 (92.3%/7.7%)	0.543
Hypertension as comorbidity (no/yes)	27/26 (50.9%/49.1%)	6/7 (46.2%/53.8%)	0.757
Clinical appearance on admission:			
Headache (no/yes)	8/45 (15.1%/84.9%)	0/13 (0%/100%)	0.135
Nausea (no/yes)	28/25 (52.8%/47.2%)	7/6 (53.8%/46.2%)	0.948
Vomiting (no/yes)	29/24 (54.7%/45.3%)	8/5 (61.5%/38.5%)	0.657
Altered conscience (no/yes)	21/32 (39.6%/60.4%)	5/8 (38.5%/61.5%)	0.939
Coma (no/yes)	49/4 (92.5%/7.5%)	11/2 (84.6%/15.4%)	0.378
Arterial blood pressure (hypotension/hypertension)	11/42 (20.8%/79.2%)	3/10 (23.1%/76.9%)	0.854
Neck rigidity (no/yes)	20/33 (37.7%/62.3%)	3/10 (23.1%/76.9%)	0.320
GCS (Mean ± SD, Median [IQR])	11.38 ± 3.065, 13 [5]	10.08 ± 4.291, 12 [7]	0.457
GCS (≤8/>8)	12/41 (22.6%/77.4%)	3/10 (23.1%/76.9%)	0.973
Duration of symptoms in hours, before admission (Mean ± SD, Median [IQR])	23.151 ± 25.582, 6 [22.75]	23.923 ± 38.300, 3 [37.5]	0.231
Duration of symptoms in hours, before admission (<6 h/6–12 h/12–24 h)	34/1/18 (64.2%/1.9%/34%)	7/3/3 (53.8%/23.1%/23.1%)	0.016
Time from onset of symptoms to EE, in hours (<2/2–4/4–6/6–12/>12 h)	10/19/9/2/13 (18.9%/35.8%/17%/3.8%/24.5%)	3/1/3/3/3 (23.1%/7.7%/23.1%/23.1%/23.1%)	0.085
Time from onset of symptoms to medication, in hours (Mean ± SD, Median [IQR])	38.481 ± 102.952, 6 [13.5]	24.154 ± 38.179, 4 [37.5]	0.342
Duration of fluoroscopy in EE (Mean ± SD, Median [IQR])	27.26 ± 6.346, 27 [10]	31.69 ± 6.33, 30 [11]	0.027 *
Aneurysm size (<5 mm/5–10 mm/11–25 mm)	16/30/7/0 (30.2%/56.6%/13.2%/0%)	2/6/5/0 (15.4%/46.2%/38.5%/0%)	0.095
Aneurysm location (ACI/ACM/ACA/ACP/AB)	22/7/19/2/3 (41.5%/13.2%/35.8%/3.8%/5.7%)	3/3/4/2/1 (23.1%/23.1%/30.8%/15.4%/7.7%)	0.396
Aneurysm height (Mean ± SD, Median [IQR])	7.108 ± 4.031, 6.72 [4.67]	8.634 ± 4.485, 7.08 [6.57]	0.211
Aneurysm width (Mean ± SD, Median [IQR])	5.816 ± 2.996, 4.45 [4.3]	7.079 ± 4.103, 6.29 [5.09]	0.314
Aneurysm neck (Mean ± SD, Median [IQR])	2.871 ± 1.004, 2.70 [1.23]	4.761 ± 4.424, 3.80 [4.56]	0.589
Cerebral vasospasm (no/yes)	29/24 (54.7%/45.3%)	4/9 (30.8%/69.2%)	0.122

Table 1. Cont.

Risk Factors	Patients Alive (n = 53)	Death Outcome (n = 13)	p Value
Hydrocephalus (no/yes)	42/11 (79.2%/20.8%)	10/3 (76.9%/23.1%)	0.854
Brain edema (no/yes)	20/33 (37.7%/62.3%)	4/9 (30.8%/69.2%)	0.640
Intracerebral or intracerebellar hematoma (no/yes)	32/21 (60.4%/39.6%)	10/3 (76.9%/23.1%)	0.266
Intraventricular hemorrhage (no/yes)	30/23 (56.6%/43.4%)	0/13 (0%/100%)	0.000 *
Hemorrhage in IV ventricle (no/yes)	40/13 (75.5%/24.5%)	6/7 (46.2%/53.8%)	0.039
HHS (Mean ± SD, Median [IQR])	2.96 ± 1.255, 3 [2]	2.69 ± 1.182, 3 [2]	0.463
FS (Mean ± SD, Median [IQR])	3.09 ± 0.883, 3 [2]	3.85 ± 0.376, 3 [2]	0.004 *
Mechanical ventilation (no/yes)	39/14 (73.6%/26.4%)	2/11 (15.4%/84.6%)	0.000 *
Liquor evacuation with lumbar puncture (no/yes)	44/9 (83%/17%)	8/5 (61.5%/38.5%)	0.090
Ventriculoperitoneal shunt (no/yes)	47/6 (88.7%/11.3%)	10/3 (76.9%/23.1%)	0.268
Duration of hospitalization (Mean ± SD, Median [IQR])	32.207 ± 19.018, 30 [25]	19.385 ± 14.847, 17 [13]	0.005 *

*—statistically significant; Abbreviations: ACI—a.carotis interna, ACM—a.cerebri media, ACA—cerebri anterior, ACP—a.cerebri posterior, AB = a.basillaris, GCS—Glasgow Coma Scale, HHS—Hunt and Hesse scale, FS—Fisher scale, DM—Diabetes mellitus. The Mann–Whitney U test was performed for continuous variables and a Chi-squared test was performed for categorical variables.

Table 2. Laboratory results of study population.

Risk Factors	Patients Alive (n = 53)	Death Outcome (n = 13)	p Value
WBC before EE (Mean ± SD, Median [IQR])	12.041 ± 3.902, 11 [5.36]	11.438 ± 3.192, 10 [5.85]	T = 0.994
WBC on day of EE (Mean ± SD, Median [IQR])	12.466 ± 4.048, 10.9 [5.71]	12.301 ± 2.879, 10 [4.86]	0.929
WBC after EE (Mean ± SD, Median [IQR])	12.773 ± 3.902, 11.8 [6.35]	12.409 ± 2.532, 11.8 [3.65]	0.929
PLT before EE (Mean ± SD, Median [IQR])	255.49 ± 101.461, 200.1 [142]	209 ± 52.075, 195 [64]	0.124
PLT on day of EE (Mean ± SD, Median [IQR])	247.11 ± 95.082, 220.2 [116]	197.15 ± 46.737, 180 [44]	0.082
PLT after EE (Mean ± SD, Median [IQR])	245.62 ± 104.585, 210 [104]	185.62 ± 41.422, 160 [58]	0.044 *
INR before EE (Mean ± SD, Median [IQR])	1.084 ± 0.084, 1.07 [0.132]	1.186 ± 0.219, 1.10 [0.232]	0.153
INR on day of EE (Mean ± SD, Median [IQR])	1.095 ± 0.078, 1.00 [0.115]	1.158 ± 0.163, 1.10 [0.212]	0.313
INR after EE (Mean ± SD, Median [IQR])	1.087 ± 0.173, 0.90 [0.093]	1.138 ± 0.102, 1.05 [0.123]	0.116
Urea before EE (Mean± SD, Median [IQR])	5.632 ± 1.994, 5.5 [2.9]	6.554 ± 3.728, 5.8 [5]	0.741
Urea on day of EE (Mean ± SD, Median [IQR])	5.523 ± 2.131, 5.5 [2.8]	6.585 ± 3.778, 5.8 [5.5]	0.583

Table 2. *Cont.*

Risk Factors	Patients Alive (n = 53)	Death Outcome (n = 13)	*p* Value
Urea after EE (Mean ± SD, Median [IQR])	5.370 ± 2.374, 5.0 [2.9]	6.869 ± 3.892, 6.2 [5.7]	0.269
CRP before EE (=or↓/↑)	13/40 (24.5%/75.5%)	4/9 (30.8%/69.2%)	0.645
WBC before EE (=or↓/↑)	13/40 (24.5%/75.5%)	4/9 (30.8%/69.2%)	0.645
Ly before EE (=or↓/↑)	47/6 (88.7%/11.3%)	13/0 (100%/0%)	0.203
PMF before EE (=or↓/↑)	47/6 (88.7%/11.3%)	9/4 (69.2%/30.8%)	0.080
RBC before EE (=or↓/↑)	51/2 (96.2%/3.8%)	13/0 (100%/0%)	0.477
HGB before EE (=or↓/↑)	33/0 (100%/0%)	33/0 (100%/0%)	N/A
HCT before EE (=or↓/↑)	52/1 (98.1%/1.9%)	13/0 (100%/0%)	0.618
PLT before EE (=or↓/↑)	48/5 (90.6%/9.4%)	13/0 (100%/0%)	0.249
Glucose before EE (=or↓/↑)	24/29 (45.3%/54.7%)	4/9 (30.8%/69.2%)	0.343
Urea before EE (=or↓/↑)	45/8 (84.9%/15.1%)	9/4 (69.2%/30.8%)	0.189
Potassium before EE (=or↓/↑)	53/0 (100%/0%)	13/0 (100%/0%)	N/A
Sodium before EE (=or↓/↑)	53/0 (100%/0%)	11/2 (84.6%/15.4%)	0.004
Proteins before EE (=or↓/↑)	47/6 (88.7%/11.3%)	13/0 (100%/0%)	0.203
PT before EE (=or↓/↑)	26/27 (49.1%/50.9%)	4/9 (30.8%/69.2%)	0.235
INR before EE (=or↓/↑)	35/18 (66%/34%)	8/5 (61.5%/38.5%)	0.760
PT% before EE (=or↓/↑)	48/5 (90.6%/9.4%)	13/0 (100%/0%)	0.249
APTT before EE (=or↓/↑)	50/3 (94.3%/5.7%)	12/1 (92.3%/7.7%)	0.783
CRP on day of EE (=or↓/↑)	22/31 (41.5%/58.5%)	3/10 (23.1%/76.9%)	0.220
WBC on day of EE (=or↓/↑)	17/36 (32.1%/67.9%)	3/10 (23.1%/76.9%)	T = 0.527
Ly on day of EE (=or↓/↑)	47/6 (88.7%/11.3%)	13/0 (100%/0%)	0.203
PMF on day of EE (=or↓/↑)	49/4 (92.5%/7.5%)	11/2 (84.6%/15.4%)	0.378
RBC on day of EE (=or↓/↑)	51/2 (96.2%/3.8%)	13/0 (100%/0%)	0.477
HGB on day of EE (=or↓/↑)	52/1 (98.1%/1.9%)	13/0 (100%/0%)	0.618
HCT on day of EE (=or↓/↑)	53/0 (100%/0%)	12/1 (92.3%/7.7%)	0.042
PLT on day of EE (=or↓/↑)	52/1 (98.1%/1.9%)	13/0 (100%/0%)	0.618
Glucose on day of EE (=or↓/↑)	22/31 (41.5%/58.5%)	3/10 (23.1%/76.9%)	0.220
Urea on day of EE (=or↓/↑)	47/6 (88.7%/11.3%)	9/4 (69.2%/30.8%)	0.080
Potassium on day of EE (=or↓/↑)	53/0 (100%/0%)	13/0 (100%/0%)	N/A
Sodium on day of EE (=or↓/↑)	53/0 (100%/0%)	11/2 (84.6%/15.4%)	0.004
Proteins on day of EE (=or↓/↑)	52/1 (98.1%/1.9%)	13/0 (100%/0%)	0.618
PT on day of EE (=or↓/↑)	30/23 (56.6%/43.4%)	6/7 (46.2%/53.8%)	0.498
INR on day of EE (=or↓/↑)	31/22 (58.5%/41.5%)	6/7 (46.2%/53.8%)	0.422
PT% on day of EE (=or↓/↑)	53/0 (100%/0%)	12/1 (92.3%/7.7%)	0.042
APTT on day of EE (=or↓/↑)	51/2 (96.2%/3.8%)	12/1 (92.3%/7.7%)	0.543
CRP after EE (=or↓/↑)	26/27 (49.1%/50.9%)	2/11 (15.4%/84.6%)	0.028
WBC after EE (=or↓/↑)	21/32 (39.6%/60.4%)	2/11 (15.4%/84.6%)	T = 0.100
Ly after EE (=or↓/↑)	48/5 (90.6%/9.4%)	13/0 (100%/0%)	0.249
PMF after EE (=or↓/↑)	50/3 (94.3%/5.7%)	10/3 (76.9%/23.1%)	0.050

Table 2. Cont.

Risk Factors	Patients Alive (n = 53)	Death Outcome (n = 13)	p Value
RBC after EE (=or↓/↑)	52/1 (98.1%/1.9%)	13/0 (100%/0%)	0.618
HGB after EE (=or↓/↑)	52/1 (98.1%/1.9%)	13/0 (100%/0%)	0.618
HCT after EE (=or↓/↑)	53/0 (100%/0%)	13/0 (100%/0%)	N/A
PLT after EE (=or↓/↑)	50/3 (94.3%/5.7%)	13/0 (100%/0%)	0.380
Glucose after EE (=or↓/↑)	36/17 (67.9%/32.1%)	0/13 (0%/100%)	0.000
Urea after EE (=or↓/↑)	48/5 (90.6%/9.4%)	7/6 (53.8%/46.2%)	0.001
Potassium after EE (=or↓/↑)	53/0 (100%/0%)	12/1 (92.3%/7.7%)	0.042
Sodium after EE (=or↓/↑)	53/0 (100%/0%)	8/5 (61.5%/38.5%)	0.000
Proteins after EE (=or↓/↑)	47/6 (88.7%/11.3%)	13/0 (100%/0%)	0.203
PT after EE (=or↓/↑)	38/15 (71.7%/28.3%)	5/8 (38.5%/61.5%)	0.024
INR after EE (=or↓/↑)	38/15 (71.7%/28.3%)	6/7 (46.2%/53.8%)	0.080
PT% after EE (=or↓/↑)	53/0 (100%/0%)	13/0 (100%/0%)	N/A
APTT after EE (=or↓/↑)	52/1 (98.1%/1.9%)	8/5 (61.5%/38.5%)	0.000

*—statistically significant; N/A—non-applicable, Abbreviations: EE—endovascular embolization, WBC—white blood cell count, PLT—platelet count, INR—international normalized ratio, CRP—C-reactive protein; (=or↓/↑)—normal or not elevated/elevated, Ly—lymphocyte count, PMF—polymorphonuclear cell count, RBC—red blood cell count, HGB—hemoglobin level, HCT—hematocrit, MCV—mean corpuscular volume, MCH—mean corpuscular hemoglobin, PCT—plateletcrit, PT—prothrombin time, PT%—prothrombin activity, APTT—activated partial thromboplastin time. For the sake of clarity, the Mann–Whitney U test was performed for continuous variables and a Chi-squared test was performed for categorical variables.

The results of the univariate logistic regression for the death outcome are depicted in Table 3.

Table 3. Univariate analysis of factors associated with intrahospital mortality.

Risk Factors	p Value	Crude Odds Ratio	Confidence Interval (95%)
Age	0.025	1.077 *	1.009–1.149
Gender	0.317	1.923	0.534–6.921
FS score	0.016	5.450 *	1.364–21.769
Hemorrhage in IV ventricle (yes/no)	0.046	3.590 *	1.021–12.620
Cerebral vasospasm (yes/no)	0.130	2.719	0.744–9.936
Mechanical ventilation (yes/no)	0.001	15.321 *	3.015–77.862
Hospitalization length	0.035	0.940 *	0.888–0.996
INR before EE (cont.)	0.039	468.871 *	1.367–160,817.788
CRP after EE (=or↓/↑)	0.041	5.296 *	1.069–26.233
Urea after EE (=or↓/↑)	0.004	8.229 *	1.974–34.294
Urea on day of EE (=or↓/↑)	0.092	3.481	0.815–14.876
PT after EE (=or↓/↑)	0.030	4.053 *	1.142–14.392
APTT after EE (=or↓/↑)	0.003	32.500 *	3.350–315.337
Urea before EE (mmol/L)	0.227	1.158	0.913–1.468
Urea on day of EE (mmol/L)	0.186	1.164	0.930–1.456
Urea after EE (mmol/L)	0.091	1.197	0.972–1.475

CRP—C-reactive protein; EE—endovascular embolization; (=or↓/↑)—normal or not elevated/elevated; PT—prothrombin time; APTT—activated partial thromboplastin time; INR—international normalized ratio; *—statistically significant.

After adjustment, the following factors were associated with in-hospital mortality: a delayed ischemic neurological deficit, the presence of blood in the fourth cerebral ventricle, the length of hospitalization, and an elevated urea value after endovascular intervention (Table 4). The strength of the relationship prevailed similar to that after the univariate analysis. Also, there was no change in the direction of influence. The estimates of the coefficient of determination according to the Cox–Snell and Nagelkerke tests were 0.368 and 0.595, respectively. Also, the Hosmer–Lemeshow test demonstrated that the observed rate of intrahospital mortality matched the expected rate of the same phenomenon ($\chi^2 = 6.770$, $p = 0.453$). Within the multivariate logistic regression, the examination of the interactions between the variables did not yield significant results.

Table 4. Multivariate analysis of factors associated with intrahospital mortality.

Risk Factors	p Value	Adjusted Odds Ratio	Confidence Interval (95%)
Age	0.152	1.076	0.973–1.189
Urea after EE (mmol/L)	0.036 *	12.657	1.187–134.913
Delayed ischemic neurological deficit	0.045 *	16.278	1.065–248.748
Hemorrhage in IV ventricle	0.028 *	12.128	1.307–112.575
Aneurysm size	0.476	1.709	0.392–7.460
Duration of hospitalization	0.036 *	0.916	0.844–0.994

EE—endovascular embolization; *—statistically significant.

4. Discussion

Examining the death outcome in patients with ASAH who were treated with endovascular embolization, it was shown that four factors are related to this outcome; namely, a delayed ischemic neurologic deficit, hemorrhage in the fourth cerebral ventricle, the length of hospitalization, and elevated urea after endovascular embolization. It was shown that if a patient develops a delayed ischemic neurologic deficit, the chances of a fatal outcome increase by 16.3 times. The presence of blood in the fourth cerebral ventricle, which was visualized on the initial CT scan, increased the chance of a fatal outcome by 12 times. The statistical results showed that an increase in the length of hospitalization reduced intrahospital mortality by 0.9 times, or, better said, the surviving patients had a longer treatment time compared to the non-survivors, who died early on. An increase in the value of urea above the reference values after an endovascular procedure increased the chance of the patient's death by 12.6 times.

So far, the following risk factors for death in patients with subarachnoid hemorrhage have been described in various studies: age, large aneurysms, cerebral ischemia as a consequence of vasospasm, vasospasm, a poor clinical picture on admission, brain edema, and intraventricular hemorrhage [23–25]. The intrahospital mortality of the patients with ASAH in one of the studies was 18% [26], which is close to our result. Another study with a smaller number of patients showed higher in-hospital mortality of 23% [27]. There were also studies with a significantly lower mortality rate (6%), but with a higher rate of poor clinical outcome (30%) that included severe disability, the vegetative state of the patient, and death [28].

It has also been shown that the presence of cerebral ischemia ($p = 0.039$), symptomatic vasospasm ($p = 0.039$), and pneumonia ($p = 0.006$) are connected with a poor outcome in ASAH patients after endovascular treatment [29].

Massive subarachnoid hemorrhage and massive intraventricular hemorrhage are strong prognostic factors for the occurrence of a lethal outcome in ASAH [27]. This can be explained by the fact that intraventricular hemorrhage is associated with the occurrence of numerous complications, such as ventriculitis, fever, and hydrocephalus, which also significantly increase the mortality rate [30]. Previous research has shown that the presence of blood in the fourth cerebral ventricle is prognostic of a poor outcome in patients with

SAH [31], which supports our result, which speaks of a strong relationship with this diagnostic sign, as it increased the chances of death by 12 times. This result is very important because the initial brain CT is indispensable in all patients with suspected subarachnoid hemorrhage, and, therefore, special attention should be paid to the presence of blood in the fourth cerebral ventricle in the context of a poor prognostic factor.

A study of poor outcomes and primarily death in patients with aneurysmal subarachnoid hemorrhage showed that with the increasing age of the patients with ASAH, the risk of death and other poor outcomes increased [32]. Our results showed a significant relationship between patient age and mortality only in the univariate logistic regression, but not in the final model.

The role of cerebral vasospasm, both angiographic and symptomatic, a delayed ischemic neurological deficit, and delayed cerebral ischemia in the occurrence of death has been investigated, but conflicting results have been published. A delayed ischemic neurologic deficit was shown to be the cause of death in 36% of patients, while single associations between poor outcome and angiographic vasospasm, neurologic deterioration, and brain ischemia were demonstrated ($p < 0.0001$) [28]. Examining three entities within delayed cerebral ischemia proved that symptomatic vasospasm without the development of ischemia, symptomatic CVS and ischemia, as well as delayed ischemia without cerebral vasospasm, individually showed a significant relationship with the development of a fatal outcome ($p = 0.095$, $p = 0.004$, $p = 0.000$), while in the multivariate regression model they lost their significance [26]. The results of this study showed that a delayed ischemic neurological deficit was a strong predictor for in-hospital mortality. In this regard, it is necessary to pay extra attention to potential neurological deterioration in order to diagnose delayed ischemic neurological deficit in time and to prevent further progression and development of delayed cerebral ischemia, which is a known risk factor for death in subarachnoid hemorrhage, with drug therapy [23]. The reason for these conflicting results may be the constant progress of endovascular procedures used for the treatment of ruptured aneurysms, which have great benefits for patients [23,26].

Very few studies have so far examined laboratory results as a risk factor for the occurrence of death in ASAH. In our research, the results of the laboratory diagnostics showed the importance of elevated urea levels after endovascular embolization of a ruptured aneurysm as a strong predictor of death in these patients. It is important to monitor kidney function and creatinine and urea levels in ASAH patients, considering that patients at risk for developing renal failure have twice the chance of death [33]. Also, untreated renal dysfunction is the strongest predictor for in-hospital mortality in ASAH ($p < 0.001$), while acute kidney injury is a confirmed risk factor ($p = 0.028$) [33]. There are no clear pathophysiological mechanisms to explain renal damage in ASAH, but the influence of hemodynamic instability that develops after aneurysm rupture, as well as potential nosocomial infections or the onset of shock, is suspected [34]. Still, a recent study investigated the urea/creatinine ratio in non-traumatic subarachnoid hemorrhage patients and revealed that the ratio is a risk factor for increased intrahospital mortality in these patients. The authors proposed several mechanisms to explain this, including (i) a body stress response leading to unstable brain and kidney circulation and (ii) dehydration that happens early in subarachnoid hemorrhage due to consciousness disorder or dysphagia [35]. Other research investigated the urea/creatinine ratio in ASAH patients with a sample size of 66 patients, like our study. It was mentioned that the urea/creatinine ratio may be a potential marker for catabolism due to critical illness. Also, it was demonstrated that the ratio had increased early values as a risk factor for poor outcome after one year, while greater critical values were connected with DCI, as well as DCI-related infarctions [35]. Both of these studies investigated the urea/creatinine ratio and suggested further research on this marker, which is in concordance with our results. The role of angiography and contrast media use should also be investigated in further studies as a possible factor that can contribute to renal dysfunction. Further research on kidney function and creatinine and urea levels in ASAH patients is needed in order to explain pathophysiological mechanisms. We propose further studies analyzing intrahospital mortality in ASAH patients treated with an endovascular approach, including a larger sample size.

This study has some limitations. It was a unicentric study with a relatively small sample size. Due to the small sample, it was possible to simultaneously test only up to 10 variables in the multivariate logistic regression, which increased the chances of a statistical type 2 error.

5. Conclusions

From the obtained results, we can conclude that a delayed ischemic neurologic deficit is the strongest predictor of intrahospital mortality in ASAH patients. Also, it is important to pay attention to the intraventricular hemorrhage on the initial head CT scan, along with monitoring kidney function and elevated urea values after endovascular aneurysm embolization, since they have been shown to be a significant risk factor for intrahospital mortality in ASAH patients.

Author Contributions: Conceptualization, V.O., N.Z. and F.D.; methodology, V.O., N.Z. and F.D.; software, N.Z.; validation, V.O., N.Z. and F.D.; formal analysis, V.O., N.Z., T.P. and M.O.; investigation, S.J., D.M., E.C., B.J., J.J.N., J.A.N., M.A., M.O., N.P., M.N. and T.P.; resources, V.O., S.J., D.M., E.C., B.J., J.J.N., J.A.N., M.A., M.O., N.P. and M.N.; data curation, V.O., S.J., D.M., B.J., J.J.N., J.A.N., M.A., M.O., N.P., M.N. and T.P.; writing—original draft preparation, V.O., N.Z., S.J., D.M., E.C., B.J., J.J.N., J.A.N., M.A., M.O., N.P., M.N., T.P. and F.D.; writing—review and editing, V.O., N.Z. and F.D.; visualization, V.O., N.Z., S.J., D.M., E.C., B.J., J.J.N., J.A.N., M.A., M.O., N.P., M.N., T.P. and F.D.; supervision, V.O. and N.Z.; project administration, V.O. and N.Z. All authors have read and agreed to the published version of the manuscript.

Funding: This research received no external funding.

Institutional Review Board Statement: The study was conducted according to the guidelines of the Declaration of Helsinki, and approved by the Ethics Committee of University Clinical Center Kragujevac, 01-10138 from 10 August 2016.

Informed Consent Statement: Informed consent was obtained from all subjects involved in the study.

Data Availability Statement: The datasets used and analyzed during the current study are made available from the corresponding author on reasonable request.

Acknowledgments: Our study was supported by the Ministry of Science, Technological Development and Innovations of the Republic of Serbia, no.451-03-47/2023-01/200111.

Conflicts of Interest: The authors declare no conflicts of interest.

References

1. Pegoli, M.; Mandrekar, J.; Rabinstein, A.A.; Lanzino, G. Predictors of excellent functional outcome in aneurysmal subarachnoid hemorrhage. *J. Neurosurg.* **2015**, *122*, 414–418. [CrossRef] [PubMed]
2. Watson, E.; Ding, D.; Khattar, N.K.; Everhart, D.E.; James, R.F. Neurocognitive outcomes after aneurysmal subarachnoid hemorrhage: Identifying inflammatory biomarkers. *J. Neurol. Sci.* **2018**, *394*, 84–93. [CrossRef] [PubMed]
3. Milinis, K.; Thapar, A.; O'Neill, K.; Davies, A.H. History of Aneurysmal Spontaneous Subarachnoid Hemorrhage. *Stroke* **2017**, *48*, e280–e283. [CrossRef] [PubMed]
4. Muehlschlegel, S. Subarachnoid Hemorrhage. *Continuum* **2018**, *24*, 1623–1657. [CrossRef] [PubMed]
5. Ciurea, A.V.; Palade, C.; Voinescu, D.; Nica, D.A. Subarachnoid hemorrhage and cerebral vasospasm—Literature review. *J. Med. Life* **2013**, *6*, 120–125. [PubMed]
6. Macdonald, R.L.; Schweizer, T.A. Spontaneous subarachnoid haemorrhage. *Lancet* **2017**, *389*, 655–666. [CrossRef]
7. Mahaney, K.B.; Todd, M.M.; Torner, J.C.; INHAST Investigators I. Variation of patient characteristics, management, and outcome with timing of surgery for aneurysmal subarachnoid hemorrhage. *J. Neurosurg.* **2011**, *114*, 1045–1053. [CrossRef]
8. Rose, M.J. Aneurysmal subarachnoid hemorrhage: An update on the medical complications and treatments strategies seen in these patients. *Curr. Opin. Anaesthesiol.* **2011**, *24*, 500–507. [CrossRef]
9. Guglielmi, G.; Vinuela, F.; Sepetka, I.; Macellari, V. Electrothrombosis of saccular aneurysms via endovascular approach. Part 1: Electrochemical basis, technique, and experimental results. *J. Neurosurg.* **1991**, *75*, 1–7. [CrossRef]
10. McDougall, C.G.; Spetzler, R.F.; Zabramski, J.M.; Partovi, S.; Hills, N.K.; Nakaji, P.; Albuquerque, F.C. The Barrow Ruptured Aneurysm Trial. *J. Neurosurg.* **2012**, *116*, 135–144. [CrossRef]

11. Spetzler, R.F.; McDougall, C.G.; Zabramski, J.M.; Albuquerque, F.C.; Hills, N.K.; Russin, J.J.; Partovi, S.; Nakaji, P.; Wallace, R.C. The barrow ruptured aneurysm trial: 6-year results. *J. Neurosurg.* **2015**, *123*, 609–617. [CrossRef] [PubMed]
12. Molyneux, A.; Kerr, R.; Stratton, I.; Sandercock, P.; Clarke, M.; Shrimpton, J.; Holman, R.; International Subarachnoid Aneurysm Trial (ISAT) Collaborative Group. International Subarachnoid Aneurysm Trial (ISAT) of neurosurgical clipping versus endovascular coiling in 2143 patients with ruptured intracranial aneurysms: A randomised trial. *Lancet* **2002**, *360*, 1267–1274. [CrossRef] [PubMed]
13. Molyneux, A.J.; Kerr, R.S.; Yu, L.-M.; Clarke, M.; Sneade, M.; A Yarnold, J.; Sandercock, P. International Subarachnoid Aneurysm Trial (ISAT) of neurosurgical clipping versus endovascular coiling in 2143 patients with ruptured intracranial aneurysms: A randomised comparison of effects on survival, dependency, seizures, rebleeding, subgroups, and aneurysm occlusion. *Lancet* **2005**, *366*, 809–817. [PubMed]
14. Spetzler, R.F.; McDougall, C.G.; Albuquerque, F.C.; Zabramski, J.M.; Hills, N.K.; Partovi, S.; Nakaji, P.; Wallace, R.C. The Barrow Ruptured Aneurysm Trial: 3-year results. *J. Neurosurg.* **2013**, *119*, 146–157. [CrossRef] [PubMed]
15. Connolly, E.S., Jr.; Rabinstein, A.A.; Carhuapoma, J.R.; Derdeyn, C.P.; Dion, J.; Higashida, R.T.; Hoh, B.L.; Kirkness, C.J.; Naidech, A.M.; Ogilvy, C.S.; et al. Guidelines for the management of aneurysmal subarachnoid hemorrhage: A statement for healthcare professionals from a special writing group of the Stroke Council, American Heart Association. *Stroke* **2012**, *43*, 1711–1737. [CrossRef]
16. Diringer, M.N.; Bleck, T.P.; Hemphill, J.C., 3rd; Menon, D.; Shutter, L.; Vespa, P.; Bruder, N.; Connolly, E.S., Jr.; Citerio, G.; Gress, D.; et al. Critical care management of patients following aneurysmal subarachnoid hemorrhage: Recommendations from the Neurocritical Care Society's Multidisciplinary Consensus Conference. *Neurocrit Care* **2011**, *15*, 211–240. [CrossRef] [PubMed]
17. Larsen, C.C.; Astrup, J. Rebleeding after aneurysmal sub- arachnoid hemorrhage: A literature review. *World Neurosurg.* **2013**, *79*, 307–312. [CrossRef]
18. Long, B.; Koyfman, A.; Runyon, M.S. Subarachnoid Hemorrhage: Updates in Diagnosis and Management. *Emerg. Med. Clin. N. Am.* **2017**, *35*, 803–824. [CrossRef]
19. Neifert, S.N.; Chapman, E.K.; Martini, M.L.; Shuman, W.H.; Schupper, A.J.; Oermann, E.K.; Mocco, J.; Macdonald, R.L. Aneurysmal Subarachnoid Hemorrhage: The Last Decade. *Transl. Stroke Res.* **2021**, *12*, 428–446. [CrossRef]
20. Papadimitriou-Olivgeris, M.; Zotou, A.; Koutsileou, K.; Aretha, D.; Boulovana, M.; Vrettos, T.; Sklavou, C.; Marangos, M.; Fligou, F. Fatores de risco para mortalidade após hemorragia subaracnoidea: Estudo observacional retrospectivo [Risk factors for mortality after subarachnoid hemorrhage: A retrospective observational study]. *Braz. J. Anesthesiol.* **2019**, *69*, 448–454. [CrossRef]
21. Lozano, C.S.; Lozano, A.M.; Spears, J. The Changing Landscape of Treatment for Intracranial Aneurysm. *Can. J. Neurol. Sci.* **2019**, *46*, 159–165. [CrossRef] [PubMed]
22. Fisher, C.M.; Kistler, J.P.; Davis, J.M. Relation of cerebral vasospasm to subarachnoid hemorrhage visualized by computerized tomographic scanning. *Neurosurgery* **1980**, *6*, 1–9. [CrossRef] [PubMed]
23. Komotar, R.J.; Schmidt, J.M.; Starke, R.M.; Claassen, J.; Wartenberg, K.E.; Lee, K.; Badjatia, N.; Connolly, E.S.; Mayer, S.A. Resuscitation and critical care of poor-grade subarachnoid hemorrhage. *Neurosurgery* **2009**, *64*, 397–410. [CrossRef] [PubMed]
24. Claassen, J.; Carhuapoma, J.R.; Kreiter, K.T.; Du, E.Y.; Connolly, E.S.; Mayer, S.A. Global cerebral edema after subarachnoid hemorrhage: Frequency, predictors, and impact on outcome. *Stroke* **2002**, *33*, 1225–1232. [CrossRef] [PubMed]
25. Helbok, R.; Ko, S.-B.; Schmidt, J.M.; Kurtz, P.; Fernandez, L.; Choi, H.A.; Connolly, E.S.; Lee, K.; Badjatia, N.; Mayer, S.A.; et al. Global cerebral edema and brain metabolism after subarachnoid hemorrhage. *Stroke* **2011**, *42*, 1534–1539. [CrossRef] [PubMed]
26. Lantigua, H.; Ortega-Gutierrez, S.; Schmidt, J.M.; Lee, K.; Badjatia, N.; Agarwal, S.; Claassen, J.; Connolly, E.S.; Mayer, S.A. Subarachnoid hemorrhage: Who dies, and why? *Crit. Care* **2015**, *19*, 309. [CrossRef] [PubMed]
27. Schütz, H.; Krack, P.; Buchinger, B.; Bödeker, R.-H.; Laun, A.; Dorndorf, W.; Agnoli, A. Outcome of patients with aneurysmal and presumed aneurysmal bleeding. A hospital study based on 100 consecutive cases in a neurological clinic. *Neurosurg. Rev.* **1993**, *16*, 15–25. [CrossRef] [PubMed]
28. Vergouwen, M.D.; Ilodigwe, D.; Macdonald, R.L. Cerebral infarction after subarachnoid hemorrhage contributes to poor outcome by vasospasm-dependent and -independent effects. *Stroke* **2011**, *42*, 924–929. [CrossRef] [PubMed]
29. Zhao, B.; Yang, H.; Zheng, K.; Li, Z.; Xiong, Y.; Tan, X.; Zhong, M.; The AMPAS Study Group. Preoperative and postoperative predictors of long-term outcome after endovascular treatment of poor-grade aneurysmal subarachnoid hemorrhage. *J. Neurosurg.* **2017**, *126*, 1764–1771. [CrossRef]
30. Kramer, A.H.; Mikolaenko, I.; Deis, N.; Dumont, A.S.; Kassell, N.F.; Bleck, T.P.; A Nathan, B. Intraventricular hemorrhage volume predicts poor outcomes but not delayed ischemic neurological deficits among patients with ruptured cerebral aneurysms. *Neurosurgery* **2010**, *67*, 1044–1053. [CrossRef]
31. Longatti, P.L.; Martinuzzi, A.; Fiorindi, A.; Maistrello, L.; Carteri, A. Neuroendoscopic Management of Intraventricular Hemorrhage. *Stroke* **2004**, *35*, e35–e38. [CrossRef] [PubMed]
32. Goldberg, J.; Schoeni, D.; Mordasini, P.; Z'graggen, W.; Gralla, J.; Raabe, A.; Beck, J.; Fung, C. Survival and Outcome After Poor-Grade Aneurysmal Subarachnoid Hemorrhage in Elderly Patients. *Stroke* **2018**, *49*, 2883–2889. [CrossRef] [PubMed]
33. Zacharia, B.E.; Ducruet, A.F.; Hickman, Z.L.; Grobelny, B.T.; Fernandez, L.; Schmidt, J.M.; Narula, R.; Ko, L.N.; Cohen, M.E.; Mayer, S.A. Renal dysfunction as an independent predictor of outcome after aneurysmal subarachnoid hemorrhage: A single-center cohort study. *Stroke* **2009**, *40*, 2375–2381. [CrossRef] [PubMed]

34. Eagles, M.E.; Powell, M.F.; Ayling, O.G.S.; Tso, M.K.; Macdonald, R.L. Acute kidney injury after aneurysmal subarachnoid hemorrhage and its effect on patient outcome: An exploratory analysis. *J. Neurosurg.* **2019**, *133*, 765–772. [CrossRef]
35. Chen, Z.; Wang, J.; Yang, H.; Li, H.; Chen, R.; Yu, J. Relationship between the Blood Urea Nitrogen to Creatinine Ratio and In-Hospital Mortality in Non-Traumatic Subarachnoid Hemorrhage Patients: Based on Propensity Score Matching Method. *J. Clin. Med.* **2022**, *11*, 7031. [CrossRef]

Disclaimer/Publisher's Note: The statements, opinions and data contained in all publications are solely those of the individual author(s) and contributor(s) and not of MDPI and/or the editor(s). MDPI and/or the editor(s) disclaim responsibility for any injury to people or property resulting from any ideas, methods, instructions or products referred to in the content.

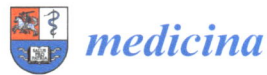

Review

Neuroimaging Modalities Used for Ischemic Stroke Diagnosis and Monitoring

Jasmin J. Nukovic [1,2,†], Valentina Opancina [3,4,5,*,†], Elisa Ciceri [4], Mario Muto [5], Nebojsa Zdravkovic [6], Ahmet Altin [7], Pelin Altaysoy [8], Rebeka Kastelic [9], Diana Maria Velazquez Mendivil [10], Jusuf A. Nukovic [1,2], Nenad V. Markovic [11], Miljan Opancina [6,12], Tijana Prodanovic [13], Merisa Nukovic [2], Jelena Kostic [14] and Nikola Prodanovic [11]

1. Faculty of Pharmacy and Health Travnik, University of Travnik, 72270 Travnik, Bosnia and Herzegovina
2. Department of Radiology, General Hospital Novi Pazar, 36300 Novi Pazar, Serbia
3. Department of Radiology, Faculty of Medical Sciences, University of Kragujevac, 34000 Kragujevac, Serbia
4. Diagnostic Imaging and Interventional Neuroradiology Unit, Department of Neurosurgery, Fondazione IRCCS Istituto Neurologico Carlo Besta, 20133 Milan, Italy
5. Diagnostic and Interventional Neuroradiology Unit, A.O.R.N. Cardarelli, 80131 Naples, Italy
6. Department of Biomedical Statistics and Informatics, Faculty of Medical Sciences, University of Kragujevac, 34000 Kragujevac, Serbia
7. Faculty of Medicine, Dokuz Eylul University, Izmir 35340, Turkey
8. Faculty of Medicine, Bahcesehir University, Istanbul 34349, Turkey
9. Faculty of Medicine, University of Ljubljana, 1000 Ljubljana, Slovenia
10. Faculty of Medicine, University of Sonora, Hermosillo 83067, Mexico
11. Department of Surgery, Faculty of Medical Sciences, University of Kragujevac, 34000 Kragujevac, Serbia
12. Military Medical Academy, Faculty of Medicine, University of Defense, 11000 Belgrade, Serbia
13. Department of Pediatrics, Faculty of Medical Sciences, University of Kragujevac, 34000 Kragujevac, Serbia
14. Department of Radiology, Medical Faculty, University of Belgrade, 11120 Beograd, Serbia
* Correspondence: valentina.opancina@gmail.com
† These authors contributed equally to this work.

Abstract: Strokes are one of the global leading causes of physical or mental impairment and fatality, classified into hemorrhagic and ischemic strokes. Ischemic strokes happen when a thrombus blocks or plugs an artery and interrupts or reduces blood supply to the brain tissue. Deciding on the imaging modality which will be used for stroke detection depends on the expertise and availability of staff and the infrastructure of hospitals. Magnetic resonance imaging provides valuable information, and its sensitivity for smaller infarcts is greater, while computed tomography is more extensively used, since it can promptly exclude acute cerebral hemorrhages and is more favorable speed-wise. The aim of this article was to give information about the neuroimaging modalities used for the diagnosis and monitoring of ischemic strokes. We reviewed the available literature and presented the use of computed tomography, CT angiography, CT perfusion, magnetic resonance imaging, MR angiography and MR perfusion for the detection of ischemic strokes and their monitoring in different phases of stroke development.

Keywords: stroke; ischemia; CT; MR; neuroimaging

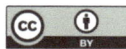

1. Introduction

Strokes are one of the global leading causes of physical or mental impairment and fatality, associated with focal CNS injury of vascular origin which precipitates neurological deficit [1]. Fundamentally, strokes are classified into hemorrhagic and ischemic strokes (ISs). ISs happen when a thrombus blocks or plugs an artery and interrupts or reduces blood supply to the brain tissue. Strokes resulting from an acute decline of vascular supply to the brain comprise a notable portion of 80% of all strokes. The predisposition aspects of these stroke subtypes are both alike and discrete. Factors such as hypertension increase susceptibility to hemorrhagic strokes, but also brings about an indirect surge in ischemic strokes that result from atherosclerosis. Moreover, hyperlipidemia, atrial fibrillation, diabetes and smoking are risk factors for intracranial and extracranial vessel atherosclerosis-originated strokes and cardioembolic strokes, respectively [2].

Treatment strategies for acute ischemic strokes (AISs) in stroke units are chiefly focused on revascularization and avoiding further neuronal injuries. Up-to-date medical care options for AISs are available, like the administration of IV tissue plasminogen activator (IV-tPA) for IV thrombolysis, as well as endovascular treatment (EVT) [3]. EVT, a minimally invasive operation also known as mechanical thrombectomy, is efficient for reanalyzing occluded blood vessels and results in better outcomes for large vessel occlusion (LVO) patients, removing the clot [4]. On the other hand, recombinant tPA-induced thrombolysis causes a reperfusion of the brain. Nonetheless, it is only effective in the first 4.5 h from onset; it can increase the chance of bleeding and is not worthwhile for larger infarcts, but it should be noted that EVT also has disadvantages such as access-site hematoma, infection, vasospasm, arterial perforation or dissection, symptomatic intracerebral hemorrhage, etc. [5]. Furthermore, drugs that are able to cross the blood–brain barrier (BBB) such as liposomes, hydrogels and nanomedicines are in clinical trials, and their potentials for AIS therapy are still being investigated. Owing to their short half-life, so far, clinical studies suggest that low doses of liposomes are sufficient for better motor function and dwindling the infarct volume [6,7]. They assist the administration of gaseous particles and certain drugs by enveloping them, shielding them from physiological events like degradation and elongating their half-lives [7]. As for hydrogels, they support the injured brain tissue structurally and benefit local regeneration. Still, there is insufficient evidence to recommend liposomes or hydrogels for clinical use.

The clinical management of strokes greatly benefits from various imaging modalities. For example, to exclude neoplasms and intracranial hemorrhages (ICHs), to determine the infarct core, which is beneficial for further therapy, to understand the extent of recoverable ischemic penumbras and to have real-time data on the vascular lumens, many subtypes of magnetic resonance imaging (MRI) and computed tomography (CT) are utilized. Deciding on the imaging modality depends on the expertise and availability of staff and the infrastructure of hospitals. MRI provides exceptional information and great sensitivity for smaller infarcts, diffusion-weighted imaging (DWI) produces accurate information on the volume of the core of the infarction and MRI is also proven to be more favorable in differentiating conditions that resemble strokes, such as convulsive attacks, migraines, venous infarctions and neoplasms. Still, CT is more extensively used, can promptly exclude acute cerebral hemorrhages and is more favorable speed-wise [8]. CT perfusion (CTP) imaging benefits the selection of AIS patients for EVT by facilitating core infarct volume calculations, necessitating less workflow in deducting the onset time of strokes that arise in patients that have no previous symptoms before waking up [9]. Aging ISs can be important in both clinical and medico-legal circumstances, and more accurate information can be provided through MRI. Acute ISs are defined as strokes which happen for between 24 h and 7 days, where the early hyperacute phase occurs between 0 and 6 h and the late hyperacute phase between 6 and 24 h. Subacute ISs occur in the time frame between 1 and 3 weeks, while chronic ISs last more than 3 weeks [10].

The aim of this article was to give information on the neuroimaging modalities used for the diagnosis of ischemic strokes and their monitoring in daily practice.

2. Methodology

2.1. Study Design

Our study is designed as a literature review.

2.2. Search Strategy

We conducted a review of the current literature, including original articles and reviews that studied various approaches of ischemic stroke diagnostic imaging. We performed extensive searches on the Google Scholar, PubMed and ScienceDirect databases to identify relevant manuscripts. As keywords, we used "stroke", "ischemic stroke", and "brain attack", "cerebrovascular accident", combined with "imaging", "neuroimaging", "diagnostic", "diagnostic modalities", "radiological modality" and "diagnosis".

2.3. Selection Criteria

Studies reporting prospective or retrospective clinical and radiological data, as well as meta-analyses involving radiological diagnostics of ischemic strokes were included. Studies not published in the English language or did not present adequate data on the neuroimaging characteristics of ischemic strokes were not included in the study. Expert opinions, book chapters and scientific meeting abstracts were also excluded.

2.4. Data Extraction

The search strategy and data extraction were performed independently by ten different authors who screened the retrieved papers for eligibility and analyzed the full-text articles that met the eligibility criteria. Data were extracted and analyzed using Microsoft Excel 2015.

3. Results

The search of the literature yielded 403 articles in total. After a thorough review and assessment of the articles, we identified and included a subset of 41 papers that provided valuable insights into the neuroimaging modalities used for ischemic stroke diagnosis and monitoring, forming the basis of our review. In Figure 1, we present the study selection process.

Over time, technical development has brought the use of different modalities in the neuroimaging area. In this paper, we will present the neuroimaging modalities used for ischemic stroke diagnosis and monitoring, summarized in Table 1, with the main advantages and disadvantages of their use.

Table 1. Summary of neuroimaging modalities used for ischemic stroke diagnosis and monitoring.

	Advantages	Disadvantages
Non-contrast CT	High availability, cost-effectiveness, and rapid image acquisition; no contrast.	Ionizing radiation. Limited in posterior fossa and small lesions, as well as hyperacute and acute IS.
CT angiography	Locates source of thrombi or emboli and the clot dimensions in order to plan the reperfusion treatment.	Ionizing radiation. Contrast contraindications.
CT perfusion	Provides an accurate delimitation of the infarct core and penumbra area and thus good selection of patients for reperfusion treatment.	Ionizing radiation. Limited availability.
MRI	No radiation; greater sensitivity than CT; better detection of small lesions in comparison to CT.	Slower than CT; higher cost; limited availability.
MR angiography	Locate source of thrombi or emboli; no contrast.	Flow-dependent images may be inaccurate, unlike CTA which presents true anatomy of vessel lumen.
MR perfusion	Assesses brain tissue perfusion level.	Higher cost; limited availability; use of contrast.

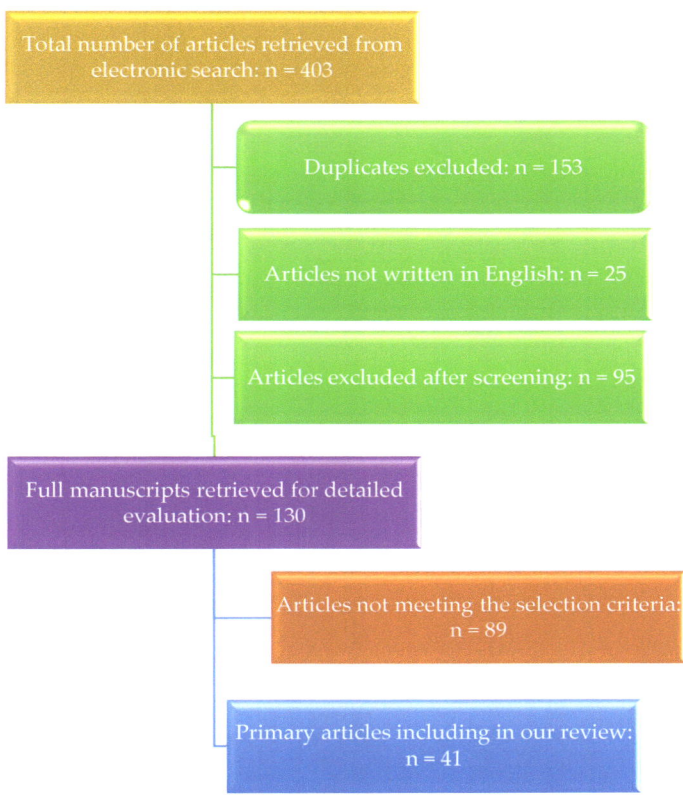

Figure 1. Study selection process.

3.1. Non-Contrast CT

Computed tomography scans play a crucial role in diagnosing and evaluating ischemic strokes. Although other imaging modalities like DWI can offer greater sensitivity and additional information that is beneficial in later stages, the high availability, cost-effectiveness and rapid image acquisition of CT scans make them particularly suitable for the early phases of the disease [10,11]. This is especially important given that treatment options like thrombolytic therapy are most effective within the first few hours of stroke onset [12]. It should be noted that differentiation between ischemic and hemorrhagic strokes through CT is not troublesome due to the fact that hemorrhagic strokes present as hyperdense collections of blood [1].

This section will focus on the different phases of ischemic strokes and their appearances on CT scans without contrast.

3.1.1. Acute Ischemic Stroke

Non-contrast computed tomography (NCCT) is a valuable tool for evaluating the initial stages of ischemic strokes. The presence of cytotoxic edema, thrombosis and cellular hypoperfusion during an ischemic event leads to observable signs on a CT scan [13–18]. These early signs are crucial for excluding intracranial hemorrhage, which is an absolute contraindication for thrombolytic therapy [14]. The most commonly seen signs include focal hypodensity, hyperdense arteries, cortical effacement, the insular ribbon sign and the obscuration of the basal ganglia [13].

The insular ribbon sign becomes evident when the insular cortex displays a reduced gray–white interface. This sign is frequently observed in middle cerebral artery (MCA) occlusions due to the insular region's limited collateral circulation from the anterior and posterior circulations [16]. It is an extremely common sign in early ischemia, presenting itself in nearly all cases [19].

The hyperdense artery sign differs from other signs in that it reveals the thrombus obstructing the artery, rather than changes in infarcted tissue [16]. While not as easily noticeable as other early signs, it is highly specific [19].

The obscuration of the basal ganglia is frequently observed in cases of acute ischemic strokes. Since the arteries supplying the basal ganglia are primarily end-arteries, they are particularly susceptible to ischemia [13]. During acute ischemic strokes, partial disappearance or reduced differentiation may be observed on NCCT [16]. In cases where the occlusion is present in the more distal parts of the arteries, the basal ganglia might remain unaffected. Some studies indicate that only 16% of patients exhibit this sign [19].

Cortical (hemispherical) sulcal effacement is a relatively common sign, occurring in 33% of cases [20]. It indicates a partially superficial infarct, characterized by reduced contrast in the cortical sulci [18]. This phenomenon is caused by edema in the ischemic cortex [13]. When observed as an isolated sign, it indicates a better prognosis for intravenous thrombolytic therapy [19–21].

Focal hypodensity is a result of increased water content due to cytotoxic edema. It may present as reduced gray–white matter differentiation. While this sign is present in up to 60% of ischemic stroke cases [9], its identification can be challenging, with sensitivities for recognizing MCA territory hypodensity ranging between 60% and 85% [19].

3.1.2. Aspects Score

The Alberta Stroke Program Early CT Score (ASPECTS) is a quantitative approach for identifying early stroke signs. It was developed to evaluate highly acute cases (within 3 h of symptom onset) and estimate the success rate of thrombolytic therapy [22]. Although initially designed for the anterior circulation, other models have been developed, such as pc-ASPECTS, which is used for the posterior circulation [23–25].

Compared to previous approaches, such as the 1/3 of MCA territory rule, ASPECTS is favored by physicians due to its higher diagnostic agreement across specialties [23–25].

The ASPECTS value ranges from 0 to 10. A total of 10 points indicate a normal CT scan, while 0 points suggest diffuse ischemic changes throughout the MCA territory. To calculate the ASPECTS value, starting from 10 points, one point is subtracted for each marked area affected by ischemic changes, such as hypoattenuation and swelling. These areas encompass the MCA territories M1, M2, M3, the insula, lentiform nucleus, caudate nucleus, internal capsule from ganglionic axial slices, and M4, M5 and M6 from the supraganglionic axial slices [23,24].

It is important to note that older studies examined only two cuts—one at the level of the basal ganglia and the other from the supraganglionic area [24]. Since then, common practice has changed, and typically, all axial slices are examined [22].

The relationship between treatment outcomes and the ASPECTS value has been a subject of long-standing debate. Earlier studies suggested a dichotomy between patients with a score higher than seven, who responded to treatment, and those with a lower score, who did not [25]. Recent studies indicate a linear relationship between a patient's ASPECTS score and their response to treatment. However, a distinct cutoff point for when thrombolytic therapy becomes unviable has not yet been established, so caution should be exercised when making treatment decisions based solely on the ASPECT score [22]. Nevertheless, the ASPECTS score remains a strong predictor of functional outcomes, providing information about potential hemorrhagic transformation, recovery and response to treatment [26].

3.1.3. Subacute Phase

A challenging aspect of NCCT imaging in diagnosing subacute ischemic strokes is a phenomenon known as "CT Fogging." This fogging effect can be described as the attenuation of affected tissue returning to a "normal" state (similar to healthy brain matter) during the second and third weeks after symptom onset [27].

CT fogging is typically attributed to multiple factors, one of which is the reduction of edema and mass effect during the recovery phase [28]. Another contributing factor may be the extravasation of liquids, leading to increased blood flow and subsequently causing the fogging effect. This concept is supported by the fact that newly formed and unstable blood vessels lack a functional BBB, potentially causing contrast medium leakage if applied [29]. Studies suggest that applying a contrast medium reveals infarcted tissue during the second and third weeks, which is the usual time window for CT fogging [27].

Since CT fogging is a common occurrence (approximately 54% of cases), accurately diagnosing subacute ischemic strokes using only NCCT may be challenging. Infarcted tissue may become isodense; lesions may be underestimated, or even overlooked entirely. Consequently, ruling out a stroke cannot be easily achieved, especially if the patient presents with symptoms; in such cases, CT with contrast should be considered [28–30].

3.1.4. Chronic Phase

As necrotic brain tissue is reabsorbed, infarcted brain tissue is replaced by cerebrospinal fluid (CSF), resulting in hypodensity. Adjacent subarachnoid and ventricular spaces may enlarge due to the negative pressure resulting from tissue loss. The infarcted area becomes clearly visible at this stage [31].

During this stage, NCCT is typically employed to monitor the recovery period and measure therapeutic success. Given that CT imaging primarily reflects structural changes in brain tissue, metrics such as infarct size are observed and correlated with clinical outcomes [32].

3.2. CT Angiography

In the context of an ischemic stroke, CT angiography (CTA) is used to localize the site of arterial occlusion [33] and the clot dimensions in order to plan the reperfusion treatment in an efficient way and re-establish brain circulation as early as possible [34]. Since it is accurate for the detection or large thrombi in proximal cerebral arteries [35], this particular type of occlusion can be resistant to the enzymatic breakdown from IV thrombolytic therapy [35,36]. It is important to mention that the contrast required for this study requires a wait of at least five minutes after the simple CT is performed [37].

For the study and interpretation of CT angiography, it is important to understand the division of vascular territories. This classification contains many divisions, starting with anterior and posterior circulation; the anterior cerebral artery (ACA), middle cerebral artery (MCA) and internal carotid artery (ICA) are part of the anterior circulation, whilst the posterior cerebral artery (PCA), cerebellar arteries, vertebral artery (VA) and basilar artery (BA) constitute the posterior circulation [38,39]. The ICA originates the anterior circulation vessels and is divided into four portions: cervical, petrous, cavernous and supraclinoid. On the other side, it has very particular occlusive patterns: stump, spearhead and streak/elongation; from these patterns, stumps are the most common in the cervical portion of the ICA and can be accompanied by calcifications. Streaks are the most frequent in terminus occlusion and spearheads are more common in the occlusion of the cavernous portion [40].

The ACA territory involves the medial frontal gyrus, superior frontal gyrus, the anterior part of the cingulate, the middle part of the cingulate and the corpus callosum; it also extends to the precuneus and splenium posteriorly [38]. For practical purposes, the ACA is divided in three main segments [41]:

A1: Horizontal/pre-communicating artery, which goes along the ipsilateral optic nerve and chiasm [41].

A2: Vertical/post-communicating artery. It goes into the interhemispheric fissure specifically anterior to the lamina terminalis [41].

A3: Pericallosal. It terminates in the choroid plexus [41].

The borders of the territory of the MCA extend from the superior frontal sulcus to the middle occipital gyrus; some of the structures involved in the territory are the anterior portion of the middle frontal gyrus, the angular gyrus and posterior involvement from the parietal lobe, inferior occipital gyrus, putamen, globus pallidus and the insula [38]. For the radiological study of the MCA, the artery is divided in four segments [42]:

M1: Sphenoidal or horizontal segment; it has its origin in the bifurcation of the carotid artery and extends laterally in the axial plane to the Sylvian fissure. It eventually divides into two trunks that, when they reach the limen insulae, turn 90 degrees. This turn is known as the genu.

M2: Insular segment. It begins its trajectory at the genu from the previous segment, composed of the trunks and its branches that circulate in the insulae, directed to the insular circular sulcus in its most distant part to make another turn to surround the opercula.

M3: Opercular segment. It originates from the circular sulcus's most distal part; the branches go along the temporal and frontoparietal opercula until the lateral edge of the Sylvian fissure.

M4: Cortical segments. They begin in the lateral edge of the Sylvian fissure, where the branches make another turn to an inferior or superior direction towards the cortical surface, where they terminate [42].

The VA is divided into extracranial and intracranial segments; its branches supply the medulla and spinal cord anterior surfaces. Besides originating the PICA and the BA at the conjunction of the intracranial portion, the BA perforating branches irrigate the brain stem; besides that, the BA originates the SCA, AICA and PCA [43].

The cerebellum is irrigated by the SCA, AICA and PICA; specifically, the SCA and AICA originate from the BA, the AICA supplies anterior–inferior cerebellum, whilst the SCA vascularizes the superior vermis and superior cerebellum. On the other hand, the PICA irrigates the lower vermis, lower medulla and posterior–inferior cerebellum [43].

The PCA constitutes the terminal branch of the BA; in its territory, the lateral border is delimited to the lateral part of the frontal gyrus and extends to the inferior occipital gyrus, middle occipital gyrus and superior occipital sulcus. This territory includes interhemispheric surfaces of the occipital lobe such as the lingual gyrus, calcarine gyrus and lower half of the cuneus; it also includes the thalamus and midbrain [38]. The PCA also has four segments [39]:

P1: Pre-communicating segment. It extends from the end of the basilar artery (BA) and ends in the posterior communicating artery (PCOM).

P2: Post-communicating segment. It has its origin at the PCOM and ends when it enters the quadrigeminal cistern.

P3: Quadrigeminal. This follows the course of the quadrigeminal cistern.

P4: Cortical. This goes along the calcarine fissure and becomes the calcarine artery [39].

Another aspect that needs to be evaluated in CT angiography is the percentage of blockage in the artery, where stenosis is defined as a narrowing of the vessel, while occlusion refers to a total blockage; the severity of the stenosis will be classified according to the percentage, where <50% is mild stenosis, >50–<70 is moderate stenosis, 70–89% is severe stenosis and 90–99% is very severe stenosis [44].

For reperfusion therapy, CT angiography has clinical relevance in selecting the type of treatment that patients will receive for ischemic strokes, since a key point in the selection is the size and location of the occlusion site [35,36]. Large and proximal arterial occlusions (ICA, M1, M2 or BA) can be associated with negative outcomes and a need for extended care, besides having lower recanalization rates with IV thrombolysis; therefore, a mechanical thrombectomy would represent a better option for these patients [45].

3.3. CT Perfusion

Besides being a diagnostic tool, CT perfusion plays an important role when it comes to selecting patients that could be candidates for reperfusion therapy [46], since it is capable of determining the following variants: mean time transit (MTT), time to peak (TTP), cerebral blood flow (CBF) and cerebral blood volume (CBV). It provides an accurate delimitation of the infarct core and penumbra area; this way, the areas that can be saved can be visualized [47]. However, it is important to take into account the limitations of this technique, such as the overestimation of the infarct core and a 50% false negative rate for lacunar strokes [48].

The information that CT perfusion seeks to capture is the dynamic of a contrast bolus passing through brain tissue, which includes its increase, peak and decrease in the area of interest, in order to obtain a quantification of the tissue with hypoperfusion. The following parameters are representative of different aspects of the blood flow that goes into the brain [47]:

CBF: Describes the blood flow volume of blood streaming into a unit of brain mass throughout a unit of time that is measured in mL/100 g/min.

CBV: Refers to the vascularized fraction of a tissue, reported in millimeters/100 g.

MTT: Represents the time it takes, on average, for the contrast bolus to cross the capillary beds; the MTT unit is in absolute seconds. This variant in particular is dependent on the two previous variants (CBF and CBV) since it is calculated by the formula MTT = CBV/CBF.

TTP: Reports the average time that the contrast medium takes to reach its highest level in the area of interest [47].

To this day, there is no standardized classification between the different processors to define the core and penumbra, since vendors establish their variations to define infarct cores and penumbras in their software [49]. However, it is the match or mismatch between the CBV and CBF with the MTT and TTP that will determine if the area is a penumbra or infarct core; this means that, if all the variants match on having altered levels, as indicated in Table 2, it is classified as an infarct. On the other hand, if there is a mismatch because the CBV or CBF only have mild alterations but the MTT and TTP are increased, the phenomenon is classified as a penumbra, since it is considered that there is salvageable tissue left [8].

Table 2. CT perfusion variant thresholds for penumbra and infarct core.

Variant	CBF	CBV	MTT	TTP
Penumbra	12–20 mL/100 g/min	>2 mL/100 g	145%	Increased
Infarct core	<10–12 mL/100 g/min	<2 mL/100 g	145%	Increased

CT perfusion allows patients who are outside the time window for reperfusion therapy (>4.5 h for intravenous thrombolysis and >6 h for mechanical thrombectomy (MT)) to have the opportunity to receive treatment, if there is a penumbra area left that is viable [47,50]. Under the criteria for CT perfusion, an MT can be performed in patients with an infarct core of ≤70 mL and large vessel occlusion [36]. The use of CT, CT angiography and CT perfusion in daily practice (experience from the Stroke Center, AORN Cardarelli, Naples, Italy) is presented in Figure 2.

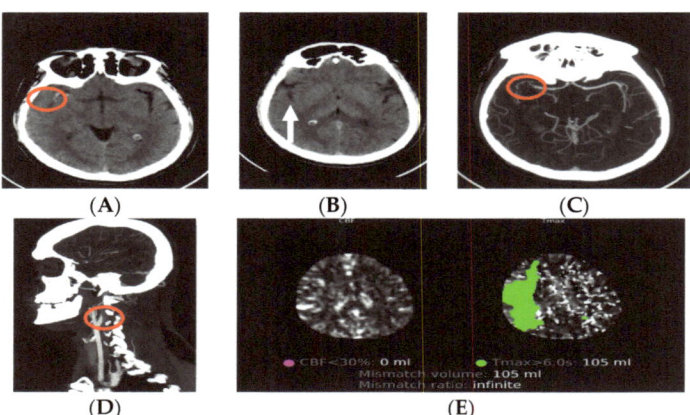

Figure 2. Patient, male, 48 years old, presented with left hemiplegia and dysarthria at the emergency department, after which a neurologist ordered CT diagnostics. (**A,B**) Non-contrast CT which shows MCA hyperdensity (red circle), loss of right insular ribbon (white arrow) and ASPECT 9. (**C,D**) CT angiography, axial and sagittal, showing tandem occlusion of origin of R-ICA (dissection) and R-MCA (both in red circles). (**E**) CT perfusion showing mismatch volume of 105 mL.

3.4. MRI in Ischemic Stroke

Magnetic resonance imaging is a non-invasive imaging modality that can be used to study the body's soft tissues [51,52]. To visualize the internal organization of an anatomical region, MRI takes advantage of the magnetic properties of the hydrogen nuclei from water molecules [52]. Although MRI is more specific and sensitive than CT, it is not commonly used for the initial diagnosis of an acute ischemic stroke. MRI is a less frequently used option as a primary imaging modality, mostly due to its greater price, extended scan time, lack of availability and more difficult workflow. The use of MRI in the initial assessment of acute ischemic strokes is limited and reserved only for unique indications. However, after the emergency setting, brain MRI can give more precise diagnostic information to improve further care [53].

Specific parts of the brain are visualized using different MRI sequences [52]. T1- and T2-weighted imaging (T1WI and T2WI) are the two MRI sequences that are most frequently used [54]. These two conventional MRI sequences, together with non-contrast CT, represent a standard imaging protocol in the imaging of a stroke and have been used mainly to exclude hemorrhages [55]. In T1WI, fluid or water-containing tissues appear dark, while fatty tissues appear bright. In T2WI, fatty tissues appear dark, and fluid or water-containing tissues appear bright [52]. The gradient-echo T2* (GRE T2*wi) sequence is a common additional MRI sequence that gives a correct assessment of hemorrhagic alteration [56,57]. Susceptibility-weighted imaging (SWI) sequences are akin to the GRE T2*wi sequence, but has better sensitivity to detect hemorrhages. Fluid attenuation inversion recovery (FLAIR) is another MRI sequence that is akin to T2WI, with the only exception being that the cerebrospinal fluid appears darker while abnormalities stay bright [52]. FLAIR imaging most importantly helps to establish the age of infarctions, and its essential clinical use is to recognize acute ischemic infarcts within therapeutic intervention time windows [58]. Diffusion-weighted MR imaging (DWI) is a sequence that recognizes the movement of water molecules [52]. It is frequently used in the diagnosis of acute brain infarctions because of its ability to reveal cytotoxic edema [59]. Ischemic brain tissue appears as a bright area or a spot on the image as a result of restricted water movement in the cells [54]. The apparent diffusion coefficient (ADC) quantitatively expresses the degrees of diffusion, and its lowered values indicate a restriction in diffusion [55,59]. However, DWI may be, at times, incapable of identifying small infarcts and can misidentify reversible injuries as irreversible. To improve image accuracy, DWI is frequently used in conjunction with perfusion-weighted imaging (PWI). PWI measures perfusions of the cerebrum using the evaluation of hemodynamic parameters like mean transit time, cerebral blood flow and cerebral blood volume [52]. The DWI/PWI mismatch concept has been used to define the presence of hypoperfused ischemic penumbra in PWI and the infarct core in DWI [52,60,61]. It has been tested as a thrombolysis selection marker and can also provide a prediction of the final infarct area, which can be used to reduce variability between cases in studying the treatment outcome [62]. The time-of-fight (TOF) sequence is used for depicting the level of proximal vessel occlusion. It has high sensitivity and specificity to detect blood flow absences; however, there is a risk of artifacts due to the MR signal being generated by blood flow [63,64]. Another disadvantage is that it is not able to give a direct visualization of the thrombus [63]. The location of occlusions can be misidentified because of lower sensitivity to slow flow, or the stenosis degree can be overestimated when there are hemodynamic changes present [63,65]. Analyzing the intensities of the signal in different sequences (DWI, ADC and FLAIR) can help to differentiate between different stages of ischemic strokes [17].

3.4.1. Early Hyperacute

Because of a decrease in the ADC, DWI can detect ischemic tissue alterations from a matter of minutes to a couple of hours following arterial occlusion. Hyperintense tissue or increased DWI signals and reductions in the ADC mean irreversible ischemia [17]. In other MRI sequences, the affected tissue looks normal [55]. No hyperintensity in FLAIR and increased signals in DWI suggest that the stroke happened less than 4.5 h prior to imaging [17]. At this stage, alterations in blood flow can be seen in MRA and thromboembolism can be detected using SWI [66].

3.4.2. Late Hyperacute

A signal with elevated T2 intensity is usually detected after six hours. The signal is initially more prominent in FLAIR and not in the conventional T2 sequence. Over the next few days, these changes continue to aggravate. The decrease in T1 becomes evident after 16 h and carries on [55]. Twenty-four hours after occlusion, 90% of infarctions can be seen in T2WI, but only 50% are detected in T1WI. Furthermore, T1WI and T2WI have presented a high false negative rate within the initial 24 h after stroke onset. However, when combing data from T1WI, T2WI and DWI, they greatly correlate with the histology of tissue [55].

3.4.3. Acute

The ADC values are initially reduced; later, they start to pseudonormalize, and after the first week, the ADC values start to rise [17,55]. The infarcted parenchyma continues to exhibit a high DWI signal. In FLAIR and T2, the infarction area remains hyperintense, with T2 signals gradually intensifying during the first four days. T1 signals stay low. When using T1 C+, contrast enhancement of the cortex is usually seen 5 days after the onset of the stroke. Arterial and meningeal enhancements are even less frequent and can also be visible during the acute stage [55].

3.4.4. Subacute + Chronic Ischemic Strokes

As stated by International Stroke Recovery and Rehabilitation Roundtable 19, the subacute stages of ischemic strokes are indicated to be between a week and 6 months post-stroke (broken down to early and late at 3 months) and the chronic stage is affirmed to be after 6 months of onset [67]. DWI and ADC imaging modalities compared to conventional MRI and CT can present with alterations from minutes to hours. The hyperdensity seen in DWI images starts to diminish after a week, while the ADC values are lessened upon the onset of ischemia, and after 7–10 days, images begin to appear brighter, resulting in a relatively normal ADC, also referred to as the "pseudonormalization of ADC". This sign can help to distinguish acute infarcts from subacute and chronic infarcts; the latter appear to be more hypodense in DWI and more hyperdense in ADC images with time [68].

DWI in the subacute phases may remain hyperintense for longer through the means of the firmly elevated T2/FLAIR signals, an effect called the "T2 shine through" [67]. Brighter DWI images result from T2 taking longer to be cleansed from tissues, not from the restriction of diffusion, which, if that were the case, would be proven through ADC hypointensity [69]. Likewise, the "Fogging phenomenon" is seen in T2 sequences of cerebral infarctions in nearly half of patients between 1 and 5 weeks, with a median of 10 days after lesion onset, marked by the cortical appearance almost returning to normal [67,70]. FLAIR sequences promote the bright appearance of ischemic areas through the suppression of cerebrospinal fluid intensity with prolonged T2. The intensity of FLAIR images reach their maximum in chronic infarcts [67,71]. Contrast enhancement in cortical regions may carry on for 2–4 months [71]. High T1-weighted image signals detected in the hyperacute phases start to transform into hypointense signals after 16 days, parenchymal enhancement is prevalent following BBB breakdown and cortical intrinsic laminar necrosis-induced hyperintensity may also be seen [67,71,72]. The spot of vessel occlusion determined through MRA, which has contrast-enhanced and non-contrast-enhanced techniques, may benefit the prediction of the final outcome associated with infarction and penumbra generation [15,73]. For monitoring of the final infarct range after 1 to 3 months, T1- and T2-weighted images are utilized [15].

The use of CT, CT angiography and CT perfusion, combined with MRI in daily practice (experience from the Stroke Center, AORN Cardarelli, Naples, Italy), is presented in Figure 3.

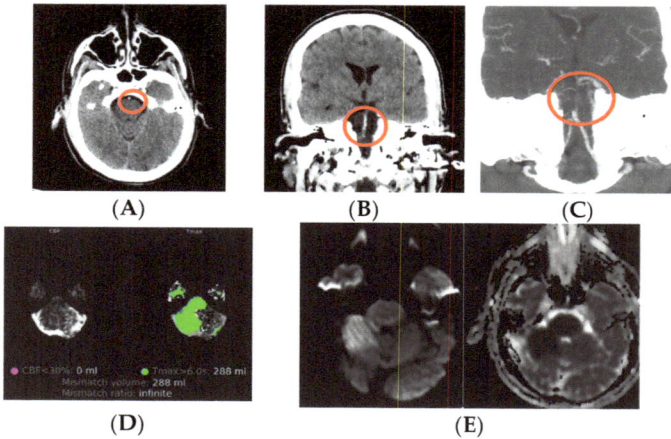

Figure 3. Male patient, 45 years old, presented with vertigo and disorientation at the emergency department, after which a neurologist ordered neuroimaging. (**A**,**B**) Non-contrast CT shows hyperdense basilar artery (red circle). (**C**) CT angiography shows occlusion of basilar artery. (**D**). CT perfusion shows mismatch volume of 288 mL and marks ischemia zone. (**E**) MRI in sequences DWI and ADC show restricted diffusion in the right cerebellar region, marking acute ischemia.

3.5. MR Angiography

Even though CTA is used as the gold standard for the detection of large vessel occlusion in acute strokes, MR angiography (MRA) is more than beneficial in patients with contraindications of intravenous contrast media used in CTA. However, MRA images are flow-dependent and may be inaccurate, unlike CTA, which presents the true anatomy of the vessel lumen [74].

MRA has benefits in the determination of stenosis severity, as well as vascular occlusion and collateral flow in AIS patients. Contrast-enhanced MRA and 3D time-of-flight (TOF) are useful for distinctions between surgical and non-surgical carotid stenosis. Three-dimensional TOF MRA has high accuracy in the evaluation of proximal stenosis/occlusions (unlike distal), while the 2D phase contrast MRA technique has an important place in the evaluation of Willis circle collateral flow schemes [75].

3.6. Magnetic Resonance Perfusion Imaging

MR perfusion (MRP) assesses brain tissue perfusion levels. It creates perfusion maps, CBF, CBV, MTT and time to peak/time to maximum. [74]. In most MTP protocols, gadolinium is applied i.v., after which GRE T2*wi is performed, although sometimes T1-WI. However, evidence from the literature suggests that CTP has a better determination of penumbra compared to MRP. Trials have shown that MRP is beneficial for the determination of patients with less chances of undesirable outcomes after reperfusion treatment, having Tmax > 8 s as a threshold [76].

4. Future Directions

The future of neuroimaging lies in artificial intelligence. It is a promising field, since it increases efficiency and reduces errors, which are particularly significant in pathological entities such as acute ISs when timing is important for treatment options and, consequently, outcome. MRI consumes time and is not available in all stroke units, and artificial intelligence suggests the use of compressed sensing since it gives a scan with a singular viewpoint. The optimization between magnetic resonance imaging and compressed sensing is one of the most promising neuroimaging applications, with important implications in strokes. Also, the development of new software which provide an automatic ASPECT score and quantitative assessment of CT perfusion have enormous clinical benefits, since they reduce time consumption and help to assess proper candidates for thrombectomy [77]. Ethical considerations need to be assessed in this field in the future, as well as more clinical studies.

5. Conclusions

The use of neuroimaging in ischemic stroke patients is crucial in order for patients to receive the correct diagnosis and receive optimal treatment in a timely manner. To this day, CT and MRI have been proven to have high specificity in ischemic stroke patients, alongside CT and MR angiography and CT and MR perfusion techniques. Each of the techniques provide valuable information for clinicians in terms of the stroke type and cause, its location, size, core and penumbra, collateral flow, etc., which are of great importance for choosing the best treatment option and achieving optimal outcomes. The future of neuroimaging lies in the hands of artificial intelligence, whose solutions will aid in increased efficiency and reduced errors for all medical professionals working with stroke patients.

Author Contributions: Conceptualization, J.J.N., V.O. and N.P.; methodology, J.J.N., V.O. and N.P.; software, J.J.N. and V.O.; validation, J.J.N. and V.O.; formal analysis, J.J.N. and V.O.; investigation, J.J.N., V.O., E.C., M.M., N.Z., A.A., P.A., R.K., D.M.V.M., J.A.N., N.V.M., M.O., T.P., M.N., J.K. and N.P.; resources, E.C. and M.M.; data curation, J.J.N., V.O., E.C., M.M., N.Z., A.A., P.A., R.K., D.M.V.M., J.A.N., N.V.M., M.O., T.P., M.N., J.K. and N.P.; writing—original draft preparation, J.J.N., V.O., E.C., M.M., N.Z., A.A., P.A., R.K., D.M.V.M., J.A.N., N.V.M., M.O., T.P., M.N., J.K. and N.P.; writing—review and editing, J.J.N., V.O., E.C., M.M., N.Z., A.A., P.A., R.K., D.M.V.M., J.A.N., N.V.M., M.O., T.P., M.N., J.K. and N.P.; visualization, J.J.N. and V.O.; supervision, J.J.N. and V.O.; project administration, J.J.N., V.O., E.C., M.M., N.Z. and N.P. All authors have read and agreed to the published version of the manuscript.

Funding: This research received no external funding.

Institutional Review Board Statement: Not applicable.

Informed Consent Statement: Not applicable.

Data Availability Statement: Data supporting the reported results are available on request from the corresponding authors.

Conflicts of Interest: The authors declare no conflict of interest.

References

1. Sacco, R.L.; Kasner, S.E.; Broderick, J.P.; Caplan, L.R.; Connors, J.J.; Culebras, A.; Elkind, M.S.; George, M.G.; Hamdan, A.D.; Higashida, R.T.; et al. An updated definition of stroke for the 21st century: A statement for healthcare professionals from the American Heart Association/American Stroke Association. *Stroke* **2013**, *44*, 2064–2089. [CrossRef] [PubMed]
2. Boehme, A.K.; Esenwa, C.; Elkind, M.S. Stroke Risk Factors, Genetics, and Prevention. *Circ. Res.* **2017**, *120*, 472–495. [CrossRef] [PubMed]
3. Maier, O.; Menze, B.H.; von der Gablentz, J.; Häni, L.; Heinrich, M.P.; Liebrand, M.; Winzeck, S.; Basit, A.; Bentley, P.; Chen, L.; et al. A public evaluation benchmark for ischemic stroke lesion segmentation from multispectral MRI. *Med. Image Anal.* **2017**, *35*, 250–269. [CrossRef] [PubMed]
4. Xiong, Y.; Wakhloo, A.K.; Fisher, M. Advances in Acute Ischemic Stroke Therapy. *Circ. Res.* **2022**, *130*, 1230–1251. [CrossRef] [PubMed]
5. Nael, K.; Sakai, Y.; Khatri, P.; Prestigiacomo, C.J.; Puig, J.; Vagal, A. Imaging-based Selection for Endovascular Treatment in Stroke. *Radiographics* **2019**, *39*, 1696–1713. [CrossRef] [PubMed]
6. Tian, X.; Fan, T.; Zhao, W.; Abbas, G.; Han, B.; Zhang, K.; Li, N.; Liu, N.; Liang, W.; Huang, H.; et al. Recent advances in the development of nanomedicines for the treatment of ischemic stroke. *Bioact. Mater.* **2021**, *6*, 2854–2869. [CrossRef]
7. Bruch, G.E.; Fernandes, L.F.; Bassi, B.L.; Alves, M.T.R.; Pereira, I.O.; Frézard, F.; Massensini, A.R. Liposomes for drug delivery in stroke. *Brain Res. Bull.* **2019**, *152*, 246–256. [CrossRef] [PubMed]
8. El-Koussy, M.; Schroth, G.; Brekenfeld, C.; Arnold, M. Imaging of acute ischemic stroke. *Eur. Neurol.* **2014**, *72*, 309–316. [CrossRef] [PubMed]
9. You, S.H.; Kim, B.; Kim, B.K.; Park, S.E. Fast MRI in Acute Ischemic Stroke: Applications of MRI Acceleration Techniques for MR-Based Comprehensive Stroke Imaging. *Investig. Magn. Reson. Imaging* **2021**, *25*, 81–92. [CrossRef]
10. Allen, L.M.; Hasso, A.N.; Handwerker, J.; Farid, H. Sequence-specific MR imaging findings that are useful in dating ischemic stroke. *Radiographics* **2012**, *32*, 1285–1297, discussion 1297–1299. [CrossRef]
11. Potter, C.A.; Vagal, A.S.; Goyal, M.; Nunez, D.B.; Leslie-Mazwi, T.M.; Lev, M.H. CT for Treatment Selection in Acute Ischemic Stroke: A Code Stroke Primer. *Radiographics* **2019**, *39*, 1717–1738. [CrossRef] [PubMed]
12. Powers, W.J.; Derdeyn, C.P.; Biller, J.; Coffey, C.S.; Hoh, B.L.; Jauch, E.C.; Johnston, K.C.; Johnston, S.C.; Khalessi, A.A.; Kidwell, C.S.; et al. American Heart Association Stroke Council. 2015 American Heart Association/American Stroke Association Focused Update of the 2013 Guidelines for the Early Management of Patients with Acute Ischemic Stroke Regarding Endovascular Treatment: A Guideline for Healthcare Professionals from the American Heart Association/American Stroke Association. *Stroke* **2015**, *46*, 3020–3035. [CrossRef] [PubMed]
13. Vojinovic, R.; Opancina, V. The Role of Computed Tomography in Evaluation of The Acute Ischemic Stroke. *Med. Časopis* **2016**, *50*, 139–143. [CrossRef]
14. Hughes, R.E.; Tadi, P.; Bollu, P.C. TPA Therapy. In *StatPearls*; StatPearls Publishing: Treasure Island, FL, USA, 2023. Available online: https://www.ncbi.nlm.nih.gov/books/NBK482376/ (accessed on 23 July 2023).
15. Rekik, I.; Allassonnière, S.; Carpenter, T.K.; Wardlaw, J.M. Medical image analysis methods in MR/CT-imaged acute-subacute ischemic stroke lesion: Segmentation, prediction and insights into dynamic evolution simulation models. A critical appraisal. *Neuroimage Clin.* **2012**, *1*, 164–178. [CrossRef] [PubMed]
16. Leiva-Salinas, C.; Wintermark, M. Imaging of acute ischemic stroke. *Neuroimaging Clin. N. Am.* **2010**, *20*, 455–468. [CrossRef] [PubMed]
17. Lin, M.P.; Liebeskind, D.S. Imaging of Ischemic Stroke. *Continuum* **2016**, *22*, 1399–1423. [CrossRef] [PubMed]
18. Radhiana, H.; Syazarina, S.O.; Shahizon Azura, M.M.; Hilwati, H.; Sobri, M.A. Non-contrast Computed Tomography in Acute Ischaemic Stroke: A Pictorial Review. *Med. J. Malays.* **2013**, *68*, 93–100.
19. Marks, M.P.; Holmgren, E.B.; Fox, A.J.; Patel, S.; von Kummer, R.; Froehlich, J. Evaluation of early computed tomographic findings in acute ischemic stroke. *Stroke* **1999**, *30*, 389–392. [CrossRef]
20. Scott, J.N.; Buchan, A.M.; Sevick, R.J. Correlation of neurologic dysfunction with CT findings in early acute stroke. *Can. J. Neurol. Sci.* **1999**, *26*, 182–189. [CrossRef]
21. Pop, N.O.; Tit, D.M.; Diaconu, C.C.; Munteanu, M.A.; Babes, E.E.; Stoicescu, M.; Popescu, M.I.; Bungau, S. The Alberta Stroke Program Early CT score (ASPECTS): A predictor of mortality in acute ischemic stroke. *Exp. Ther. Med.* **2021**, *22*, 1371. [CrossRef]
22. Cagnazzo, F.; Derraz, I.; Dargazanli, C.; Lefevre, P.-H.; Gascou, G.; Riquelme, C.; Bonafe, A.; Costalat, V. Mechanical thrombectomy in patients with acute ischemic stroke and ASPECTS ≤ 6: A meta-analysis. *J. NeuroInterv. Surg.* **2020**, *12*, 350–355. [CrossRef] [PubMed]
23. Puetz, V.; Dzialowski, I.; Hill, M.D.; Demchuk, A.M. The Alberta Stroke Program Early CT Score in clinical practice: What have we learned? *Int. J. Stroke* **2009**, *4*, 354–364. [CrossRef] [PubMed]
24. Pexman, J.H.W.; Barber, P.A.; Hill, M.D.; Sevick, R.J.; Demchuk, A.M.; Hudon, M.E.; Hu, W.Y.; Buchan, A.M. Use of the Alberta Stroke Program Early CT Score (ASPECTS) for assessing CT scans in patients with acute stroke. *AJNR Am. J. Neuroradiol.* **2001**, *22*, 1534–1542. [PubMed]
25. Tei, H.; Uchiyama, S.; Usui, T.; Ohara, K. Posterior circulation ASPECTS on diffusion-weighted MRI can be a powerful marker for predicting functional outcome. *J. Neurol.* **2010**, *257*, 767–773. [CrossRef] [PubMed]

26. Barber, P.A.; Demchuk, A.M.; Zhang, J.; Buchan, A.M. Validity and reliability of a quantitative computed tomography score in predicting outcome of hyperacute stroke before thrombolytic therapy. ASPECTS Study Group. Alberta Stroke Programme Early CT Score. *Lancet* **2000**, *355*, 1670–1674. [CrossRef] [PubMed]
27. Schröder, J.; Thomalla, G. A Critical Review of Alberta Stroke Program Early CT Score for Evaluation of Acute Stroke Imaging. *Front. Neurol.* **2017**, *7*, 245. [CrossRef] [PubMed]
28. Becker, H.; Desch, H.; Hacker, H.; Pencz, A. CT fogging effect with ischemic cerebral infarcts. *Neuroradiology* **1979**, *18*, 185–192. [CrossRef]
29. Skriver, E.B.; Olsen, T.S. Transient disappearance of cerebral infarcts on CT scan, the so-called fogging effect. *Neuroradiology* **1981**, *22*, 61–65. [CrossRef]
30. Liu, H.M. Neovasculature and blood-brain barrier in ischemic brain infarct. *Acta Neuropathol.* **1988**, *75*, 422–426. [CrossRef]
31. Bahn, M.M.; Oser, A.B.; Cross, D.T. 3rd. CT and MRI of stroke. *J. Magn. Reson. Imaging* **1996**, *6*, 833–845. [CrossRef]
32. Saver, J.L.; Johnston, K.C.; Homer, D.; Wityk, R.; Koroshetz, W.; Truskowski, L.L.; Haley, E.C. Infarct volume as a surrogate or auxiliary outcome measure in ischemic stroke clinical trials. The RANTTAS Investigators. *Stroke* **1999**, *30*, 293–298. [CrossRef] [PubMed]
33. Mäkelä, T.; Öman, O.; Hokkinen, L.; Wilppu, U.; Salli, E.; Savolainen, S.; Kangasniemi, M. Automatic CT Angiography Lesion Segmentation Compared to CT Perfusion in Ischemic Stroke Detection: A Feasibility Study. *J. Digit. Imaging* **2022**, *35*, 551–563. [CrossRef] [PubMed]
34. Polito, V.; La Piana, R.; Del Pilar Cortes, M.; Tampieri, D. Assessment of clot length with multiphase CT angiography in patients with acute ischemic stroke. *Neuroradiol. J.* **2017**, *30*, 593–599. [CrossRef] [PubMed]
35. Power, S.; McEvoy, S.H.; Cunningham, J.; Ti, J.P.; Looby, S.; O'Hare, A.; Williams, D.; Brennan, P.; Thornton, J. Value of CT angiography in anterior circulation large vessel occlusive stroke: Imaging findings, pearls, and pitfalls. *Eur. J. Radiol.* **2015**, *84*, 1333–1344. [CrossRef] [PubMed]
36. Ontario Health (Quality). Automated CT Perfusion Imaging to Aid in the Selection of Patients with Acute Ischemic Stroke for Mechanical Thrombectomy: A Health Technology Assessment. *Ont. Health Technol. Assess. Ser.* **2020**, *20*, 1–87.
37. Ramos, M.M.; Giadas, T.C. Vascular assessment in stroke codes: Role of computed tomography angiography. *Radiologia* **2015**, *57*, 156–166. [CrossRef]
38. Kim, D.-E.; Schellingerhout, D.; Ryu, W.-S.; Lee, S.-K.; Jang, M.U.; Jeong, S.-W.; Na, J.-Y.; Park, J.E.; Lee, E.J.; Cho, K.-H.; et al. Mapping the Supratentorial Cerebral Arterial Territories Using 1160 Large Artery Infarcts. *JAMA Neurol.* **2019**, *76*, 72–80. [CrossRef] [PubMed]
39. Kuybu, O.; Tadi, P.; Dossani, R.H. Posterior Cerebral Artery Stroke. In *StatPearls*; StatPearls Publishing: Treasure Island, FL, USA, 2022.
40. Jolugbo, P.; Ariëns, R.A. Thrombus Composition and Efficacy of Thrombolysis and Thrombectomy in Acute Ischemic Stroke. *Stroke* **2021**, *52*, 1131–1142. [CrossRef] [PubMed]
41. Tahir, R.A.; Haider, S.; Kole, M.; Griffith, B.; Marin, H. Anterior Cerebral Artery: Variant Anatomy and Pathology. *J. Vasc. Interv. Neurol.* **2019**, *10*, 16–22.
42. Medrano-Martorell, S.; Pumar-Pérez, M.; González-Ortiz, S.; Capellades-Font, J. A review of the anatomy of the middle cerebral artery for the era of thrombectomy: A radiologic tool based on CT angiography and perfusion CT. *Radiologia* **2021**, *63*, 505–511. [CrossRef]
43. Salerno, A.; Strambo, D.; Nannoni, S.; Dunet, V.; Michel, P. Patterns of ischemic posterior circulation strokes: A clinical, anatomical, and radiological review. *Int. J. Stroke* **2022**, *17*, 714–722. [CrossRef] [PubMed]
44. Patel, P.B.; LaMuraglia, G.M.; Lancaster, R.T.; Clouse, W.D.; Kwolek, C.J.; Conrad, M.F.; Cambria, R.P.; Patel, V.I. Severe contralateral carotid stenosis or occlusion does not have an impact on risk of ipsilateral stroke after carotid endarterectomy. *J. Vasc. Surg.* **2018**, *67*, 1744–1751. [CrossRef] [PubMed]
45. Young, J.Y.; Schaefer, P.W. Acute ischemic stroke imaging: A practical approach for diagnosis and triage. *Int. J. Cardiovasc. Imaging* **2016**, *32*, 19–33. [CrossRef] [PubMed]
46. Chiu, A.H.; Phillips, T.J.; Phatouros, C.C.; Singh, T.P.; Hankey, G.J.; Blacker, D.J.; McAuliffe, W. CT perfusion in acute stroke calls: A pictorial review and differential diagnoses. *J. Med. Imaging Radiat. Oncol.* **2016**, *60*, 165–171. [CrossRef] [PubMed]
47. Václavík, D.; Volný, O.; Cimflová, P.; Švub, K.; Dvorníková, K.; Bar, M. The importance of CT perfusion for diagnosis and treatment of ischemic stroke in anterior circulation. *J. Integr. Neurosci.* **2022**, *21*, 92. [CrossRef] [PubMed]
48. Boned, S.; Padroni, M.; Rubiera, M.; Tomasello, A.; Coscojuela, P.; Romero, N.; Muchada, M.; Rodríguez-Luna, D.; Flores, A.; Rodríguez, N.; et al. Admission CT perfusion may overestimate initial infarct core: The ghost infarct core concept. *J. Neurointerv. Surg.* **2017**, *9*, 66–69. [CrossRef] [PubMed]
49. Peerlings, D.; van Ommen, F.; Bennink, E.; Dankbaar, J.W.; Velthuis, B.K.; Emmer, B.J.; Hoving, J.W.; Majoie, C.B.L.M.; Marquering, H.A.; de Jong, H.W.A.M. Probability maps classify ischemic stroke regions more accurately than CT perfusion summary maps. *Eur. Radiol.* **2022**, *32*, 6367–6375. [CrossRef] [PubMed]
50. Feil, K.; Reidler, P.; Kunz, W.G.; Küpper, C.; Heinrich, J.; Laub, C.; Müller, K.; Vöglein, J.; Liebig, T.; Dieterich, M.; et al. Addressing a real-life problem: Treatment with intravenous thrombolysis and mechanical thrombectomy in acute stroke patients with an extended time window beyond 4.5 h based on computed tomography perfusion imaging. *Eur. J. Neurol.* **2020**, *27*, 168–174. [CrossRef]

51. Ghadimi, M.; Sapra, A. Magnetic Resonance Imaging Contraindications. In *StatPearls*; StatPearls Publishing: Treasure Island, FL, USA, 2023.
52. Kakkar, P.; Kakkar, T.; Patankar, T.; Saha, S. Current approaches and advances in the imaging of stroke. *Dis. Model. Mech.* **2021**, *14*, dmm048785. [CrossRef]
53. Lee, H.; Yang, Y.; Liu, B.; Castro, S.A.; Shi, T. Patients with Acute Ischemic Stroke Who Receive Brain Magnetic Resonance Imaging Demonstrate Favorable In-Hospital Outcomes. *J. Am. Heart Assoc.* **2020**, *9*, e016987. [CrossRef]
54. Tedyanto, E.H.; Tini, K.; Pramana, N.A.K. Magnetic Resonance Imaging in Acute Ischemic Stroke. *Cureus* **2022**, *14*, e27224. [CrossRef] [PubMed]
55. Wey, H.-Y.; Desai, V.R.; Duong, T.Q. A review of current imaging methods used in stroke research. *Neurol. Res.* **2013**, *35*, 1092–1102. [CrossRef] [PubMed]
56. Cao, C.; Liu, Z.; Liu, G.; Jin, S.; Xia, S. Ability of weakly supervised learning to detect acute ischemic stroke and hemorrhagic infarction lesions with diffusion-weighted imaging. *Quant. Imaging Med. Surg.* **2022**, *12*, 321–332. [CrossRef] [PubMed]
57. Adam, G.; Ferrier, M.; Patsoura, S.; Gramada, R.; Meluchova, Z.; Cazzola, V.; Darcourt, J.; Cognard, C.; Viguier, A.; Bonneville, F. Magnetic resonance imaging of arterial stroke mimics: A pictorial review. *Insights Imaging* **2018**, *9*, 815–831. [CrossRef] [PubMed]
58. Meshksar, A.; Villablanca, J.P.; Khan, R.; Carmody, R.; Coull, B.; Nael, K. Role of EPI-FLAIR in patients with acute stroke: A comparative analysis with FLAIR. *AJNR Am. J. Neuroradiol.* **2014**, *35*, 878–883. [CrossRef] [PubMed]
59. Ulu, E.; Ozturk, B.; Atalay, K.; Okumus, I.B.; Erdem, D.; Gul, M.K.; Terzi, O. Diffusion-Weighted Imaging of Brain Metastasis: Correlation of MRI Parameters with Histologic Type. *Turk. Neurosurg.* **2022**, *32*, 58–68. [CrossRef] [PubMed]
60. Xu, K.; Gu, B.; Zuo, T.; Xu, X.; Chen, Y.-C.; Yin, X.; Feng, G. Predictive value of Alberta stroke program early CT score for perfusion weighted imaging—Diffusion weighted imaging mismatch in stroke with middle cerebral artery occlusion. *Medicine* **2020**, *99*, e23490. [CrossRef] [PubMed]
61. Heo, H.Y.; Tee, Y.K.; Harston, G.; Leigh, R.; Chappell, M.A. Amide proton transfer imaging in stroke. *NMR Biomed.* **2023**, *36*, e4734. [CrossRef]
62. Mandeville, E.T.; Ayata, C.; Zheng, Y.; Mandeville, J.B. Translational MR Neuroimaging of Stroke and Recovery. *Transl. Stroke Res.* **2017**, *8*, 22–32. [CrossRef]
63. Le Bras, A.; Raoult, H.; Ferré, J.-C.; Ronzière, T.; Gauvrit, J.-Y. Optimal MRI sequence for identifying occlusion location in acute stroke: Which value of time-resolved contrast-enhanced MRA? *AJNR Am. J. Neuroradiol.* **2015**, *36*, 1081–1088. [CrossRef]
64. Boujan, T.; Neuberger, U.; Pfaff, J.; Nagel, S.; Herweh, C.; Bendszus, M.; Möhlenbruch, M.A. Value of Contrast-Enhanced MRA versus Time-of-Flight MRA in Acute Ischemic Stroke MRI. *AJNR Am. J. Neuroradiol.* **2018**, *39*, 1710–1716. [CrossRef] [PubMed]
65. Wang, Q.; Wang, G.; Sun, Q.; Sun, D.-H. Application of MAGnetic resonance imaging compilation in acute ischemic stroke. *World J. Clin. Cases* **2021**, *9*, 10828–10837. [CrossRef] [PubMed]
66. Li, X.; Su, F.; Yuan, Q.; Chen, Y.; Liu, C.-Y.; Fan, Y. Advances in differential diagnosis of cerebrovascular diseases in magnetic resonance imaging: A narrative review. *Quant. Imaging Med. Surg.* **2023**, *13*, 2712–2734. [CrossRef] [PubMed]
67. Gaillard, F.; Hacking, C.; Sharma, R.; Worsley, C.; Saber, M.; Anan, R.A.; Bell, D.; Murphy, A.; Deng, F.; Baba, Y.; et al. Ischemic Stroke. Available online: Radiopaedia.org (accessed on 13 August 2023).
68. Dmytriw, A.A.; Sawlani, V.; Shankar, J. Diffusion-Weighted Imaging of the Brain: Beyond Stroke. *Can. Assoc. Radiol. J.* **2017**, *68*, 131–146. [CrossRef] [PubMed]
69. Gaillard, F.; Petrovic, A.; Bell, D.; Knipe, H.; Goel, A.; Mudgal, P.; St-Amant, M. T2 Shine through. Available online: Radiopaedia.org (accessed on 14 August 2023).
70. Gaillard, F.; Saber, M.; Murphy, A.; Bell, D.; Thurston, M.; Di Muzio, B. Fogging Phenomenon (Cerebral Infarct). Available online: Radiopaedia.org (accessed on 14 August 2023).
71. Isla, L.G.; Márquez, I.G.; Naranjo, P.P.; Paniza, M.R.; Ventura, J.M.; Rubia, L.D.; Conesa, M.F. Magnetic resonance imaging of ischemic stroke and its correlation with multimodal computed tomography. In Proceedings of the European Congress of Radiology-ECR 2020, Vienna, Austria, 15–19 July 2020. [CrossRef]
72. Kraniotis, P.; Solomou, A. Subacute cortical infarct: The value of contrast-enhanced FLAIR images in inconclusive DWI. *Radiol. Bras.* **2019**, *52*, 273–274. [CrossRef] [PubMed]
73. Non Contrast Enhanced MR Angiography. Available online: Radiopaedia.org (accessed on 14 August 2023).
74. Kamalian, S.; Lev, M.H. Stroke Imaging. *Radiol. Clin. N. Am.* **2019**, *57*, 717–732. [CrossRef] [PubMed]
75. Vu, D.; González, R.G.; Schaefer, P.W. Conventional MRI and MR Angiography of Stroke. In *Acute Ischemic Stroke*; Springer: Berlin/Heidelberg, Germany, 2006. [CrossRef]
76. Kurz, K.D.; Ringstad, G.; Odland, A.; Advani, R.; Farbu, E.; Kurz, M.W. Radiological imaging in acute ischaemic stroke. *Eur. J. Neurol.* **2016**, *23* (Suppl. 1), 8–17. [CrossRef] [PubMed]
77. Monsour, R.; Dutta, M.; Mohamed, A.Z.; Borkowski, A.; Viswanadhan, N.A. Neuroimaging in the Era of Artificial Intelligence: Current Applications. *Fed. Pract.* **2022**, *39* (Suppl. 1), S14–S20. [CrossRef] [PubMed]

Disclaimer/Publisher's Note: The statements, opinions and data contained in all publications are solely those of the individual author(s) and contributor(s) and not of MDPI and/or the editor(s). MDPI and/or the editor(s) disclaim responsibility for any injury to people or property resulting from any ideas, methods, instructions or products referred to in the content.

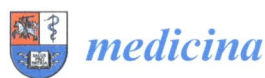

Article

High-Resolution Computed Tomography in Middle Ear Cholesteatoma: How Much Do We Need It?

Eugen Horatiu Stefanescu [1], Nicolae Constantin Balica [1], Sorin Bogdan Motoi [2], Laura Grigorita [3], Madalina Georgescu [4,*] and Gheorghe Iovanescu [1]

1. Department of Otolaryngology, Victor Babeș University of Medicine and Pharmacy, 300041 Timișoara, Romania; stefanescu@umft.ro (E.H.S.); balica@umft.ro (N.C.B.); giovanescu@umft.ro (G.I.)
2. Department of Radiology and Medical Imaging, Victor Babeș University of Medicine and Pharmacy, 300041 Timișoara, Romania; motoi.sorin@umft.ro
3. Department of Anatomy and Embriology, Victor Babeș University of Medicine and Pharmacy, 300041 Timișoara, Romania; grigorita.laura@umft.ro
4. Discipline of General Surgery and Qualified Care in Surgical Specialties, Carol Davila University of Medicine and Pharmacy, 050474 București, Romania
* Correspondence: madalina.georgescu@umfcd.ro

Citation: Stefanescu, E.H.; Balica, N.C.; Motoi, S.B.; Grigorita, L.; Georgescu, M.; Iovanescu, G. High-Resolution Computed Tomography in Middle Ear Cholesteatoma: How Much Do We Need It? *Medicina* **2023**, *59*, 1712. https://doi.org/10.3390/medicina59101712

Academic Editor: Giuseppe Magliulo

Received: 25 August 2023
Revised: 20 September 2023
Accepted: 21 September 2023
Published: 25 September 2023

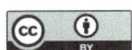

Copyright: © 2023 by the authors. Licensee MDPI, Basel, Switzerland. This article is an open access article distributed under the terms and conditions of the Creative Commons Attribution (CC BY) license (https://creativecommons.org/licenses/by/4.0/).

Abstract: *Background and Objectives*: The diagnosis of cholesteatoma is usually clinic, and the only efficient treatment is surgical. High-resolution computed tomography (HRCT) is not considered absolutely necessary for the management of an uncomplicated cholesteatoma, but unsuspected situations from a clinical point of view can be discovered using the scans, warning the surgeon. Our objective is to compare HRCT scan information with intraoperative findings in patients with cholesteatoma and analyze the usefulness of a preoperative HRCT scan from a surgical point of view. *Materials and Methods*: This is a prospective descriptive study conducted in the Department of Otolaryngology, Victor Babes University of Medicine and Pharmacy Timisoara, Romania, from May 2021 to April 2022. It was carried out on 46 patients with a clinical diagnosis of cholesteatoma who were consequently operated on in our department. All patients received full clinical and audiological examinations. In all cases, an HRCT scan was performed preoperatively as a mandatory investigation. Preoperative HRCT scans were analyzed, and their findings were compared to the intraoperative notes. The two sets of observations were analyzed using standard statistical methods. *Results*: Extensive cholesteatoma was the most common type of disease, involving 46% of the patients, followed by pars flaccida cholesteatoma (35%) and pars tensa cholesteatoma (19%). Eroded scutum was the most frequent lesion involving 70% of the patients, followed by incus erosion (67%). Comparison of the HRCT and intraoperative findings revealed a very good correlation for tegmen tympani erosion, sigmoid plate erosion, scutum and malleus erosion, and a moderate-to-good correlation for lateral semicircular canal erosion, incus and stapes erosion, and fallopian canal erosion. *Conclusions*: HRCT is a valuable tool in the preoperative assessment of cholesteatoma, helping in making surgical decisions. It can accurately predict the extent of disease and is helpful for detecting unapparent dangerous situations. However, it is not very accurate in detecting fallopian canal and stapes erosion.

Keywords: high-resolution computed tomography; cholesteatoma surgery; very good correlation

1. Introduction

When discussing a topic, we usually start with its definition. When the topic is cholesteatoma, the problems already start there, and they continue in almost every aspect; it is quite difficult to name one where there are no controversies. The old definition of "skin in the wrong place" is more misleading than helpful. Cholesteatoma is a benign cystic lesion involving the temporal bone, which is derived from an abnormal growth of keratinizing squamous epithelium [1]. It consists of an outer lining of stratified squamous epithelium, an inner keratin mass, and an external peri-matrix that produces enzymes, destroying the surrounding tissues [2]. Middle ear cholesteatoma has a higher incidence in individuals younger than 50 years of age but can occur at any age [3]. Cholesteatoma in children tends to behave in a different manner than in adults; it has a more aggressive pattern of growth and recurs more frequently.

The clinical features of cholesteatoma vary considerably, ranging from an asymptomatic disease to life-threatening complications [4]. Even if the complication rate has decreased significantly today, the danger is still there, and a warning sign of any kind is always helpful for the physician. The management of this disease is strictly surgical, continues to be a challenge for otolaryngologists, and is sometimes quite a nightmare for both patient and surgeon.

The temporal bone has a very complicated architecture and contains delicate structures like the ossicular chain, inner ear, facial nerve, and even vital ones like the internal carotid artery [3]. Cholesteatoma may damage all of them, and it also may involve adjacent structures like the dura mater, the temporal lobe of the brain, and the sigmoid sinus, leading to both extra-cranial and intra-cranial complications as local invasion is a characteristic of the disease. It is considered to be a benign lesion, but given the complications encountered, one cannot be so sure this is the right word.

There are also many anatomic variants of the structures in the middle ear, and the very narrow space inside the temporal bone makes discovering the lesions and tackling the complications quite challenging, so any preoperative information is highly appreciated [5].

HRCT of the temporal bone is one of the imaging modalities used to evaluate the extent of the disease and the lesions produced by cholesteatoma in and out of the temporal bone prior to surgery, and it is considered to be accurate as its slice thickness is usually less than 1 mm. Using special algorithms, HRCT scans offer an excellent resolution [6]. On HRCT scans, cholesteatoma appears as a soft-tissue mass in the middle ear cavity and mastoid with associated signs of surrounding bony erosion [3]. However, HRCT cannot accurately differentiate cholesteatoma from inflammatory/granulation tissue or scar tissue inside the middle ear [7]. The sinus tympani and facial recess are two hidden areas of the middle ear, and their involvement by cholesteatoma can be detected intraoperatively, especially if using an endoscope, but can also be identified preoperatively on an HRCT scan.

In attic cholesteatoma, erosion of the scutum in the coronal view can be assessed on HRCT scans, and it is a useful sign for early diagnosis [8]. Ossicular chain erosion is a common feature in cholesteatoma, which can result in more or less significant conductive hearing loss. It can vary from small erosion of the long process of the incus and incudostapedial joint, which is the most frequent situation, to complete destruction of the entire ossicular chain. The interposition of the cholesteatoma between the tympanic membrane and stapes, no matter if it is intact or if its superstructure is eroded, can improve the sound transmission to the inner ear and be deceiving regarding the patient's actual hearing level. Another dangerous site of erosion is the dome of the lateral semicircular canal (LSC), just above the second genu of the facial nerve canal. Speaking of the facial nerve canal, the most frequent portion that can be dehiscent or eroded in cases of cholesteatoma is the tympanic one, usually just above the oval window area [5]. These are some of the reasons why such preoperative "inside information" is useful for planning the surgical approach, and this can be best achieved using HRCT. Early detection and treatment of such dangerous situations have considerably reduced the morbidity and mortality of cholesteatoma [9].

The tremendous amount of information provided by the HRCT of the temporal bone has led to several studies in the literature trying to double-check the accuracy of this information by comparing it to intraoperative findings. One of the first studies to evaluate the correlation between surgical and HRCT findings in cholesteatoma was performed by Jackler in 1984 [7]. Since then, the technology behind HRCT has evolved in a spectacular manner, providing more and more details regarding the lesions in the middle ear. Most of these studies confirm a very good general correlation between HRCT and intraoperative findings, but when it comes to specific small lesions—the erosion of the stapes or a situation that can occur in normal ears as well like facial nerve canal dehiscence—this is not always the case [10–12]. The biggest limitation of these studies is the small number of patients—usually less than 100.

2. Materials and Methods

This is a prospective descriptive study conducted in the Department of Otolaryngology, Head and Neck Surgery of the Victor Babes University of Medicine and Pharmacy Timisoara, Romania, from May 2021 to April 2022. The study protocol was approved by the Ethics Committee of Victor Babes University of Medicine and Pharmacy Timisoara. The present study included 46 patients with a clinical diagnosis of chronic otitis media with cholesteatoma, in which we performed tympano-mastoid surgery, both open and closed techniques, with ossicular chain reconstruction. All patients received preoperative full clinical and audiological examination. Collected clinical data included information about tympanic cavity status (tympanic membrane, ossicles, and mucosa lesions), hearing and vestibular status, and facial nerve function. All patients underwent preoperative HRCT of the temporal bone as part of the mandatory investigations. All surgeries were performed between 3 and 8 weeks after imaging by the same surgical team under the surgical microscope. We only used the endoscope to assess the extension of the disease to sinus tympani and to check for the complete removal of the lesions. Surgical findings were recorded by the surgical team.

The choice between the open and closed technique was made on a case-by-case basis. However, whenever possible, we went for a closed technique, or we tried to obliterate the mastoid cavity. HRCT also provided information regarding the size of the mastoid, the level of the tegmen tympani, and the position of the lateral sinus, details that are crucial when choosing the type of surgery. The extent of mastoid pneumatisation is another detail that may influence the surgical approach. If the pneumatization is good, then a closed technique can be employed easily. If there is poor pneumatisation, then an open technique is preferable with or without mastoid obliteration. However, this is not the only factor to be taken into account. The location and extension of the cholesteatoma is another crucial one, and it is very well described on an HRCT.

Interpretation of preoperative HRCT images was focused on defining the following: location and extent of cholesteatoma; bony erosions of the following structures: scutum, tegmen tympani, facial nerve (FN) canal, and inner ear (LSC, promontory); and integrity of the ossicular chain. All HRCT scans were assessed by a single radiologist with over 15 years of experience in head and neck imaging.

The operative findings were compared to the radiological findings, assessing the usefulness of a preoperative HRCT scan in describing the status of the middle ear structures in cases of cholesteatoma with or without complications. Sensitivity, specificity, positive predictive value (PPV), negative predictive value (NPV) of HRCT scans, and Cohen's Kappa coefficient (to evaluate their agreement with the intraoperative findings) were calculated for the following features, considered to be of interest for surgery: scutum, tegmen tympani, sigmoid sinus plate, LSC, FN canal, malleus, incus, and stapes. For statistical analysis, we used Microsoft Excel 2013 and Statistical Package for Social Sciences (SPSS) version 26 (IBM Corp., Armonk, NY, USA). The kappa coefficient in the ranges of 0–0.40, 0.41–0.75, and 0.76–1.0 indicates poor, moderate-to-good, and very good correlation, respectively.

We did not include in the study cases with any kind of previous surgery in the same ear, cholesteatoma recurrences, and patients who were operated on later than 8 weeks after performing imaging. Written informed consent was obtained from all patients prior to data collection.

Scan Protocol

HRCT scans were obtained on GE Revolution EVO (General Electric, Boston, MA, USA), a 128-slice CT scanner. The patient was lying in the supine position. The topogram was made in the lateral incidence, which includes the area between the tip of the mastoid and the arcuate eminence of the temporal bone as the lower and upper scanning point, respectively; scanning was not performed with an inclined gantry.

Axial projections were obtained by serial 1 mm sections of the temporal bone with the plane along the line joining the infra-orbital rim and external auditory meatus, perpendicular to the table with 20×0.625 collimation. The images were reconstructed using the high-resolution bone algorithm in the axial plane with 0.625 mm section thickness and a field of view (FOV) of 100–110 mm, with a matrix size of 512×512. The effective amperage in the tube was modulated according to the patient's age: between 130 mAs (for a newborn) and 400 mAs (for an adult). The voltage in the tube was between 110 and 140 kV, usually 120 kV.

The acquisition was in the spiral mode, which ensures a better reformation in the coronal and sagittal plane. The reconstruction in the axial plane is the basic one and includes sections parallel to the lateral semicircular canal; simultaneously with the reconstruction in the three planes, a set of images in the axial plane with a thickness of 2 mm was also obtained, which helps to visualize the tissue structures within the cholesteatoma as a whole.

The administration of the contrast substance was not always indicated in cholesteatoma involving the middle ear, but it becomes mandatory in situations where there is a suspicion of evolution towards complication: abscesses, coalescent otomastoiditis, and sigmoid sinus thrombosis.

3. Results

Chronic otitis media with cholesteatoma represents 41% of the chronic otitis media cases operated in our department in 2022. There were 46 patients enrolled in our study, including 6 children ages 8 to 15 years old. The oldest patient was 73 years old. The mean age of our patients was 37.3 ± 10.8 years. The largest number of cases, 19 (41%), were in the 31–40-year-old group, and among them 11 (57%) were male and 8 (43%) were female. There was generally a slight male preponderance in our study population—24 (52%) male and 22 (48%) female patients—with a male/female ratio of 1.09:1. Extensive cholesteatoma was the most commonly encountered type, detected in 21 patients (46%), and followed by pars flaccida cholesteatoma encountered in 16 patients (35%) and pars tensa cholesteatoma in 9 patients (19%).

The erosion of the scutum was the most common lesion, but only by a narrow margin, and was found in 32 patients (70%). The other destructive lesions were eroded incus, mainly the long process, in 31 patients (67%), eroded malleus in 21 patients (46%), eroded stapes in 14 patients (30%), significantly thinned/eroded tegmen tympani in 10 patients (22%), dehiscent/eroded facial nerve canal in 8 cases (17%), lateral semicircular canal fistula in 4 cases (9%), and eroded sigmoid sinus plate in 3 cases (7%). The patients enrolled in this study presented the following complications: two patients with facial nerve palsy (grade III and IV House–Brackmann, respectively) and four patients with vertigo. All the patients with vertigo were correctly assessed from an imaging point of view. There was an extra case described as having a lateral semicircular canal fistula on HRCT scans, which was not confirmed during surgery. When analyzing alterations of tegmen tympani, we considered both erosion and thinning together as their clinical and surgical significance is comparable.

Table 1 shows the sensitivity, specificity, positive predictive and negative predictive values, and correlation levels for the considered HRCT findings.

Table 1. Accuracy of preoperative HRCT in detecting cholesteatoma lesions.

HRCT Findings	Sensitivity	Specificity	PPV	NPV	Correlation
Tegmen tympani erosion/thinning	90.0	88.8	69.2	96.9	0.97
Sigmoid plate erosion	100	97.6	75.0	100	0.87
Malleus erosion	85.7	96.0	94.7	88.8	0.82

Table 1. Cont.

HRCT Findings	Sensitivity	Specificity	PPV	NPV	Correlation
Scutum erosion	87.5	92.8	96.5	76.4	0.76
LSC erosion	75.0	97.6	75.0	97.6	0.68
Incus erosion	80.6	86.6	92.5	68.4	0.62
Stapes erosion	57.1	84.3	61.5	81.8	0.44
Facial canal dehiscence/erosion	50.0	92.1	57.0	89.7	0.42

The greatest correlation between imaging and surgery was in the detection of the tegmen tympani erosion/thinning (kappa = 0.97). We also obtained a very good imaging-surgical correlation in the detection of sigmoid sinus plate dehiscence (kappa = 0.87), malleus erosion (kappa = 0.82), and scutum erosion (kappa = 0.76). We obtained moderate-to-good results in detecting lateral semicircular canal dehiscence (kappa = 0.68), incus erosion (kappa = 0.62), stapes erosion (kappa = 0.44), and facial nerve canal dehiscence (kappa = 0.42). There was no poor imaging-surgical correlation for any of the investigated lesions in our study. The poorest correlation was in facial nerve canal dehiscence/erosion (kappa = 0.42) and stapes erosion (kappa = 0.44). The best correlation was in cases with extensive and severe lesions, as it was expected preoperatively.

4. Discussion

The ability of HRCT to detect cholesteatoma and its complications prior to surgery is well known. It is especially helpful in detecting minimal erosion of the ossicular chain and other dangerous areas like the tegmen tympani, lateral semicircular canal, and fallopian canal [10]. Such information is very useful when discussing with the patient and getting informed consent for surgery. It is still worth remembering that HRCT cannot accurately differentiate cholesteatoma from granulation tissue and cholesterol granuloma, which are also encountered in chronic suppurative otitis media. All our cases had a clinical diagnosis of cholesteatoma prior to imaging, so this was not our main concern, but cholesteatoma was confirmed, and its extension was accurately described on imaging.

Age—In our study, we found that the majority of patients were aged between 31 and 40 years of age, involving 19 (41%) cases. In other studies, a much younger age prevalence of less than 30 years of age was observed [11,12].

Gender prevalence—In the present study, the majority of patients were male (52%), but only by a thin margin, with a male-to-female ratio of 1.09: 1. Kemppainen et al. also reported that cholesteatoma was more frequent in men under the age of 50 years [13]. Other studies reported a much higher male predominance, with a male/female ratio of 1.39:1 [14].

Location and extent of cholesteatoma—In our study, extensive cholesteatoma was the most commonly encountered type, detected in 46% of patients, followed by pars flaccida cholesteatoma in 35% of patients and pars tensa cholesteatoma present in 19% of patients. The same prevalence was observed in the study performed by Gomma et al., where extensive cholesteatoma was detected in 35.7% of patients. Also commonly detected was the pars flaccida type [12]. In other studies, the most frequently encountered type was pars flaccida cholesteatoma: a study on 30 cholesteatoma cases showed lesions in the epitympanum in 73.3% of patients, followed by mesotympanum [15], and in another one pars flaccida cholesteatoma was described in 50.7% of cases, followed by extensive cholesteatoma in 30.1% of patients [16]. Pars tensa cholesteatoma was the least encountered type in most of the studies.

Accurate assessment of the extension of the lesions may provide crucial information regarding the most suitable surgical approach considering the given anatomy of the middle ear and mastoid. It is notorious for the controversy among the surgeons supporting either the open or the closed technique in the treatment of cholesteatoma. However, the closed technique might be extremely difficult in some temporal bones, and this can be foreseen in imaging. There are also situations in which an open technique is not required because of the limited extension of cholesteatoma [17].

From a surgical point of view, the accuracy in detecting lesions of the delicate structures of the middle ear presents great importance, and this is why several aspects regarding this topic deserve some comments.

Scutum erosion—It is considered to be an early sign of pars flaccida cholesteatoma, but it does not appear in all cases. In our study, it was detected in 32 cases (70%) with a sensitivity of 87.5% and a specificity of 92.8%. The correlation was still very good but borderline (kappa = 0.76). In another study, the scutum was eroded in 55.5% of the cholesteatoma cases [16]. Rai et al. reported scutum erosion in 65% of the patients [18]. The PPV was very good in our study (96.5%). In other studies, scutum erosion was accurately predicted in 91% of cases [19,20]. However, Sunitha reported no imaging-surgical correlation for scutum erosion [21]. Suat Keskin believes that differences between imaging and intraoperative findings regarding scutum erosion may be due to inappropriate angles of the coronal sections [22]. From a surgical point of view, the erosion of the scutum may influence the approach to the ossicular chain, especially to the incus and malleus.

Sinus plate erosion—In our study, erosion of the sigmoid sinus plate was described on HRCT in four cases, but intraoperatively, only three cases had sinus plate erosion, so only 75% of cases were accurately detected by HRCT with relatively lower sensitivity when compared to other studies. In a study by Dutta et al., HRCT sensitivity was 100%, and specificity was also 100% for sinus plate erosion [11]. C Shah reported the sensitivity and specificity of HRCT in detecting sigmoid erosion to be 91.7% and 95.25%, respectively [17]. Kanotra et al. reported the sensitivity, specificity, and positive and negative predictive value to be 100% [23]. Sinus plate erosion is quite a rare occurrence, and this can explain why there are such differences between studies. Knowing that the sinus plate is eroded requires special attention and careful exploration of the region, even if there are no clinical signs of sigmoid sinus pathology. It can also alert the surgeon and prevent the inadvertent opening of the sinus wall with massive bleeding and prolonged surgical time.

Tegmen tympani erosion/thinning—We evaluated erosion and significant thinning of the tegmen tympani together, but not all studies did so. This is probably one reason why we obtained such good specificity and sensitivity compared to others. HRCT finding shows eroded/thinned tegmen tympani in 13 cases, but intraoperatively, it was present in 9 cases out of the total of 46 (19%) with a sensitivity of 90% and specificity of 88.8%. Another study identified tegmen tympani erosion in 38% of the cases [16]. In a study performed by Jamal et al., tegmen tympani erosion was seen in 30% of the patients [24]. Kanotra et al. reported a sensitivity of 100% in detecting tegmen tympani erosion by HRCT, which was higher than the current study [23]. A high specificity rate of 95% was reported by Gerami et al. [25]. A poor sensitivity rate of HRCT in detecting tegmen tympani erosion was reported by Jackler et al. [9] and O'Reilly et al. [26], while a moderate sensitivity rate was described by Vlastarakos et al. [27] and Chee and Tan [10]. From a surgical point of view, it is invaluable information for the dissection of the cholesteatoma matrix away from that area, even in the absence of dura-related complications. The poor imaging-surgical correlation for tegmen tympani erosion is probably due to the partial volume of both the tympanic cavity and cerebral soft tissue [22].

Lateral semicircular canal erosion—This structure may be eroded by cholesteatoma, especially in its dome region on the medial wall of the epitympanum, close to the second genu of the facial nerve [3]. In our study, we found four cases (9%) of an LSC fistula. Other studies noted an LSC fistula in just 4.7% of the cases and even lower (4% of the patients) [16,28]. In our study, HRCT scans assessed the LSC fistula cases with a sensitivity of 75% and specificity of 97.6%. In a study performed by Gaurano et al. on 64 patients, there were four cases (6.3%) that had labyrinthine fistula found on HRCT, but only three (4.7%) were confirmed intraoperatively [19]. Usually, HRCT accurately predicts lateral semicircular canal fistula with excellent sensitivity and good specificity. Mafee et al., Chee et al., and Rocher et al. reported HRCT to be 100% sensitive in detecting lateral semicircular canal fistula [3,10,20]. Knowing in advance about the suspicion and location of the fistula is very important for the surgeon as dissection of the matrix of the cholesteatoma in that area has to be performed very carefully, avoiding unnecessary manipulation and suction. The closure of the fistula is of utmost importance for inner ear function.

FN Canal dehiscence/erosion—Fallopian canal dehiscence/erosion is a relatively common finding in cholesteatoma affecting the middle ear, usually occurring in the tympanic portion of the facial nerve canal [8,29]. We found facial nerve canal dehiscence/erosion in eight patients (17%). In another study, facial canal dehiscence was observed in 34.9% of the cholesteatoma cases [16]. The study by Jamal et al. reported facial canal dehiscence in 30% of the patients [24]. The sensitivity and specificity obtained in our study were 50% and 92.1%, respectively, with a moderate-to-poor correlation between imaging and surgery (kappa = 0.42). Other studies presented similar observations with a sensitivity ranging from 33.3% to 83% and specificity between 60% and 97%. It is well known that the Fallopian canal can be so thin as to appear dehiscent on a CT scan [30]. It is good to remember that the fallopian canal may be dehiscent even in a healthy ear. The detection of the facial nerve dehiscence/erosion on imaging should influence the decision and timing of surgery, being a good reason to operate earlier and alert the surgeon when working in that area. One should always consider the proximity of the stapes and facial nerve, especially when dissecting the cholesteatoma matrix off these structures.

Ossicular chain—It is usually involved by cholesteatoma of the middle ear, even if not always eroded or discontinued. This situation presents great importance for the surgeon as he/she has to drill and dissect a lot around the ossicular chain. Touching the ossicular chain during drilling might generate severe SNHL and should be avoided at any cost. We found ossicular chain erosion in 37 out of 46 patients (80%). Incus was the most eroded ossicle, found in 67% of the patients in our study. In another study, incus was found to be eroded in 60.3% of the cases, followed by malleus in 58.7% and stapes in 47.6% of the patients [16]. Manik et al. also showed incus to be the most commonly affected ossicle in 70% of the patients, followed by malleus in 42% and stapes in 34% of the patients [31]. In our study, the most accurate information was regarding the erosion of the malleus, the head of the malleus being the most affected site, with a sensitivity of 85.7% and a specificity of 96% (kappa = 0.82). It was followed by erosion of the incus, with a sensitivity of 80.6 and specificity of 86.6% (kappa = 0.62). Other authors observed comparable sensitivity of 87% and 85%, respectively [11,18]. The stapes is the least eroded ossicle in most of the studies. However, the poorest imaging-surgical correlation was regarding stapes erosion. In our study, sensitivity was 57.1%, and specificity was 84.3% (kappa = 0.44), which is borderline between moderate and poor correlation. Other authors also reported poor radiologic-surgical correlation in stapes erosion and stated that the small size of the bone may be the cause of poor detection on HRCT scans [32,33]. However, if an ossicle is involved by the cholesteatoma, it has to be removed, no matter if it is eroded or not. The only exception is the stapes footplate, in which case the cholesteatoma matrix should be carefully dissected off the structure. Anything else can and should be removed, so preoperative information regarding the erosion of the malleus, incus, and even stapes superstructure is not essential for the ossicular chain reconstruction. The only unknown factor is which type of prosthesis should be used for the reconstruction of the sound transmission mechanism, and this depends on the status of the stapes superstructure—present and functional or absent/eroded. Either way, the stapes footplate needs to be mobile. However, you can always use a total ossicular replacement prosthesis (TORP) even if the stapes superstructure is intact by bypassing it.

HRCT is still considered the best available imaging method to describe the cholesteatoma of the middle ear, benefiting both the patient and the surgeon. Early diagnosis of cholesteatoma is also crucial, and there are important findings that can alert the physician, such as erosion of the scutum. MRI is another useful tool in cholesteatoma patient evaluation. Its main role is especially in the follow-up of patients with previous surgery since recurrence or residual cholesteatoma can be well detected, avoiding the risk of unnecessary revision surgery (second look operation). Preoperatively, MRI is also very useful in detecting intracranial complications. In both these circumstances, MRI is more helpful than HRCT.

This study demonstrated a good-to-excellent correlation between temporal bone HRCT findings and intraoperative lesions, particularly in tegmen tympani erosion, sigmoid plate dehiscence, malleus erosion, and scutum erosion. Our findings contrast with other reports, which showed an excellent radio-surgical correlation for the stapes (kappa = 0.94) and semicircular canals (kappa = 0.80), but poorer for the tegmen tympani erosion/thinning (kappa = 0.65) and facial nerve canal (kappa = 0.3) [10]. Rocher and colleagues revealed a good-to-excellent correlation for the scutum erosion and the lateral semicircular canal dehiscence (kappa > 0.75) and a good correlation for tegmen tympani erosion (k = 0.6) but a poor correlation for the facial nerve canal dehiscence (kappa < 0.4) [20].

The very good correlation between the findings on HRCT scans and intra-operative lesions may determine a higher degree of suspicion for unexpected problems during surgery and may improve the success rate of cholesteatoma surgery. The limitations and errors in interpretation may be improved by newer imaging technology.

The main limitation of this study consists of the small number of patients included and the small number of dangerous lesions encountered: eroded tegmen tympany in nine cases (19%), lateral semicircular canal fistula in four cases (9%), and eroded sigmoid sinus plate in three cases (7%).

5. Conclusions

The results of the present study indicate that HRCT is a most valuable preoperative imaging modality to evaluate cholesteatoma of the middle ear, playing an important role and guiding surgical management. HRCT scans can accurately predict the extent of the disease and are helpful in detecting erosion of the tegmen tympani, lateral semicircular canal fistulas, sigmoid sinus plates, and ossicular chain erosion with considerably high sensitivity and specificity. Accurate information on cholesteatoma lesions that are offered to the surgeon by means of HRCT allows for more limited procedures to be performed when eradicating the disease while preserving the function of the middle and inner ear and can alert the surgeon over dangerous but "silent" complications making him operate early. However, this imaging technique is not yet able to accurately distinguish between cholesteatoma and granulation tissue and cannot accurately detect facial nerve dehiscence/erosion and stapes erosion. Considering the characteristics—more aggressive and more prone to recurrences—cholesteatoma in children should deserve a separate study regarding the correlation between HRCT and intraoperative findings but on a more significant number of cases.

Author Contributions: The authors contributed to this article as follows: conceptualization, E.H.S.; methodology, E.H.S., N.C.B. and S.B.M.; software, L.G.; validation, E.H.S., N.C.B., M.G. and G.I.; investigation, E.H.S., M.G. and S.B.M.; data curation, E.H.S., S.B.M. and L.G.; writing—E.H.S. and L.G.; writing—review and editing, E.H.S., M.G. and S.B.M.; supervision, N.C.B. and G.I.; project administration, N.C.B. and G.I. All authors have read and agreed to the published version of the manuscript.

Funding: This research received no external funding.

Institutional Review Board Statement: This study was conducted in accordance with the Declaration of Helsinki and approved by the Ethics Committee of the Victor Babeş University of Medicine and Pharmacy (Nr. 57/9 September 2020).

Informed Consent Statement: Informed consent was obtained from all subjects involved in this study.

Data Availability Statement: Data supporting reported results can be found in the archives of the Department of Otolaryngology and Department of Radiology and Medical Imaging of the Victor Babes University of Medicine and Pharmacy Timisoara.

Conflicts of Interest: The authors declare no conflict of interest.

References

1. Olszewska, E.; Wagner, M.; Bernal-Sprekelsen, M.; Ebmeyer, J.; Dazert, S.; Hildmann, H.; Sudhoff, H. Etiopathogenisis of cholesteatoma. *Eur. Arch. Oto-Rhino-Laryngol. Head Neck* **2004**, *261*, 6–24. [CrossRef] [PubMed]
2. Ashutosh, R.; Soumit, M.; Yati, R.D.; Rezaul, K. Pre-operative HRCT of middle ear pathology with particular reference to intra-operative findings in cholesteatoma. *Int. J. Acad. Med. Pharm.* **2023**, *5*, 2303–2307.
3. Mafee, M.F.; Levin, B.C.; Applebaum, E.L.; Campos, C.F. Cholesteatoma of the middle ear and mastoid. *Otolaryngol. Clin. N. Am.* **1988**, *21*, 265–268. [CrossRef]
4. Lan, M.Y.; Lien, C.F.; Liao, W.H. Using high resolution computed tomography to evaluate middle ear cleft aeration of postoperative cholesteatoma ears. *J. Chin. Med. Assoc.* **2003**, *66*, 217–223. [PubMed]
5. Meyer, T.A.; Strunker, J.R.; Chester, L.; Lambert, P.R. Cholesteatoma. In *Head and Neck Surgery Otolaryngology*, 4th ed.; Bailey, B.J., Johnson, J.T., Eds.; Lippincott Williams and Wilkins: Philadelphia, PA, USA, 2006; Volume 2, pp. 2081–2091.
6. Bagul, M. High-resolution Computed Tomography Study of Temporal Bone Pathologies. *Headache* **2016**, *32*, 26–66.
7. Jackler, R.K.; Dillon, W.P.; Schindler, R.A. Computed tomography in suppurative ear disease: A correlation of surgical and radiographic findings. *Laryngoscope* **1984**, *94*, 746–752. [CrossRef] [PubMed]
8. Mohammadi, G.H.; Naderpour, M.; Mousaviagdas, M. Ossicular Erosion in Patients Requiring Surgery for Cholesteatoma. *Iran. J. Otorhinol. Gol.* **2012**, *24*, 125–128.
9. Vivek, R.; Gunasekaran, P.; Sethurajan, S.; Adaikappan, M. Evaluation of HRCT temporal bone and pathologies. *J. Evol. Med. Dent. Sci.* **2014**, *3*, 12118–12127.
10. Chee, N.C.; Tan, T.Y. The value of preoperative high resolution CT scans in cholesteatoma surgery. *Singap. Med. J.* **2001**, *2*, 155–159.
11. Datta, G.; Mohan, C.; Mahajan, M.; Mendiratta, V. Correlation of preoperative HRCT findings with surgical findings in unsafe CSOM. *J. Dent. Med. Sci.* **2014**, *13*, 120–125. [CrossRef]
12. Gomaa, M.A.; Karim, A.R.A.A.; Ghany, H.S.A.; Elhiny, A.A.; Sadek, A.A. Evaluation of temporal bone cholesteatoma and the correlation between high resolution computed tomography and surgical finding. *Clin. Med. Insights Ear Nose Throat* **2013**, *6*, 21–28. [CrossRef]
13. Kemppainen, H.; Puhakka, H.J.; Sipila, M.M.; Manninen, M.P.; Karma, P.H. Epidemiology and etiology of middle ear cholesteatoma. *Acta Otolaryngol.* **1999**, *119*, 568–572. [PubMed]
14. Khavasi, P.; Bhargavi, K.; Malashetti, S.P.; Yasha, C. Acquired cholesteatoma in children: Presentation, complications and management. *Int. J. Otorhinolaryngol. Head Neck Surg.* **2018**, *4*, 1017–1022. [CrossRef]
15. Jacob, A.; Sreedhar, S.; Choolakkaparambu, A.; Anwar, S.; Bashir Nalakath, K. Utility of high resolution computed tomography in pre-operative evaluation of cholesteatoma. *Int. J. Otorhinolaryngol. Head Neck Surg.* **2020**, *6*, 1278. [CrossRef]
16. Zaman, S.U.; Rangankar, V.; Muralinath, K.; Shah, V.; Gowtham, K.; Pawar, R. Temporal Bone Cholesteatoma: Typical Findings and Evaluation of Diagnostic Utility on High Resolution Computed Tomography. *Cureus* **2022**, *14*, e22730. [CrossRef] [PubMed]
17. Shah, C.; Shah, P.; Shah, S. Role of HRCT Temporal Bone in Pre Operative Evaluation of Choesteatoma. *Int. J. Med. Sci. Public Health* **2014**, *3*, 69–72. [CrossRef]
18. Rai, T. Radiological study of the temporal bone in chronic otitis media: Prospective study of 50 cases. *Indian J. Otol.* **2014**, *20*, 48. [CrossRef]
19. Gaurano, J.L.; Joharjy, I.A. Middle ear cholesteatoma: Characteristic CT findings in 64 patients. *Ann. Saudi Med.* **2004**, *24*, 442–447.
20. Rocher, P.; Carlier, R.; Attal, P.; Doyon, D.; Bobin, S. Contribution and role of the scanner in the preoperative evaluation of chronic otitis. radiosurgical correlation apropos of 85 cases. *Ann. D'oto-Laryngol. Chir. Cervico Faciale Bull. La Soc. D'oto-Laryngol. Des Hop. Paris* **1995**, *112*, 317–323.
21. Sunita, M.; Sambandan, A. Importance of Pre-Operative HRCT Temporal Bone in chronic suppurative otitis media. *Odisha J. Otorhinolaryngol. Head Neck Surg.* **2015**, *9*, 10–13.
22. Keskin, S.; Çetin, H.; Töre, H.G. The correlation of temporal bone CT with surgery findings in evaluation of chronic inflammatory diseases of the middle ear. *Eur. J. Gen. Med.* **2011**, *8*, 24–30. [CrossRef]
23. Kanotra, S.; Gupta, R.; Gupta, N.; Sharma, R.; Gupta, S.; Kotwal, S. Correlation of high-resolution computed tomography temporal bone findings with intra-operative findings in patients with cholesteatoma. *Indian J. Otol.* **2015**, *21*, 280.
24. Jamal, S.; Rahman, A.; Mohan, C.; Srivastava, A. Is pre-operative HRCT temporal bone findings consistent with tympano-mastoid surgical findings. *Int. J. Health Clin. Res.* **2020**, *3*, 104–109.
25. Gerami, H.; Naghavi, E.; Wahabi-Moghadam, M.; Forghanparast, K.; Akbar, M.H. Comparison of preoperative computerized tomography scan imaging of temporal bone with the intra-operative findings in patients undergoing mastoidectomy. *Saudi Med. J.* **2009**, *30*, 104–108. [PubMed]
26. O'reilly, B.J.; Chevretton, E.B.; Wylie, I.; Thakkar, C.; Butler, P.; Sathanathan, N.; Morrison, G.A.; Kenyon, G.S. The value of CT scanning in chronic suppurative otitis media. *J. Laryngol. Otol.* **1991**, *105*, 990–994. [CrossRef]
27. Vlastarakos, P.V.; Kiprouli, C.; Pappas, S.; Xenelis, J.; Maragoudakis, P.; Troupis, G.; Nikolopoulos, T.P. CT scan versus surgery: How reliable is the preoperative radiological assessment in patients with chronic otitis media? *Eur. Arch. Oto-Rhino-Laryngol.* **2012**, *269*, 81–86. [CrossRef] [PubMed]
28. Dashottar, S.; Bucha, A.; Sinha, S.; Nema, D. Preoperative temporal bone HRCT and intra-operative findings in middle ear cholesteatoma: A comparative study. *Int. J. Otorhinolaryngol. Head Neck Surg.* **2018**, *5*, 77. [CrossRef]

29. Ozbek, C.; Tuna, E.; Ciftci, O.; Yazkan, O.; Ozdem, C. Incidence of fallopian canal dehiscence at surgery for chronic otitis media. *Eur. Arch. Otorhinolaryngol.* **2009**, *266*, 357–362. [CrossRef]
30. Yetiser, S.; Tosun, F.; Kazkayasi, M. Facial nerve paralysis due to chronic otitis media. *Otol. Neurotol.* **2002**, *23*, 580–588. [CrossRef]
31. Manik, S.; Dabholkar, Y.; Bhalekar, S.; Velankar, H.; Chordia, N.; Saberwal, A. Sensitivity and specificity of high resolution computed tomography (HRCT) of temporal bone in diagnosing cholesteatoma and its correlation with intraoperative findings. *Indian J. Otolaryngol. Head Neck Surg.* **2021**, *73*, 25–29. [CrossRef]
32. Sreedhar, S.; Pujary, K.; Agarwal, A.C.; Balakrishnan, R. Role of high-resolution computed tomography scan in the evaluation of cholesteatoma: A correlation of high-resolution computed tomography with intra-operative findings. *Indian J. Otol.* **2015**, *21*, 103.
33. Rogha, M.; Hashemi, S.M.; Mokhtarinejad, F.; Eshaghian, A.; Dadgostar, A. Comparison of Preoperative Temporal Bone CT with Intraoperative Findings in Patients with Cholesteatoma. *Iran. J. Otorhinolaryngol.* **2014**, *26*, 7–12. [PubMed]

Disclaimer/Publisher's Note: The statements, opinions and data contained in all publications are solely those of the individual author(s) and contributor(s) and not of MDPI and/or the editor(s). MDPI and/or the editor(s) disclaim responsibility for any injury to people or property resulting from any ideas, methods, instructions or products referred to in the content.

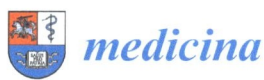

Article

A Cone Beam Computed Tomography-Based Investigation of the Frequency and Pattern of Radix Entomolaris in the Saudi Arabian Population

Muhammad Qasim Javed [1,*], Swati Srivastava [1], Badi Baen Rashed Alotaibi [1], Usman Anwer Bhatti [2], Ayman M. Abulhamael [3] and Syed Rashid Habib [4]

1. Department of Conservative Dental Sciences, College of Dentistry, Qassim University, P.O. Box 1162, Buraidah 51452, Qassim, Saudi Arabia; s.kumar@qu.edu.sa (S.S.); bb.alotaibi@qu.edu.sa (B.B.R.A.)
2. Department of Operative Dentistry, Islamic International Dental College, Riphah International University, Islamabad 44000, Pakistan; usman.anwer@riphah.edu.pk
3. Department of Endodontics, Faculty of Dentistry, King Abdulaziz University, P.O. Box 80209, Jeddah 21589, Saudi Arabia; amahmad4@kau.edu.sa
4. Department of Prosthetic Dental Sciences, College of Dentistry, King Saud University, P.O. Box 60169, Riyadh 11545, Saudi Arabia
* Correspondence: m.anayat@qu.edu.sa

Abstract: *Background and Objectives*: An understanding of the anatomical complexity of teeth is a significant factor for a successful endodontic treatment outcome. The aim of this study was to explore the frequency and pattern of distribution of radix entomolaris (RE) in mandibular first molars (MFMs) of a Saudi Arabian subpopulation using CBCT scans. *Materials and Methods*: This study was conducted at dental clinics of Qassim University from February to May 2023 by evaluating CBCT scans that were previously obtained for diagnostic purposes. Scans of Saudi national patients with bilaterally present MFMs and fully formed root apices were included. Conversely, scans with one/or two missing MFMs, MFMs with incomplete root apices, full- or partial-coverage prosthesis, endodontic treatment, and associated radicular resorption were excluded from study. A total of 303 CBCT scans with 606 bilateral MFMs were analyzed by two calibrated evaluators for the presence of, and type according to Song's typolgy of RE. The data were analyzed using SPPS-24. The descriptive variables were documented as frequencies and percentages. The chi-square test was used to determine the association between the prevalence of RE with the gender, jaw side and age group. Both inter-rater and intra-rater agreements were estimated for detecting and classifying RE using Cohen's kappa test. *Results*: The sample had 63.7% males and 36.3% females. The prevalence of RE was 6.6%, with Song's type III (57.5%) as the most common variant. Absolute agreement was noted between the raters about the presence of RE and very strong agreement was noted for the classification of the RE. *Conclusions*: RE is an uncommon finding among the mandibular first molars of the Saudi population without any gender and quadrant predilection. The clinicians' knowledge of the presence and Song's type of RE may contribute towards the enhancement of endodontic treatment outcomes.

Keywords: cone beam computed tomography; cross-sectional studies; diagnostic imaging; dentistry; endodontics; mandibular molars; prevalence; radix entomolaris; root canal anatomy; three-dimensional imaging

Citation: Javed, M.Q.; Srivastava, S.; Alotaibi, B.B.R.; Bhatti, U.A.; Abulhamael, A.M.; Habib, S.R. A Cone Beam Computed Tomography-Based Investigation of the Frequency and Pattern of Radix Entomolaris in the Saudi Arabian Population. *Medicina* **2023**, *59*, 2025. https://doi.org/10.3390/medicina59112025

Academic Editors: Bruno Chrcanovic, Romica Cergan, Adrian Costache and Mihai Dumitru

Received: 29 October 2023
Revised: 15 November 2023
Accepted: 15 November 2023
Published: 17 November 2023

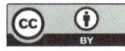

Copyright: © 2023 by the authors. Licensee MDPI, Basel, Switzerland. This article is an open access article distributed under the terms and conditions of the Creative Commons Attribution (CC BY) license (https://creativecommons.org/licenses/by/4.0/).

1. Introduction

Successful endodontic treatment (ET) relies on various factors, including an anatomic understanding of the teeth and root canal system (RCS), which serves as the anatomical foundation for ET [1,2]. Failing to identify a single root canal during ET can result in the development of secondary or persistent apical periodontitis (AP) [3]. The first permanent teeth to appear in the oral cavity are the mandibular first molars (MFMs). These teeth, often referred to as the "key of the occlusion", possess various pits and fissures on the occlusal surface, making self-cleaning a challenging process. As a result, individuals with a higher susceptibility to tooth decay are more prone to requiring ET for MFMs [4–6].

The cleaning and shaping of the RCS in the MFMs pose a great challenge due to the unpredictability of its morphological characteristics [7–9]. The typical shape of MFMs is described as having two roots and two canals in the mesial root, with one or two canals in the distal root [1]. Nevertheless, there are various deviations in the canal structure of mandibular molars, one being the presence of an extra distolingual root and canal [10], as well as the existence of a third canal in the mesial root known as the middle mesial canal [11]. The existence of additional root and complex root anatomy holds clinical significance as it can impact various dental procedures, such as prosthetic restorations, apical surgery, extraction, intentional replantation, and ET [12,13].

The understanding of the anatomical complexity of mandibular molars has improved over time. Modern imaging techniques like cone beam computed tomography (CBCT) have substantially increased the identification of various morphological variations like accessory middle mesial canals, distolingual roots, and distobuccal roots [14–17]. The existence of an additional root, referred to as radix entomolaris, at the distolingual aspect is an important variation. While this extra root has been associated with a notable ethnic characteristic in Asian countries, its prevalence in other regions of the world remains uncertain [7]. The accessory distolingual root was first discovered by Carabelli in 1844 [18]. It was later named radix entomolaris (RE) by Bolk in 1915 [19]. Typically, RE is characterized by its curvature and relatively shorter length compared to other roots, and may either be fused or separate from the main distal root [20]. Generally, RE is shorter than the distobuccal root, but in some cases, it may be completely separate from the DB root or fused with it [21]. Such anatomic nuances pose a serious challenge in root canal treatment for clinicians. For instance, the orifice of the RE is hard to locate without an appropriate modification of the access cavity, and when left untreated, these canals become a major cause of post-treatment disease due to microbial contamination [22,23]. Thus, a knowledge of the regional prevalence of distolingual roots is of great clinical significance to indigenous clinicians.

The presence of RE is a variable occurrence among different populations. A recent meta-analysis concluded a 5.6% global prevalence of this peculiar anatomic feature [24]. Studies of certain East Asian ethnic groups report a frequency as high as 32% [7]. In contrast, there are reports of zero percent prevalence in other ethnicities [14]. Several theories try to explain the etiology and the race-related high prevalence of this trait [14,16]. One such idea is the possible hereditary role of these three-rooted mandibular first molars, but this is still debatable due to a lack of adequate evidence [14–19].

Among the Saudi population, there is a paucity of CBCT-based evidence on the distribution of RE. Al-Alawi and colleagues reported a 4.3% presence of RE, while Mashyakhy et al. described a 2.9% prevalence [25,26]. The difference in the reports and the lack of high-quality CBCT-based studies warrant further investigation of this anomaly. Moreover, this morphological feature demonstrates a mixed topologic tendency, with no consensus on the bilateral occurrence or side predilection (left vs. right side) [14]. Hence, the objective of this study was to explore the frequency and pattern of distribution of radix entomolaris in mandibular first molars of a Saudi Arabian subpopulation using CBCT scans.

2. Materials and Methods

2.1. Study Design

This cross-sectional research was carried out following the recommendations for cross-sectional epidemiologic studies on root canal configuration and roots utilizing CBCT scans [27] after obtaining approval from the Dental Ethical Review Board at Qassim University, Saudi Arabia (Approval No.: EA/m-2019-3023).

2.2. Study Settings

The study was conducted at the dental clinics of Qassim University Medical City (QUMC) from February to May 2023.

2.3. Sample Size Calculation

The sample size was calculated using a Scalex sample size calculator [28]. With 5% precision, a 6.07% expected prevalence and a 95 confidence level, a minimum of 88 CBCT scans with 176 bilateral MFMs were calculated as an adequate sample size [29].

2.4. Participants

The CBCT scans of only Saudi national patients were included in the study by screening the patients' files for nationality. Data acquisition was conducted in accordance with the American Association of Endodontists' position statement [30]. The included CBCT scans were taken from 2019 to 2023 for different reasons, including the planning of treatment for endodontics, dental implants, dento-facial trauma, and orthodontic management and were obtained from the archives of the Oral Radiology Department at QUMC, Saudi Arabia. These CBCT scans were acquired using the Sirona Galileos comfort machine (Beinshiem, Germany). It had a voxel size of 160 μm and a field of view of 15 × 15 cm, and the scans were observed with GALILEOS viewer software version 1.8.

2.4.1. Inclusion Criteria

Scans of Saudi national patients having bilaterally present MFMs with fully formed root apices and recorded gender/age information in patients' files were included in the study.

2.4.2. Exclusion Criteria

Scans with one/or two missing MFMs, MFMs with incomplete root apices, full- or partial-coverage prosthesis, ET, and associated radicular resorption were excluded from the study.

2.5. Variables

The prevalence of RE (primary outcome) and frequency of an additional canal in the main distal root, the concurrent occurrence of RE in PMFMs and permanent mandibular second molars (PMSMs), and the simultaneous presence of RE in PMFMs and a C-shaped canal in PMSMs (secondary outcomes) were determined by two endodontists with 12 years of experience (M.Q.J. and S.S.)

2.6. Calibration

The two evaluators were calibrated using 15 CBCT scans that were excluded from the study. Both inter-rater and intra-rater agreements were estimated for detecting and classifying RE using Cohen's kappa test. The intra-rater reliability test was conducted after evaluating 15 CBCT scans two times at a fifteen-day interval.

2.7. Data Sources and Measurements

The patients' ages and genders were also documented on the data collection sheet during data collection. The assessment method of CBCT scans comprised a distal aspect assessment of MFMs in three dimensions (axial, coronal, and sagittal) after 3D alignment of the roots' long axis with the visualization software's reference lines. Both evaluators were permitted to adjust tools and visualization settings (filters and noise reduction) to enhance the quality of the image. The RE (yes/no) presence was documented as suggested by Calberson and De Moor [16,17]. Moreover, the REs were classified according to Song's classification [20].

2.8. Statistical Methods

The data were exported to SPPS-24 (IBM Corp, 32, Armonk, NY, USA) from the Excel sheet. The descriptive variables were documented as frequencies and percentages. The chi-square test was used to determine the association between the prevalence of RE and the gender, jaw side and age group.

3. Results

A total of 543 CBCT scans were screened. In the final analysis, 240 CBCT scans were excluded, with one (109 scans) and two (131 scans) missing mandibular first molars. The final sample consisted of 303 CBCT scans with 606 bilaterally present mandibular first molars (Figure 1). The male to female ratio of the sample was 1.75:1, with 193 males (63.7%) and 110 females (36.3%). The mean age of the patients was 30.95 ± 11.61 years, with a range from 11 to 66 years. Absolute agreement was noted between the raters about the presence of RE and very strong agreement was noted during the classification of the RE (Cohen's kappa: 0.98, $p < 0.05$). Moreover, intra-rater reliability was found to be 1.00 for the presence and classification of RE.

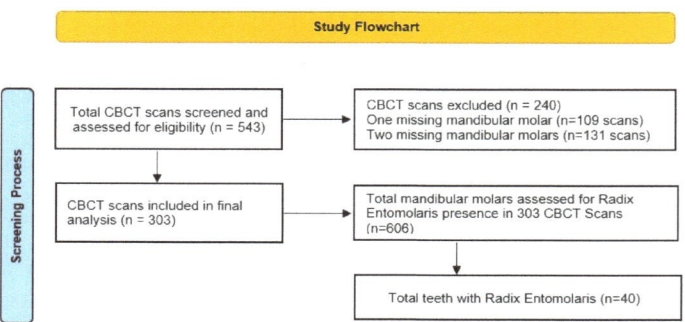

Figure 1. Flowchart depicting the screening process during the study.

The overall prevalence of radix entomolaris (RE) was 6.6%, with no significant difference between genders (Table 1). When comparing quadrants, RE was more prevalent on the right side, but the difference was not statistically significant (Table 2). Table 3 highlights the prevalence of RE according to age groups, with the highest prevalence recorded in the 11–30 year age group and the lowest in the 51–70 year age group. A detailed analysis of the unilateral or bilateral presence of RE in relation to gender is demonstrated in Table 4. The presence of RE was either unilateral or bilateral, with comparable frequencies between genders. Type III (57.5%) was the most common variant of radix entomolaris, followed by type I (25%) and type II (17.5%) (Figure 2), whereas the small type (0%) and conical type (0%) were not identified in the study sample. Table 5 depicts the distribution of RE according to Song's classification.

Table 1. Gender-wise prevalence of radix entomolaris and description of the total number of roots in mandibular first molars.

		Radix Entomolaris N (%)			p-Value *
		Absent	Present	Total	
Gender	Male	362 (93.8)	24 (6.2)	386 (63.7)	
	Female	204 (92.7)	16 (7.3)	220 (36.3)	0.62
Total		566 (93.4)	40 (6.6)	606 (100)	

* Chi-Square.

Table 2. Prevalence of radix entomolaris in mandibular first molars by quadrant.

		Radix Entomolaris N (%)			p-Value *
		Absent	Present	Total	
Tooth Type	Mandibular Left First Molar	286 (94.4)	17 (5.6)	303 (50)	0.33
	Mandibular Right First Molar	280 (92.4)	23 (7.6)	303 (50)	
Total		566 (93.4)	40 (6.6)	606 (100)	

* Chi-Square.

Table 3. Prevalence of radix entomolaris in mandibular first molars according to age groups.

		Radix Entomolaris N (%)			p-Value *
		No	Yes	Total	
Age Group	11–30	337	18	355 (58.6)	0.07
	31–50	191	16	207 (34.2)	
	51–70	38	6	44 (7.3)	
Total		566 (93.4)	40 (6.6)	606 (100)	

* Chi-Square.

Table 4. Radix entomolaris (distolingual root) prevalence in mandibular first molars by gender and jaw quadrant ($n = 606$).

Gender	Quadrant Side	No. of Patients	No. of Teeth	Radix Entomolaris
Male	Bilateral	8	16	16 (2.64%)
	Unilateral	8	8	8 (1.32%)
	Total	16	24	24 (3.96%)
Female	Bilateral	6	12	12 (1.98%)
	Unilateral	4	4	4 (0.66%)
	Total	10	16	16 (2.64%)
Grand Total		26	40	40 (6.6%)

Table 5. Song's classification of radix entomolaris ($n = 40$).

Song's Classification of Radix Entomolaris	Frequency (%)
Type 1	10 (25)
Type 2	7 (17.5)
Type 3	23 (57.5)
Small type	0 (0)
Conical type	0 (0)

During the sample analysis, a few additional observations were made. When the anatomy of the main distal root was examined, only one tooth in a female patient with RE had a second distal canal in the main distal root. None of the lower second molars adjacent to the first molars with RE showed a C-shaped canal anatomy. One patient with a bilateral radix in the lower first molars also had a bilateral radix in the adjacent lower second molars. In comparison, another patient with a unilateral radix in the lower first molars had a unilateral radix in the adjacent lower second molar (Figure 3).

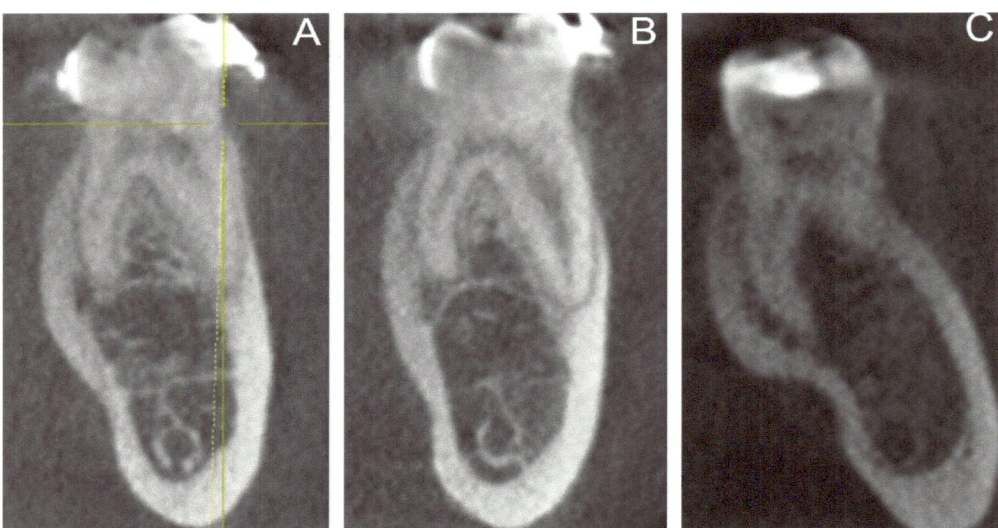

Figure 2. Coronal section of a CBCT image indicating the three variants of radix entomolaris according to Song et al.: (**A**) type 1, (**B**) type 2 and (**C**) type 3.

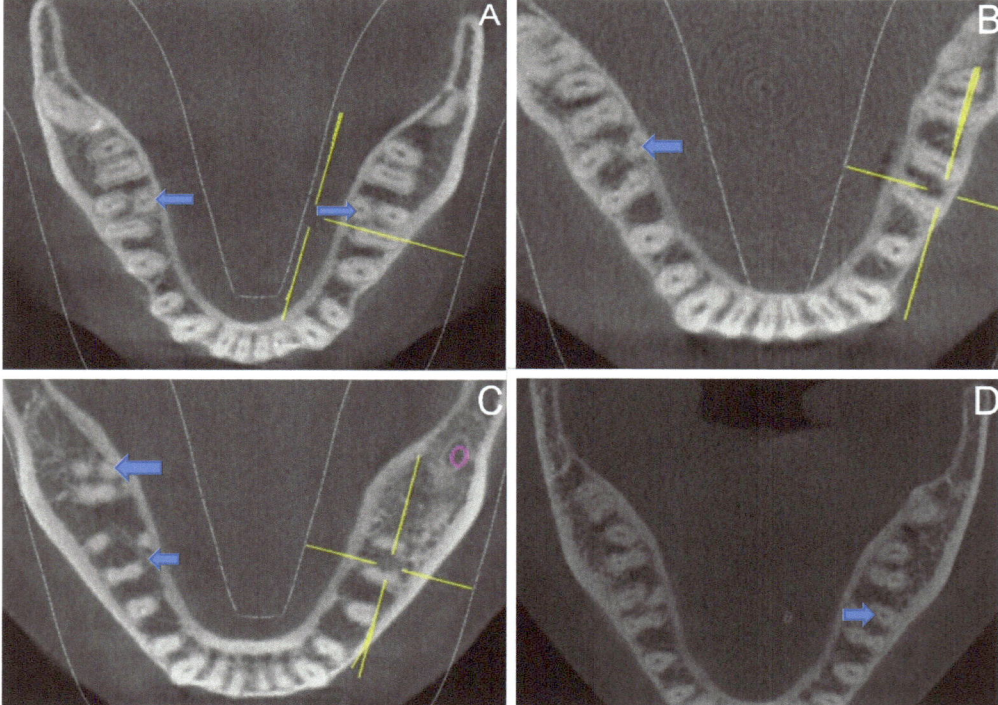

Figure 3. Axial sections of CBCT images indicating (blue arrows) (**A**) bilateral RE in MFM, (**B**) unilateral RE in MFM, (**C**) unilateral RE in MFM and MSM, and (**D**) an additional distal canal in the main distal root.

4. Discussion

The prevalence of RE is presently an issue of debate, primarily due to the discrepancies in occurrence rates amongst diverse populations. Amongst Caucasians, Africans, Eurasians, and Indians, it has been reported that RE constitutes less than 5% of the population, whereas in populations of Mongol ancestry, such as Chinese, Eskimos, and Native Americans, the frequency of RE ranges from 5% to as high as 40% [10,17,31,32].

In the present study, the overall prevalence of RE was found to be 6.6%. Our results show a slightly higher prevalence compared with the previous investigations performed in Saudi Arabia, where a proportion of 2.3% was shown by Younes et al. using extracted teeth, 5.97% was recorded by Al-Nazhan using clinical and radiographical evaluations, and 6% was recorded by Bahammam and Bahammam using extracted teeth [30,33,34]. These variations might be due to the investigation method applied. In previous studies, RE was recognized with a visual examination of extracted teeth or through periapical radiographs. However, in the present research, CBCT scans might have led to a better visualization of the roots and a higher prevalence. CBCT offers the advantage of visualizing an area from three different planes—sagittal, coronal, and axial—resulting in the elimination of the superimposition of anatomical structures, as documented [35,36]. In Asian populations of Mongol ancestry, RE is a prevalent morphological feature, with a high frequency of appearance. Research studies report a frequency exceeding 20% in some and over 30% in others [7,20,37,38]. In India, the incidence of a third root ranges from 4.5% to 13.3% [39], while in Africa, it is lower at 3.1% [40]. Conversely, in Caucasian populations, RE is considered rare, with a frequency lower than 10% [41]. This global variation in the occurrence of RE was also confirmed in a recent meta-analysis [42].

We also found that although the prevalence of RE was slightly higher in females (7.3%) than in males (6.2%), the result was not statistically significant (Table 1). Findings from other studies suggest a similar trend with no statistically significant difference in prevalence between either gender [7,9,39].

In a quadrant-wise comparison, we found that the prevalence of RE on the right side was 7.6% and on the left side it was 5.6% (Table 2). However, the result was not statistically significant. It is worth highlighting that a statistically significant association was observed in populations with a high prevalence of supernumerary roots, with a right-sided preponderance [20,43,44]. On the contrary, some researchers have documented a preference for a left-side localization [45,46]. However, there has been a relatively low frequency of reports regarding the left-sided predominance.

An age-wise comparison of the RE prevalence did not show a statistically significant difference in our study. The prevalence of RE was lowest (7.3%) among the 51–70-year-old group and highest (58.6%) among the 11–30-year-old group. Our findings are in corroboration with Talabani et al. [47], who found no statistically significant association between the age group and RE. Moreover, age-related changes in the tooth cannot interfere with the detection of RE.

The bilateral prevalence of RE in males was 2.6%, whereas in females, it was 1.98% (Table 3). These findings are in agreement with Hosseini et al. [48]. However, the present outcome falls notably below the report by Qiao et al. [49], who conducted a study on the occurrence of RE (76.87%) among MFMs in a population from Western China. This difference highlights the importance of conducting thorough clinical and radiological assessments for individuals having RE on one or both sides.

The morphological classification of RE was originally established by De Moor et al. in 2004 [17], who categorized it into three types (types I, II, and III) based on the curvature of the DL root. The classification used in this study was based on the morphological anatomy of RE by Song et al., which was a modification of De Moors' classification [20]. This study found that type III had the highest occurrence rate at 57.5%, followed by type I at 25% and type II at 17.5%. De Moor et al. reported a prevalence rate of 61.6% for the type III morphological anatomy [17], while another study by Chen et al. only found 28.6% for type III [49], which is lower than the 57.5% found in this study. Hence, practitioners must exercise caution when treating RE, as these roots can exhibit significant curvature that can lead to potential complications in shaping the root canal, including transportation and the creation of ledges. The underdeveloped root forms, small type, and conical type were not found in the present study but have been reported in the literature, with variations existing in different geographic locations [16,40,50]. These small and conical type roots carry an increased risk of strip perforation or over-instrumentation and should be handled cautiously by the clinician [20].

In the present investigation, we have taken note of some additional observations. Firstly, out of all the scans, only one scan of a female patient had an extra canal in the distal root, making a total of five canals in her right MFM: mesiobuccal, mesiolingual, distobuccal, distolingual, and one canal in the supernumerary root situated distolingually (RE). Secondly, we investigated the presence of a C-shaped canal in the mandibular second molar adjacent to the MFM with RE. However, none of the scans investigated showed the presence of C-shaped anatomy in the mandibular second molar. Thirdly, only one scan had a bilateral RE in the MFM and mandibular second molar. Moreover, only one scan indicated the combined presence of unilateral RE in the MFM and mandibular second molar. All these root variations differ according to ethnicity, with the C-shaped canals being more common among mandibular second molars, while RE is more common among MFMs [51].

RE is a widely discussed topic due to the variations in its frequency across different populations. Ethnicity is a leading factor that influences the presence of a third root in MFM. Such a morphological variation is often present among individuals of Asian descent of Mongol ancestry [7,20]. These findings show that the prevalence of RE is a function of the demographic and geographic characteristics of the study population. Having a comprehensive knowledge of various forms of dental morphology is an essential aspect when it comes to effective endodontic treatment. Understanding this variant is critical in ensuring a successful outcome. Therefore, endodontists must thoroughly understand dental morphology to achieve an optimal result.

Diagnostic methods like sonography can be studied for the detection of RE as an alternative to CBCT. Ultrasonography (USG) was initially employed in dentistry in 1963 to evaluate tooth vitality [52]. Since that time, ultrasound imaging has been utilized in dentistry for a range of reasons, including caries detection, muscle thickness assessment, and diagnosing temporomandibular disorders [53]. In the ultrasonographic image, the alveolar bone, when in a healthy condition, exhibits full reflection and presents itself as a white surface. Similarly, the lines representing the roots of the teeth appear even whiter and are referred to as hyperechoic [54]. The use of ultrasonography in the detection of RE can be beneficial, as the sonography imaging technique may offer numerous benefits that include efficiency, cost-effectiveness, radiation-free nature with no known biological side-effects, and practical application with better patient comfort [54]. However, the efficacy of the detection of roots decreases when the thickness of the cortical plate increases, like in the mandibular posterior region [54]. Moreover, the utilization of USG for RE detection is still at a rudimentary stage.

4.1. Strengths and Limitations

The strength of this study lies in the use of CBCT data that are far more detailed and comprehensive than two-dimensional periapical radiographs, where the distobuccal root can easily superimpose the distobuccal root, causing an underreporting of data. Moreover, the inclusion of bilateral molars allows an analysis of bilateral prevalence that was missing in previous studies. One of the main constraints of our study was the analysis of a limited sample size confined to a particular geographic location, which restricts the external validity of the results. Moreover, the male to female ratio of the study sample (1.75:1) is not representative of the actual male to female ratio of the Saudi population (1.01:1).

4.2. Future Recommendations

Future CBCT-based studies with a larger sample size and male to female ratio of the sample corresponding to the actual male to female ratio of Saudi nationals is recommended, as well as the utilization of ultrasonography and Micro-CT in future research for the detection of RE.

5. Conclusions

To conclude, radix entomolaris is an uncommon finding among the mandibular first molars of the Saudi population without any gender and quadrant predilection. Moreover, type III is the most common variant of RE in MFMs, which may exhibit an additional distal canal on rare occasions. The findings of the current study will improve clinicians' knowledge of the frequency of different Song's RE types in Saudi subpopulations. Subsequently, this may contribute to the enhancement in ET outcomes.

Author Contributions: Conceptualization, M.Q.J. and S.S.; methodology, M.Q.J.; software, B.B.R.A.; validation, A.M.A., S.R.H. and B.B.R.A.; formal analysis, B.B.R.A. and U.A.B.; investigation, M.Q.J. and S.S.; resources, S.R.H. and S.S.; data curation, M.Q.J.; writing—original draft preparation, M.Q.J., S.S., B.B.R.A. and U.A.B.; writing—review and editing, U.A.B., A.M.A. and S.R.H.; visualization, A.M.A. and U.A.B.; supervision, M.Q.J.; project administration, M.Q.J. and B.B.R.A.; funding acquisition, S.R.H. All authors have read and agreed to the published version of the manuscript.

Funding: The research was funded by the Researchers Supporting Project number RSPD2023R950, King Saud University, Riyadh, Saudi Arabia.

Institutional Review Board Statement: The current research was approved by the Dental Ethical Review Board at Qassim University, Saudi Arabia (Approval No.: EA/m-2019-3023 dated 29 September 2019).

Informed Consent Statement: Not applicable.

Data Availability Statement: Data will be made available upon request. However, CBCT scans cannot be provided due to ethical restrictions from Deanship of Scientific Research at Qassim University, Saudi Arabia.

Acknowledgments: The authors appreciate the support from the Researchers Supporting Project number RSPD2023R950, King Saud University, Riyadh, Saudi Arabia.

Conflicts of Interest: The authors have no conflict of interest to declare.

References

1. De Pablo, O.V.; Estevez, R.; Peix Sanchez, M.; Heilborn, C.; Cohenca, N. Root anatomy and canal configuration of the permanent mandibular first molar: A systematic review. *J. Endod.* **2010**, *36*, 1919–1931. [CrossRef]
2. Toru, N. Better success rate for root canal therapy when treatment includes obturation short of the apex. *Evid. Based Dent.* **2005**, *6*, 45.
3. Reuben, J.; Velmurugan, N.; Kandaswamy, D. The evaluation of root canal morphology of the mandibular first molar in an Indian population using spiral computed tomography scan: An in vitro study. *J. Endod.* **2008**, *34*, 212–215. [CrossRef]
4. Skidmore, A.E.; Bjorndal, A.M. Root canal morphology of the human mandibular first molar. *Oral Surg. Oral Med. Oral Pathol.* **1971**, *32*, 778–784. [CrossRef] [PubMed]
5. Silva, E.J.; Nejaim, Y.; Silva, A.V.; Haiter-Neto, F.; Cohenca, N. Evaluation of root canal configuration of mandibular molars in a Brazilian population by using cone-beam computed tomography: An in vivo study. *J. Endod.* **2013**, *39*, 849–852. [CrossRef]
6. Baugh, D.; Wallace, J. Middle mesial canal of the mandibular first molar: A case report and literature review. *J. Endod.* **2004**, *30*, 185–186. [CrossRef] [PubMed]
7. Gu, Y.; Lu, Q.; Wang, H.; Ding, Y.; Wang, P.; Ni, L. Root canal morphology of permanent three-rooted mandibular first molars-part I: Pulp floor and root canal system. *J. Endod.* **2010**, *36*, 990–994. [CrossRef]
8. Kim, S.Y.; Kim, B.S.; Woo, J.; Kim, Y. Morphology of mandibular first molars analyzed by cone-beam computed tomography in a Korean population: Variations in the number of roots and canals. *J. Endod.* **2013**, *39*, 1516–1521. [CrossRef]
9. Martins, J.N.; Marques, D.; Silva, E.J.N.L.; Caramês, J.; Versiani, M.A. Prevalence studies on root canal anatomy using cone-beam computed tomographic imaging: A systematic review. *J. Endod.* **2019**, *45*, 372–386. [CrossRef] [PubMed]
10. Huang, R.Y.; Cheng, W.C.; Chen, C.J.; Lin, C.D.; Lai, T.M.; Shen, E.C.; Chiang, C.Y.; Chiu, H.C.; Fu, E. Three-dimensional analysis of the root morphology of mandibular first molars with distolingual roots. *Int. Endod. J.* **2010**, *43*, 478–484. [CrossRef]

11. Nosrat, A.; Deschenes, R.J.; Tordik, P.A.; Hicks, M.L.; Fouad, A.F. Middle mesial canals in mandibular molars: Incidence and related factors. *J. Endod.* **2015**, *41*, 28–32. [CrossRef]
12. Wu, Y.C.; Su, C.C.; Tsai, Y.W.C.; Cheng, W.C.; Chung, M.P.; Chiang, H.S.; Hsieh, C.Y.; Chung, C.H.; Shieh, Y.S.; Huang, R.Y. Complicated root canal configuration of mandibular first premolars is correlated with the presence of the distolingual root in mandibular first molars: A cone-beam computed tomographic study in Taiwanese individuals. *J. Endod.* **2017**, *43*, 1064–1071. [CrossRef] [PubMed]
13. Zhang, X.; Xu, N.; Wang, H.; Yu, Q. A cone-beam computed tomographic study of apical surgery–related morphological characteristics of the distolingual root in 3-rooted mandibular first molars in a Chinese population. *J. Endod.* **2017**, *43*, 2020–2024. [CrossRef] [PubMed]
14. Abella, F.; Patel, S.; Durán-Sindreu, F.; Mercadé, M.; Roig, M. Mandibular first molars with disto-lingual roots: Review and clinical management. *Int. Endod. J.* **2012**, *45*, 963–978. [CrossRef] [PubMed]
15. Bhatti, U.A.; Muhammad, M.; Javed, M.Q.; Sajid, M. Frequency of middle mesial canal in mandibular first molars and its association with various anatomic variables. *Aust. Endod. J.* **2022**, *48*, 494–500. [CrossRef]
16. Calberson, F.L.; De Moor, R.J.; Deroose, C.A. The radix entomolaris and paramolaris: Clinical approach in endodontics. *J. Endod.* **2007**, *33*, 58–63. [CrossRef] [PubMed]
17. De Moor, R.J.; Deroose, C.A.; Calberson, F.L. The radix entomolaris in mandibular first molars: An endodontic challenge. *Int. Endod. J.* **2004**, *37*, 789–799. [CrossRef]
18. Carabelli, G. *Systemntisches Handbueh der Zahnkeilkunde*, 2nd ed.; BraumuUer und Seidel: Vienna, Austria, 1844; p. 114.
19. Bolk, L. Bemerkungen über wurzelvariationen am menschlichen unteren molaren. *Z. Morphol. Anthropol.* **1915**, *3*, 605–610.
20. Song, J.S.; Choi, H.J.; Jung, I.Y.; Jung, H.S.; Kim, S.O. The prevalence and morphologic classification of distolingual roots in the mandibular molars in a Korean population. *J. Endod.* **2010**, *36*, 653–657. [CrossRef]
21. Carlsen, O.; Alexandersen, V. Radix entomolaris: Identification and morphology. *Scan. J. Dent. Res.* **1990**, *98*, 363–373. [CrossRef]
22. Wu, W.; Guo, Q.; Tan, B.K.; Huang, D.; Zhou, X.; Shen, Y.; Gao, Y.; Haapasalo, M. Geometric Analysis of the Distolingual Root and Canal in Mandibular First Molars: A Micro-computed Tomographic Study. *J. Endod.* **2021**, *47*, 779–786. [CrossRef]
23. Costa, F.F.N.P.; Pacheco-Yanes, J.; Siqueira, J.F., Jr.; Oliveira, A.C.S.; Gazzaneo, I.; Amorim, C.A.; Santos, P.H.B.; Alves, F.R.F. Association between missed canals and apical periodontitis. *Int. Endod. J.* **2019**, *52*, 400–406. [CrossRef]
24. Martins, J.N.R.; Nole, C.; Ounsi, H.F.; Parashos, P.; Plotino, G.; Ragnarsson, M.F.; Aguilar, R.R.; Santiago, F.; Seedat, H.C.; Vargas, W.; et al. Worldwide Assessment of the Mandibular First Molar Second Distal Root and Root Canal: A Cross-sectional Study with Meta-analysis. *J. Endod.* **2022**, *48*, 223–233. [CrossRef]
25. Al-Alawi, H.; Al-Nazhan, S.; Al-Maflehi, N.; Aldosimani, M.A.; Zahid, M.N.; Shihabi, G.N. The prevalence of radix molaris in the mandibular first molars of a Saudi subpopulation based on cone-beam computed tomography. *Restor. Dent. Endod.* **2019**, *45*, e1. [CrossRef] [PubMed]
26. Mashyakhy, M.; Chourasia, H.R.; Halboub, E.; Almashraqi, A.A.; Khubrani, Y.; Gambarini, G. Anatomical variations and bilateral symmetry of roots and root canal system of mandibular first permanent molars in Saudi Arabian population utilizing cone-beam computed tomography. *Saudi Dent. J.* **2019**, *31*, 481–486. [CrossRef]
27. Martins, J.N.; Kishen, A.; Marques, D.; Silva, E.J.N.L.; Carames, J.; Mata, A.; Versiani, M.A. Preferred reporting items for epidemiologic cross-sectional studies on root and root canal anatomy using cone-beam computed tomographic technology: A systematized assessment. *J. Endod.* **2020**, *46*, 915–935. [CrossRef] [PubMed]
28. Naing, L.; Nordin, R.B.; Abdul Rahman, H.; Naing, Y.T. Sample size calculation for prevalence studies using Scalex and ScalaR calculators. *BMC Med. Res. Methodol.* **2022**, *22*, 209. [CrossRef] [PubMed]
29. Bahammam, L.A.; Bahammam, H.A. The incidence of radix entomolaris in mandibular first permanent molars in a Saudi Arabian sub-population. *JKAU Med. Sci.* **2011**, *18*, 83–90. [CrossRef]
30. AAE and AAOMR joint position statement: Use of cone beam computed tomography in endodontics 2015 update. *Oral Surg. Oral Med. Oral Pathol. Oral Radiol.* **2015**, *120*, 508–512. [CrossRef]
31. Gulabivala, K.; Aung, T.H.; Alavi, A.; Ng, Y.L. Root and canal morphology of Burmese mandibular molars. *Int. Endod. J.* **2001**, *34*, 359–370. [CrossRef] [PubMed]
32. Chen, G.; Yao, H.; Tong, C. Investigation of the root canal configuration of mandibular first molars in a Taiwan Chinese population. *Int. Endod. J.* **2009**, *42*, 1044–1049. [CrossRef]
33. Younes, S.A.; al-Shammery, A.R.; el-Angbawi, M.F. Three-rooted permanent mandibular first molars of Asian and black groups in the Middle East. *Oral Surg. Oral Med. Oral Pathol.* **1990**, *69*, 102–105. [CrossRef] [PubMed]
34. Al-Nazhan, S. Incidence of four canals in root-canal-treated mandibular first molars in a Saudi Arabian sub-population. *Int. Endod. J.* **1999**, *32*, 49–52. [CrossRef]
35. Cotton, T.P.; Geisler, T.M.; Holden, D.T.; Schwartz, S.A.; Schindler, W.G. Endodontic applications of cone-beam volumetric tomography. *J. Endod.* **2007**, *33*, 1121–1132. [CrossRef]
36. Neelakantan, P.; Subbarao, C.; Subbarao, C.V. Comparative evaluation of modified canal staining and clearing technique, cone-beam computed tomography, peripheral quantitative computed tomography, spiral computed tomography, and plain and contrast medium-enhanced digital radiography in studying root canal morphology. *J. Endod.* **2010**, *36*, 1547–1551. [PubMed]

37. Wang, Y.; Zheng, Q.H.; Zhou, X.D.; Tang, L.; Wang, Q.; Zheng, G.N.; Huang, D.M. Evaluation of the root and canal morphology of mandibular first permanent molars in a western Chinese population by cone-beam computed tomography. *J. Endod.* **2010**, *36*, 1786–1789. [CrossRef] [PubMed]
38. Zhang, R.; Wang, H.; Tian, Y.Y.; Yu, X.; Hu, T.; Dummer, P.M.H. Use of cone-beam computed tomography to evaluate root and canal morphology of mandibular molars in Chinese individuals. *Int. Endod. J.* **2011**, *44*, 990–999. [CrossRef]
39. Garg, A.K.; Tewari, R.K.; Kumar, A.; Hashmi, S.H.; Agrawal, N.; Mishra, S.K. Prevalence of three-rooted mandibular permanent first molars among the Indian Population. *J. Endod.* **2010**, *36*, 1302–1306. [CrossRef]
40. Sperber, G.H.; Moreau, J.L. Study of the number of roots and canals in Senegalese first permanent mandibular molars. *Int. Endod. J.* **1999**, *31*, 117–122. [CrossRef]
41. Torres, A.; Jacobs, R.; Lambrechts, P.; Brizuela, C.; Cabrera, C.; Concha, G.; Pedemonte, M.E. Characterization of mandibular molar root and canal morphology using cone beam computed tomography and its variability in Belgian and Chilean population samples. *Imaging Sci. Dent.* **2015**, *45*, 95–101. [CrossRef]
42. Hatipoğlu, F.P.; Mağat, G.; Hatipoğlu, Ö.; Al-Khatib, H.; Elatrash, A.S.; Abidin, I.Z.; Kulczyk, T.; Ahmed Mohamed Alkhawas, M.B.; Buchanan, G.D.; Kopbayeva, M.; et al. Assessment of the Prevalence of Radix Entomolaris and Distolingual Canal in Mandibular First Molars in 15 Countries: A Multinational Cross-sectional Study with Meta-analysis. *J. Endod.* **2023**, *49*, 1308–1318. [CrossRef]
43. Gulabivala, K.; Opasanon, A.; Ng, Y.L.; Alavi, A. Root and canal morphology of Thai mandibular molars. *Int. Endod. J.* **2002**, *35*, 56–62. [CrossRef]
44. Tu, M.G.; Tsai, C.C.; Jou, M.J.; Chen, W.L.; Chang, Y.F.; Chen, S.Y.; Cheng, H.W. Prevalence of three-rooted mandibular first molars among Taiwanese individuals. *J. Endod.* **2007**, *33*, 1163–1166. [CrossRef]
45. Loh, H.S. Incidence and features of three-rooted permanent mandibular molars. *Aust. Dent. J.* **1990**, *35*, 434–437. [CrossRef]
46. Curzon, M.E. Three-rooted mandibular permanent molars in English Caucasians. *J. Dent. Res.* **1973**, *52*, 181. [CrossRef]
47. Talabani, R.M.; Abdalrahman, K.O.; Abdul, R.J.; Babarasul, D.O.; Hilmi Kazzaz, S. Evaluation of Radix Entomolaris and Middle Mesial Canal in Mandibular Permanent First Molars in an Iraqi Subpopulation Using Cone-Beam Computed Tomography. *BioMed Res. Int.* **2022**, *2022*, 7825948. [CrossRef]
48. Hosseini, S.; Soleymani, A.; Moudi, E.; Bagheri, T.; Gholinia, H. Frequency of middle mesial canal and radix entomolaris in mandibular first molars by cone beam computed tomography in a selected Iranian population. *Caspian J. Dent. Res.* **2020**, *9*, 63–70.
49. Qiao, X.; Zhu, H.; Yan, Y.; Li, J.; Ren, J.; Gao, Y.; Zou, L. Prevalence of middle mesial canal and radix entomolaris of mandibular first permanent molars in a western Chinese population: An in vivo cone-beam computed tomographic study. *BMC Oral Health* **2020**, *20*, 224. [CrossRef] [PubMed]
50. Chen, Y.C.; Lee, Y.Y.; Pai, S.F.; Yang, S.F. The morphologic characteristics of the distolingual roots of mandibular first molars in a Taiwanese population. *J. Endod.* **2009**, *35*, 643–645. [CrossRef] [PubMed]
51. Ahmed, H.A.; Abu-Bakr, N.H.; Yahia, N.A.; Ibrahim, Y.E. Root and canal morphology of permanent mandibular molars in a Sudanese population. *Int. Endod. J.* **2007**, *40*, 766–771. [CrossRef] [PubMed]
52. Baum, G.; Greenwood, I.; Slawski, S.; Smirnow, R. Observation of internal structures of teeth by ultrasonography. *Science* **1963**, *139*, 495–496. [CrossRef] [PubMed]
53. Marotti, J.; Heger, S.; Tinschert, J.; Tortamano, P.; Chuembou, F.; Radermacher, K.; Wolfart, S. Recent advances of ultrasound imaging in dentistry—A review of the literature. *Oral Surg. Oral Med. Oral Pathol. Oral Radiol.* **2013**, *115*, 819–832. [CrossRef] [PubMed]
54. Arslan, Z.B.; Demir, H.; Berker Yıldız, D.; Yaşar, F. Diagnostic accuracy of panoramic radiography and ultrasonography in detecting periapical lesions using periapical radiography as a gold standard. *Dentomaxillofac. Radiol.* **2020**, *49*, 20190290. [CrossRef] [PubMed]

Disclaimer/Publisher's Note: The statements, opinions and data contained in all publications are solely those of the individual author(s) and contributor(s) and not of MDPI and/or the editor(s). MDPI and/or the editor(s) disclaim responsibility for any injury to people or property resulting from any ideas, methods, instructions or products referred to in the content.

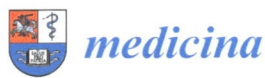 *medicina*

Case Report

Odontoma Recurrence. The Importance of Radiographic Controls: Case Report with a 7-Year Follow-Up

Josefa Alarcón Apablaza [1], Gonzalo Muñoz [1,2], Carlos Arriagada [3], Cristina Bucchi [4,5], Telma S. Masuko [6] and Ramón Fuentes [5,7,*]

1. Doctoral Program in Morphological Sciences, Faculty of Medicine, Universidad de La Frontera, Temuco 4780000, Chile; josefa.alarcon@ufrontera.cl (J.A.A.)
2. Undergraduate Research Group in Dentistry (GIPO), Faculty of Health Sciences, Universidad Autónoma de Chile, Temuco 4780000, Chile
3. Master Program in Dental Sciences, Dental School, Universidad de La Frontera, Temuco 4780000, Chile
4. Oral Biology Research Centre (CIBO-UFRO), Dental School—Facultad de Odontología, Universidad de La Frontera, Temuco 4780000, Chile; cristina.bucchi@ufrontera.cl
5. Department of Integral Adults Dentistry, Dental School, Universidad de La Frontera, Temuco 4780000, Chile
6. Department of Biomorphology, Institute of Health Sciences, Bahia Federal University (ICS-UFBA), Salvador 402331-300, Brazil; tsmasuko@uol.com.br
7. Research Center in Dental Sciences (CICO-UFRO), Dental School—Facultad de Odontología, Universidad de La Frontera, Temuco 4780000, Chile
* Correspondence: ramon.fuentes@ufrontera.cl; Tel.: +56-(452)-325-775

Citation: Alarcón Apablaza, J.; Muñoz, G.; Arriagada, C.; Bucchi, C.; Masuko, T.S.; Fuentes, R. Odontoma Recurrence. The Importance of Radiographic Controls: Case Report with a 7-Year Follow-Up. *Medicina* **2024**, *60*, 1248. https://doi.org/10.3390/medicina60081248

Academic Editors: Silvia Angeletti, Romica Cergan, Adrian Costache and Mihai Dumitru

Received: 27 June 2024
Revised: 26 July 2024
Accepted: 29 July 2024
Published: 31 July 2024

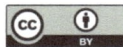

Copyright: © 2024 by the authors. Licensee MDPI, Basel, Switzerland. This article is an open access article distributed under the terms and conditions of the Creative Commons Attribution (CC BY) license (https://creativecommons.org/licenses/by/4.0/).

Abstract: Odontomas are benign tumors characterized by slow and limited growth with a rare recurrence. Odontomas are generally detected by radiographic findings in the radiopaque stage, where calcification of the tissues is observed. This article seeks to report the recurrence of a radiologically diagnosed odontoma to show the importance of radiographic controls after enucleation as a diagnostic and follow-up method. Case report: A female patient, 9 years old, attended dental care in 2020 due to malpositioned teeth. In the intraoral clinical examination, she presented stage II mixed dentition with crowding. A radiographic exam showed no associated lesions. The patient reported a history of odontoma removal and a supernumerary tooth in sextant II in 2016. Subsequently, she was referred to orthodontics, where permanent dentition with moderate anterior crowding in the maxilla and mandible was observed. The radiographic examination showed a radiopaque area compatible with odontoma, palatal to teeth 12 and 13. Conclusions: Although recurrence is rare, complete removal in the case of an odontoma is critical. This study demonstrates the importance of performing radiographic controls 5 years after enucleation of an odontoma, considering the stages of evolution.

Keywords: diagnostics; odontoma; recurrence; recidivism; complications; tomography; imaging

1. Introduction

Odontogenic tumors constitute about 3% of oral lesions [1]. Among these, odontomas are the most frequent, accounting for 22% [2,3]. The term "odontoma" was introduced by Pierre Paul Broca in 1867, referring to any tumor formed by transient or complete overgrowth of dental tissues [4]. Odontomas are classified as odontogenic tumors; however, due to their slow and limited growth, they are considered hamartomas [5–8]. They originate from an alteration of differentiated epithelial and mesenchymal odontogenic cells that can form enamel, dentin, and cementum [5,6,9]. Trauma during primary dentition, genetic factors, cell rests of Serres, and genetic mutations are accepted as possible etiological factors. Odontomas have also been associated with pathological conditions, inflammatory processes, and/or infections [4].

The World Health Organization classifies odontomas according to the degree of differentiation as (1) compound odontomas and (2) complex odontomas. The former are approximately twice as common as complex odontomas [5]. The compound odontoma is usually located in the anterior maxilla and appears radiographically as small, multiple, irregular, radiopaque, tooth-like denticles in the center of a radiolucent lesion. They consist of enamel, dentin, cementum, and pulp tissue [4,6]. The complex odontoma is usually found in the posterior mandibular region as an amorphous calcification of dental tissues arranged in an irregular pattern, with no resemblance to a tooth structure, surrounded by a thin radiolucent demarcation line [4,6,8].

The odontoma goes through stages similar to developing teeth. In the early stages, odontomas may appear radiolucent. This is due to less dense tissue, such as pulp, and areas of non-mineralized tissue. This is followed by an intermediate stage, characterized by partial calcification of the odontogenic tissues, producing a radiolucent–radiopaque picture. Finally, the most radiopaque stage is reached, in which the calcification of the dental tissues is complete. Odontoma formation begins during infancy, coinciding with the development of the natural dentition [5,10,11].

Most odontomas are asymptomatic, although there are occasionally signs and symptoms related to their presence [4]. The most frequent reason for a consultation of a patient with an odontoma is delayed tooth eruption. However, odontomas are frequently detected during routine radiographic examinations [12].

Recurrence of odontomas is very rare [5,13–16]. It is generally not recommended to perform surgical procedures for enucleation before the age of 5, due to several factors. One of the main reasons is the risk of enucleating permanent dental follicles, which could affect the normal development of permanent teeth that have not yet erupted [17,18]. Furthermore, there is an increased risk of recurrence from these tissues following surgery [13]. This is because odontomas can be closely associated with surrounding tissues, and surgery on a developing bone structure can be more complicated, increasing the likelihood that remnants of the odontoma will remain. It is very important to remove the surrounding capsule, as any remnants can increase the risk of lesion recurrence [5,13]. However, complete removal of the lesion is difficult in the early stages of development, due to odontomas being characterized by the presence of non-calcified cellular portions [13]. In light of the above, this article aims to document the recurrence of a radiologically diagnosed odontoma, to highlight the importance of radiographic controls after enucleation as a diagnostic and follow-up method.

2. Case Report

The case presentation is documented chronologically. Authorization to publish the case was obtained, with informed consent from the mother and the patient.

In 2020, a 9-year-old female patient attended dental care. The reason for consultation was tooth malpositioning. There was no indication of systemic disease or medication in the medical history. The patient reported the surgical removal of an odontoma and supernumerary in the anterosuperior sector in 2016, diagnosed radiographically (Figure 1).

The maxillary cone-beam computed tomography (CBCT) exam performed in 2016, prior to the first surgery, detected a mesiodens in an intraosseous formation, in vestibular relation to teeth 11 and 21, distoangular, with the crown in the apical position and the root in the coronal zone. In addition, multiple radiopaque masses with irregular margins compatible with an odontoma were observed in the palatal area about teeth 11, 12, and 13 (Figure 1). The odontoma and mesiodens were surgically removed in the same year as their diagnosis.

In the intraoral clinical examination performed in 2020, four years after the first surgery to remove the odontoma and mesiodens, the patient presented stage II mixed dentition with a normal eruption time and chronology. Rotation was noted in teeth 11 and 12. The panoramic X-ray (Figure 2) showed a lack of radiographic space for correct positioning of teeth 13, 33, and 43 in the dental arch, rotation of teeth 11 and 12, total root resorption of teeth 55, 65, 75, and 84, almost total root resorption in tooth 85, intraosseous evolution of teeth 17, 27, 35, 37, 45, and 47, and extraosseous evolution of teeth 13, 15, 23, 25, 33, 34, 43, and 44.

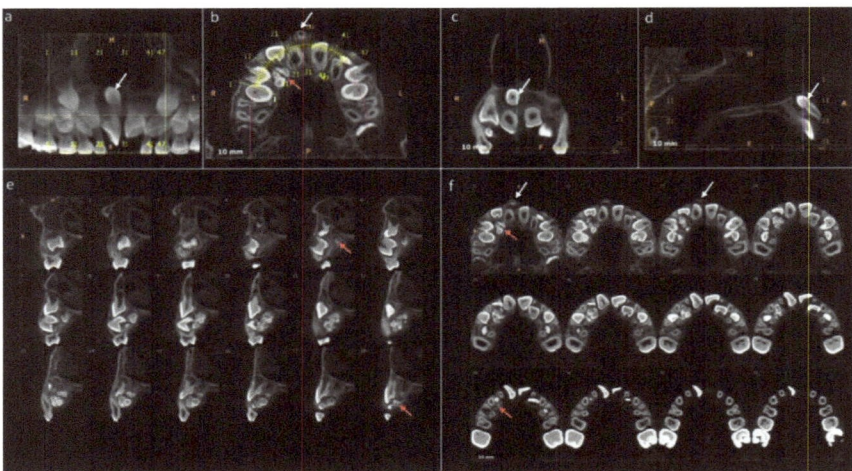

Figure 1. Cone-beam computed tomography (CBCT) of the maxilla. 2016, 6 years old, prior to first surgery. (**a**) The panoramic reconstruction shows the presence of a mesiodens supernumerary tooth between 11 and 21. (**b**) Axial section. Location of mesiodens vestibular to teeth 11 and 21. Presence of multiple denticles compatible with odontoma, in intraosseous evolution, distal to tooth 11, and palatal to teeth 12 and 13. (**c**) Coronal section. Presence of mesiodens in relation to teeth 11 and 21, surrounded by a radiolucent demarcation area. (**d**) Sagittal section. Presence of supernumerary, crown in apical position and root in coronal area. Presence of pericoronary sac. (**e**) Sagittal section. Presence of multiple radiopaque masses with irregular margins compatible with odontoma (Sections 5–18) in intraosseous evolution palatal to tooth 13. (**f**) Axial section. Presence of mesiodens (Sections 21–23) in vestibular relation to teeth 11 and 21. Presence of radiopaque masses compatible with odontoma (Sections 21–29) distal to tooth 11 and palatal to teeth 12 and 13. White arrow = mesiodens. Red arrow = odontoma.

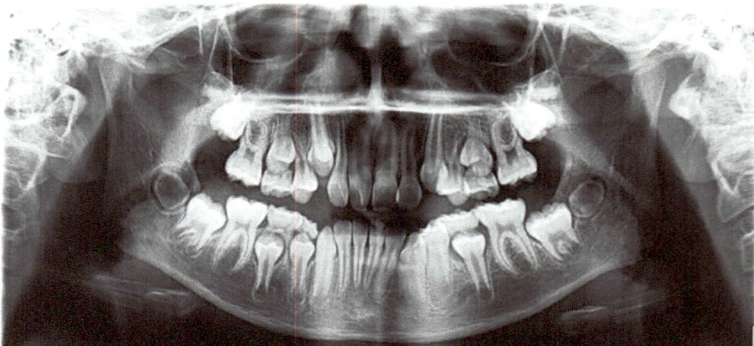

Figure 2. Panoramic X-ray. 2020, four years after the first surgery. Maxillary sinuses of ample development, shape, contour, and characteristic transparency. Stage II mixed dentition. 13, 43, and 33 lack radiographic space for a correct position in the dental arch. Third molars in intraosseous evolution.

Due to health contingencies around the SARS-CoV-2 virus, the patient postponed orthodontic treatment until 2021.

The patient attended dental care in February 2021 for corrective orthodontic treatment. Extraoral examination showed vertical and horizontal symmetry within normal parameters, lips together in the resting position, normal nasolabial and mentolabial angles, and slight lip protrusion. Intraoral examination showed permanent dentition with moderate crowding in the anterior region of the maxilla and mandible (Figure 3).

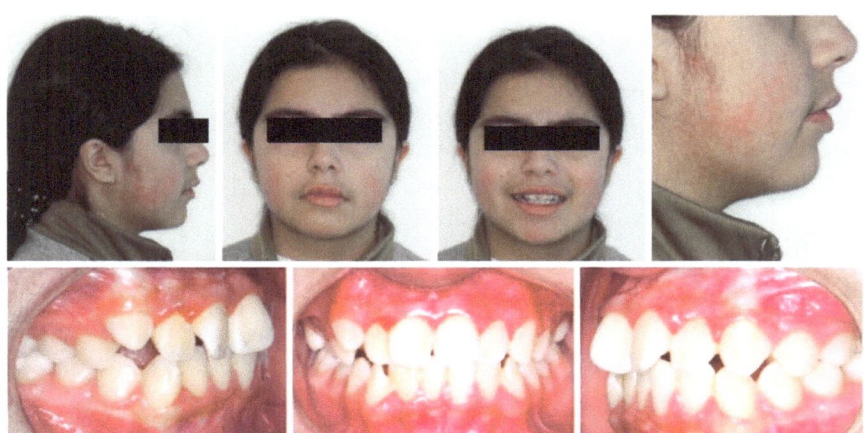

Figure 3. Extraoral and intraoral photographs for diagnosis and corrective orthodontic treatment planning.

A radiopaque element with a denticle form of intraosseous evolution was observed in the radiographic update of the diagnostic studies carried out to begin the orthodontic treatment examination, performed five years after the first surgery to remove the odontoma and mesiodens (Figure 4). CBCT was requested to confirm the finding and plan the surgical removal. A radiopaque area compatible with an odontoma was observed in relation to teeth 12 and 13 in a marked mesioangular position, microdontic, located palatal to the roots of the neighboring teeth, and in intraosseous evolution (Figure 5). The odontoma was surgically removed.

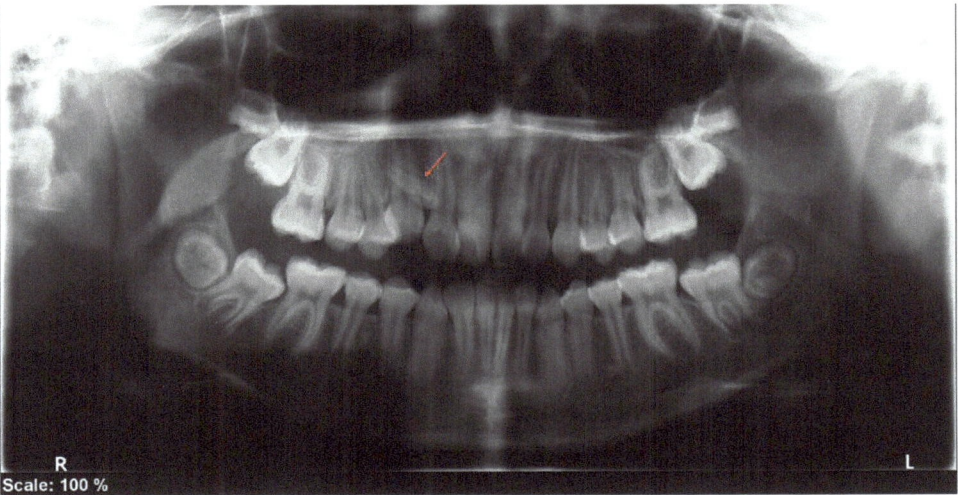

Figure 4. Panoramic X-ray. 2021, five years after the first surgery. Presence of a radiopaque element with a denticle shape in relation to teeth 12 and 13. Red arrow = odontoma.

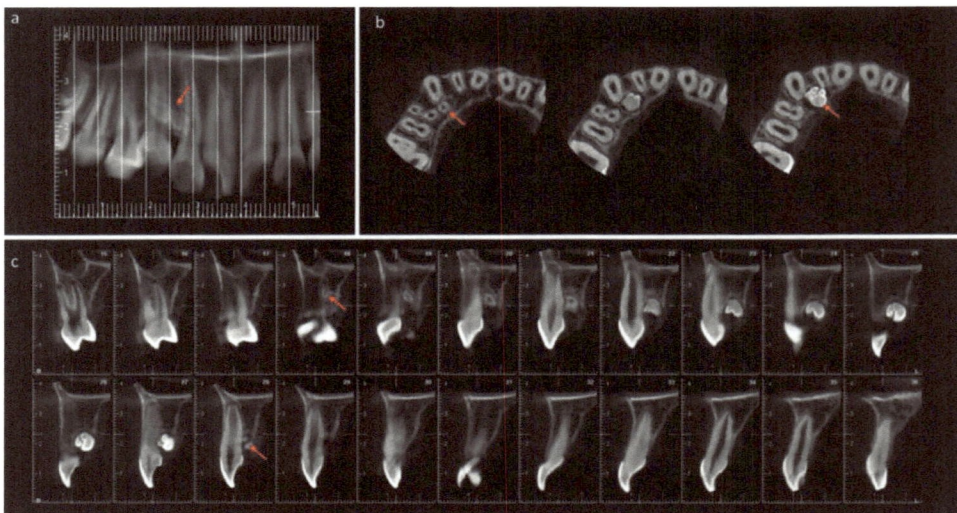

Figure 5. Cone-beam computed tomography (CBCT) of the maxilla. 2021, five years after the first surgery. (**a**) Panorex section. Presence of a radiopaque area, compatible with odontoma, overprojected to teeth 12 and 13, mesioangular. (**b**) Axial section. Multilobulated odontoma, located palatal to teeth 12 and 13, surrounded by a radiolucent demarcation line. Discrete external resorption in the cervical third of the palatal root of tooth 13. (**c**) Cross-section. Presence of odontoma (Sections 18–28) in intraosseous evolution, microdontic, mesioangular, coronal structural alteration. Palatally displaced tooth location with thinning and perforation of palatal bone cortex. The crown is located palatally and in contact with the cervical third palatal root of tooth 12 and the cervical and middle third palatal root of tooth 13. Root location is palatally displaced. Root middle third in contact with palatal root middle third of tooth 13. Pericoronary sac and periodontal ligament space of preserved thickness (scale 100%). Red arrow = odontoma.

Twenty-four months after surgical removal of the odontoma recurrence, a radiographic control was performed, where no apparent recurrence was observed (Figure 6).

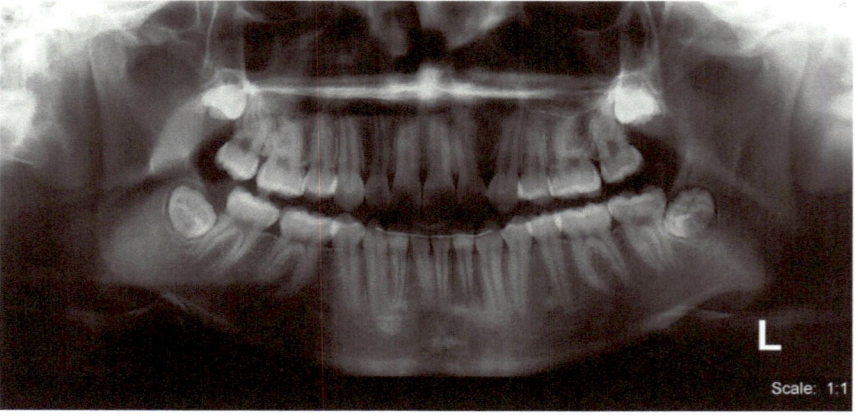

Figure 6. Panoramic X-ray. 2023, 24 months after the second surgical removal. Permanent dentition. Third molars in intraosseous evolution. Anterior mandibular splinting.

3. Literature Review

3.1. Systematic Literature Search

A review was performed on odontoma recurrence. Our review was performed according to the Preferred Reporting Items for Systematic Reviews and Meta-Analyses extension for Scoping Reviews (PRISMA-ScR) guidelines [19].

An electronic search was conducted in three digital databases (PubMed, SCOPUS, and Web of Science). The search was performed between January and March 2024. The bibliographies of potentially eligible clinical trials, case reports, case studies, and systematic reviews were also screened for additional studies that were possibly fit for inclusion. The following search equation was used in PubMed:

("Odontoma" [MeSH Terms] OR ("Odontoma" [MeSH Terms] OR "Odontoma" [All Fields] OR "odontomas" [All Fields]) OR "odontoma compound" [All Fields] OR "odontomas compound" [All Fields] OR ("tooth abnormalities" [MeSH Terms] OR ("tooth" [All Fields] AND "abnormalities"[All Fields]) OR "tooth abnormalities" [All Fields] OR "odontome" [All Fields] OR "odontomes" [All Fields]) OR "odontome*" [All Fields]) AND ("Recurrence" [MeSH Terms] OR "neoplasm recurrence, local" [MeSH Terms] OR ("reappear" [All Fields] OR "reappearance" [All Fields] OR "reappearances" [All Fields] OR "reappeared" [All Fields] OR "reappearing" [All Fields] OR "reappears" [All Fields]) OR ("recurrance" [All Fields] OR "Recurrence" [MeSH Terms] OR "Recurrence" [All Fields] OR "recurrences" [All Fields] OR "recurrencies" [All Fields] OR "recurrency" [All Fields] OR "recurrent" [All Fields] OR "recurrently" [All Fields] OR "recurrents" [All Fields]) OR ("recrudesce" [All Fields] OR "recrudesced" [All Fields] OR "recrudescent" [All Fields] OR "recrudescing" [All Fields] OR "Recurrence" [MeSH Terms] OR "Recurrence"[All Fields] OR "recrudescence" [All Fields] OR "recrudescences" [All Fields]) OR ("recrudesce" [All Fields] OR "recrudesced" [All Fields] OR "recrudescent" [All Fields] OR "recrudescing" [All Fields] OR "Recurrence" [MeSH Terms] OR "Recurrence" [All Fields] OR "recrudescence" [All Fields] OR "recrudescences" [All Fields])).

3.2. Eligibility Criteria

Observational (case reports and case series) and experimental (randomized and controlled clinical trials) studies were included where they reported odontoma recurrence. The potentially eligible articles were screened based on the inclusion criteria: studies in English or Spanish and a full text with no publication date limit. A summary of the inclusion and exclusion criteria considered in this review is given in Table 1.

Table 1. Inclusion and exclusion criteria of the scoping review.

Inclusion Criteria	Exclusion Criteria
Observational and experimental studies	Systematic literature reviews or letters to the editor
Studies that report odontoma recurrence	Studies that report only the characteristics, diagnosis, or treatment of odontoma
English or Spanish language, and full text with no publication date limit	Studies reporting another tumor

3.3. Article Selection and Data Extraction

Two independent reviewers analyzed articles obtained in the systematic search process by reviewing the titles and abstracts. The articles that met the eligibility criteria were then analyzed in their full text to confirm their relevance.

The article search and selection process is summarized in Figure 7. The total number of articles found in the databases was 502, and 1 was identified from the manual search, of which 12 were duplicates. After the initial reading by title, 223 were discarded, of which 112 were studies that reported only the characteristics, diagnosis, treatment, or surgical management of odontoma, 64 articles studied other tumors, 37 were not related to the subject under study, and 10 were systematic reviews. Subsequently, 157 studies were discarded due to the abstract, of which 76 were studies that reported only the characteristics, diagnosis, treatment, or surgical management of odontoma, 68 were not related to the subject under study, and 13 were systematic reviews. After reading the full-text articles (111 articles), 108 were excluded, of which 68 were studies that reported only the characteristics and surgical management of odontoma, 21 reported other tumors, and 19 were systematic reviews. Finally, in this review, 3 articles corresponding to observational and experimental studies that reported odontoma recurrence were included [3,7,20].

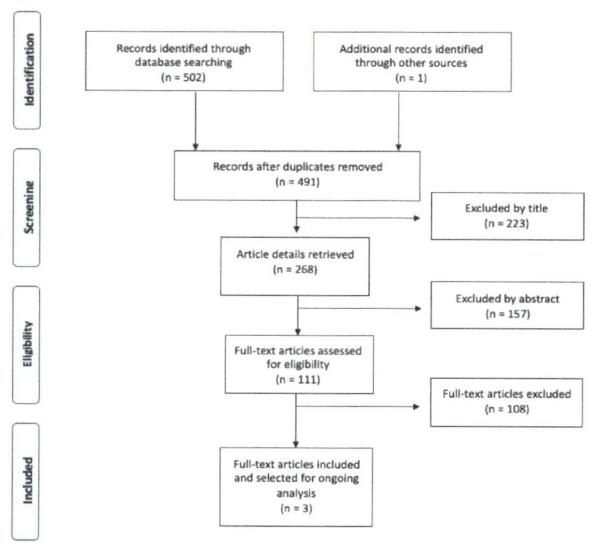

Figure 7. Flow chart for study selection.

The data were extracted from the reports of the selected cases, and information considered relevant for the analysis is shown in Table 2.

Table 2. Case reports of odontoma recurrence reported in the literature.

Study	Type of Study	Tooth Involved	Age of First Enucleation	Age of Recurrence	Diagnosis of Recurrence	Complications
Boffano, P., 2022 [3]	Multicenter study with 4 recurrences in 127 patients	Not reported	22 years on average	Not reported	Odontoma	Not reported
Tomizawa, M., 2005 [7]	Case report in 1 subject	Left maxillary primary central incisor	1 year and 8 months	6 years and 5 months	Odontoma	Delayed eruption
Matsuo, K., 2013 [20]	Case report	Second deciduous molar	3 years	7 years	Ossifying fibroma	Delayed eruption

4. Discussion

This case report describes the recurrence of a radiologically diagnosed odontoma to highlight the importance of radiographic controls after enucleation as a method of diagnosis and follow-up. Nonetheless, although the radiological approach provides valuable diagnostic information, we recognize that histopathological analysis remains the gold standard to confirm the diagnosis and ensure appropriate treatment. Omitting histopathological analysis could have significant implications, including the possibility of residual diagnostic uncertainty and the risk of not detecting other potential pathologies. To mitigate these consequences, we consider it crucial to extend the patient's follow-up time. This measure will allow continued surveillance for any possible recurrence or complications that may arise.

Conventional X-rays, such as periapical and panoramic, are often considered the gold standard in detecting and evaluating odontomas. However, CBCT is a valuable tool for ascertaining the precise location of the odontoma with respect to adjacent teeth [13,21]. Following diagnosis and localization, the treatment of choice for odontomas is surgical removal. However, special care must be taken to remove it completely to avoid recurrence [4]. Although the odontoma is a common odontogenic tumor [1], its recurrence is rare [2,3]. Only three studies were found reporting odontoma recurrence [3,7,20].

The main possibilities for recurrence are an odontoma and secondary ossifying fibroma (OF) [20]. Radiographic differentiation between an odontoma and an ossifying fibroma is crucial for the diagnosis of these lesions. Odontomas are typically radiopaque, appearing as white areas on radiographs due to their enamel and dentin content. They may show a "tooth" appearance within a mass, especially in compound odontomas, whereas complex odontomas are disorganized masses of dental tissues [4,6]. In addition, odontomas often have a well-defined halo and may be surrounded by a radiolucent capsule, indicating the presence of soft fibrous tissue around the tumor. Radiographically, a compound odontoma appears as a mixed image (radiopaque and radiolucent), which adopts a configuration of multiple clearly distinguished denticles surrounded by a radiolucent halo; and complex odontomas appear as one or multiple radiopaque masses surrounded by a radiolucent halo [4,6,22,23]. In contrast, the density of the FO mass is even; it can vary from radiolucency to a mixture of radiolucency and radiodensity, due to the presence of fibrous tissue and calcifications [24–26]. The boundary between the lesion and the surrounding bone is not clearly discernible [27]. Unlike odontomas, FO has a lytic appearance, compromising the bone and causing bone expansion. It is also common to observe root resorption and displacement of involved teeth. FO can be unilocular or multilocular [24–26]. These distinctive radiographic features allowed us to differentiate that the recurrence in this case was an odontoma, although histopathological analysis remains the gold standard to confirm the diagnosis and ensure adequate treatment

Recurrence occurs when resection is performed at the noncalcified stage of the lesion or if the resection is incomplete [3,28]. In the present report, radiographic images performed in 2016 indicated that the odontoma was in an advanced developmental stage of mineralization, as a radiopaque stage was observed, with multiple denticles. Therefore, the recurrence must have been due to a residual mass in the first enucleation [3,28] or the presence of the capsule surrounding it [5,13]. In the radiological analysis performed 4 years after the enucleation, the odontoma was at an early stage of development and was not calcified. Radiolucency makes it difficult to visualize a lesion [7], which can cause the undiagnosed recurrence of an odontoma. Here, at one year, the radiolucent lesion had progressed to a radiopaque mineralized stage, which made the recurrence diagnosis possible 5 years after enucleation of the odontoma, similar to the follow-up time of recurrences reported in the literature [3,7,20].

The follow-up time after enucleation of an odontoma is an important factor to consider. Several studies report no recurrence; however, they do not exceed 3 years of follow-up after surgical removal [2,17,29–38]. It is important to consider the stages of evolution of odontoma since, in the early stages of development, it is very difficult to diagnose [39]. In the cases reported in the literature, most odontomas appeared as well-calcified masses on the X-rays [4]. However, some cases were not diagnosed in the first radiographic examination [7]. In a retrospective study of X-rays taken at different times, Tomiwasa et al., 2005, revealed that calcification was still immature in the early stages of odontoma development with a radiolucent image being observed, making it very difficult to diagnose. This becomes very important since it is clear that, from the earliest stages, an odontoma may disturb tooth eruption and lead to complications [7].

Various complications have been reported for odontomas, such as displacement of teeth surrounding the odontoma, delayed eruption of permanent teeth [3], diastemas, displacement, rotation, crowding, rhyzolisis, periodontal lesions, or even pulp necrosis of adjacent teeth [40,41]. Therefore, although recurrence of an odontoma is very rare, it can lead to complications if not diagnosed promptly [7,41]. In the present case, due to the radiographic control, a timely diagnosis of recurrence could be made, and complications were avoided.

Early detection of an odontoma is more likely to be a radiological finding, so the need for routine radiographic analysis should be emphasized. Odontomas have been reported to have limited growth potential and a slow-growing clinical course [41]. Hence, based on the evolution time of the reported case and what is reported in the literature, a time of 5 years after enucleation of the odontoma is suggested.

This study has certain limitations. It is predicated on the presentation of a single case report, and more cases should be evaluated to draw more significant conclusions regarding the control period after odontoma removal. However, the rarity of odontoma recurrence makes obtaining larger samples difficult. Therefore, this case report provides a basis for establishing an appropriate follow-up period. It is also important to note that the diagnosis of odontomas in this study was mainly based on radiographic interpretation, which could limit the accuracy of the diagnosis compared to histological analysis. Although X-rays are a useful tool in the initial detection of odontomas, it is recognized that definitive diagnosis should ideally be confirmed by histological analysis for a more complete and accurate characterization of the lesion.

5. Conclusions

Here, the complex analysis and follow-up made it possible to confirm the recurrence of the odontoma by radiographic diagnosis. Surgical treatment obtained a satisfactory result in the medium and long term, confirmed by the periodic radiographic reevaluation protocol, which was established using a correct initial diagnosis and following the suggestions proposed in the literature.

This study guides dentists to perform radiographic controls 5 years after enucleation of an odontoma, considering the stages of evolution. This will allow for an early diagnosis in patients who do not report clinical signs or symptoms, avoid complications, and enable treatment planning according to the location and associated anatomical structures of each case.

Author Contributions: Conceptualization, J.A.A. and R.F.; methodology, J.A.A., G.M., and C.A.; validation, J.A.A. and G.M.; formal analysis, J.A.A., C.A., and G.M.; investigation, J.A.A., C.A., G.M., G.M., and R.F.; writing—original draft preparation, J.A.A., C.A., R.F., C.B., and G.M.; writing—review and editing, J.A.A., C.A., G.M., C.B., T.S.M., and R.F.; visualization, J.A.A., C.A., and G.M.; supervision, R.F. All authors have read and agreed to the published version of the manuscript.

Funding: This work was funded (partially) by the Research Department, Universidad de La Frontera, Project PP23-0008.

Institutional Review Board Statement: Not applicable.

Informed Consent Statement: Informed consent was obtained from the patient involved in this case report.

Data Availability Statement: Data is contained within the article.

Conflicts of Interest: The authors declare no conflicts of interest.

References

1. Sekerci, A.E.; Nazlim, S.; Etoz, M.; Deniz, K.; Yasa, Y. Odontogenic tumors: A collaborative study of 218 cases diagnosed over 12 years and comprehensive review of the literature. *Med. Oral. Patol. Oral. Cir. Bucal.* **2015**, *20*, e34–e44. [CrossRef] [PubMed]
2. Maltagliati, A.; Ugolini, A.; Crippa, R.; Farronato, M.; Paglia, M.; Blasi, S.; Angiero, F. Complex odontoma at the upper right maxilla: Surgical management and histomorphological profile. *Eur. J. Paediatr. Dent.* **2020**, *21*, 199–202. [CrossRef] [PubMed]
3. Boffano, P.; Cavarra, F.; Brucoli, M.; Ruslin, M.; Forouzanfar, T.; Ridwan-Pramana, A.; Rodríguez-Santamarta, T.; de Vicente, J.C.; Starch-Jensen, T.; Pechalova, P.; et al. The epidemiology and management of odontomas: A European multicenter study. *Oral. Maxillofac. Surg.* **2023**, *27*, 479–487. [CrossRef]
4. Satish, V.; Prabhadevi, M.C.; Sharma, R. Odontome: A brief overview. *Int. J. Clin. Pediatr. Dent.* **2011**, *4*, 177–185. [CrossRef] [PubMed]

5. Barba, L.T.; Campos, D.M.; Rascón, M.M.N.; Barrera, V.A.R.; Rascón, A.N. Aspectos descriptivos del odontoma: Revisión de la literatura. *Rev. Odont. Mex.* **2016**, *20*, 272–276. [CrossRef]
6. Marimuthu, M.; Prabhu, A.R.; Kalyani, P.; Murali, S.; Senthilnathan, P.; Ramani, P. Complex-compound Odontome with 526 Denticles: A Unique Case Report. *Int. J. Clin. Pediatr. Dent.* **2022**, *15*, 789–792. [CrossRef]
7. Tomizawa, M.; Otsuka, Y.; Noda, T. Clinical observations of odontomas in Japanese children: 39 cases including one recurrent case. *Int. J. Paediatr. Dent.* **2005**, *15*, 37–43. [CrossRef]
8. Wang, X.P.; Fan, J. Molecular genetics of supernumerary tooth formation. *Genesis* **2011**, *49*, 261–277. [CrossRef]
9. Mendez, G.I.; Di Bella, A.R.; Di Pascuale, S.; Schröh, C.; Masotto, A. Unusual mandibular odontoma and its resolution. Case report. *Rev. Asoc. Odontol. Argent.* **2022**, *110*, 5. [CrossRef]
10. Wood, N.K.; Goaz, P.W. *Diagnóstico Diferencial de las Lesiones Orales y Maxilofaciales*, 5th ed.; Harcourt Brace: Madrid, Spain, 1998.
11. Soluk Tekkesin, M.; Pehlivan, S.; Olgac, V.; Aksakallı, N.; Alatli, C. Clinical and histopathological investigation of odontomas: Review of the literature and presentation of 160 cases. *J. Oral. Maxillofac. Surg.* **2012**, *70*, 1358–1361. [CrossRef]
12. Falkinhoff, P.E.; García Reig, E.L. The odontomas and their implications. *Rev. Asoc. Odontol.* **2019**, *107*, 19–24. Available online: https://raoa.aoa.org.ar/revistas/?roi=1071000025 (accessed on 2 May 2024).
13. Harris Ricardo, J.; Rebolledo Cobos, M.; Díaz Caballero, A.; Carbonell Muñoz, Z. Odontoma case series. Review of literature. *Av. Odontoestomatol.* **2011**, *27*, 25–32. Available online: https://scielo.isciii.es/scielo.php?script=sci_arttext&pid=S0213-12852011000100003 (accessed on 2 May 2024). [CrossRef]
14. Waldron, A.C. Quistes y tumores odontogénicos. In *Patología Oral y Maxilofacial*, 2nd ed.; Neville, B., Ed.; WB Saunders: Filadelfia, PA, USA, 2002; pp. 631–632.
15. Mazur, M.; Di Giorgio, G.; Ndokaj, A.; Jedliński, M.; Corridore, D.; Marasca, B.; Salucci, A.; Polimeni, A.; Ottolenghi, L.; Bossù, M.; et al. Characteristics, Diagnosis and treatment of compound odontoma associated with impacted teeth. *Children* **2022**, *9*, 1509. [CrossRef] [PubMed]
16. Gervasoni, C.; Tronchet, A.; Spotti, S.; Valsecchi, S.; Palazzolo, V.; Riccio, S.; D Aiuto, A.; Azzi, L.; Di Francesco, A. Odontomas: Review of the literature and case reports. *J. Biol. Regul. Homeost. Agents.* **2017**, *31*, 119–125. [PubMed]
17. Caeiro-Villasenín, L.; Serna-Muñoz, C.; Pérez-Silva, A.; Vicente-Hernández, A.; Poza-Pascual, A.; Ortiz-Ruiz, A.J. Developmental dental defects in permanent teeth resulting from trauma in primary dentition: A systematic review. *Int. J. Environ. Res. Public. Health* **2022**, *19*, 754. [CrossRef]
18. Cahill, D.R.; Marks, S.C., Jr. Tooth eruption: Evidence for the central role of the dental follicle. *J. Oral. Pathol.* **1980**, *9*, 189–200. [CrossRef] [PubMed]
19. Page, M.J.; McKenzie, J.E.; Bossuyt, P.M.; Boutron, I.; Hoffmann, T.C.; Mulrow, C.D.; Shamseer, L.; Tetzlaff, J.M.; Akl, E.A.; Brennan; et al. The PRISMA 2020 statement: An updated guideline for reporting systematic reviews. *BMJ* **2021**, *372*, n71. [CrossRef] [PubMed]
20. Matsuo, K.; Yamamoto, N.; Morimoto, Y.; Yamashita, Y.; Zhang, M.; Ishikawa, A.; Tanaka, T.; Kito, S.; Takahashi, T. Multiple complex odontomas and subsequent occurrence of an ossifying fibroma at the same site as the removed odontoma. *J. Dent. Sci.* **2013**, *8*, 189–195. [CrossRef]
21. da Silva Rocha, O.K.M.; da Silva Barros, C.C.; da Silva, L.A.B.; de Souza Júnior, E.F.; de Morais, H.H.A.; da Costa Miguel, M.C. Peripheral compound odontoma: A rare case report and literature review. *J. Cutan. Pathol.* **2020**, *47*, 720–724. [CrossRef]
22. Martinovic-Guzmán, G.; Santorcuato-Cubillos, B.; Alister-Herdener, J.P.; Plaza-Álvarez, C.; Raffo-Solari, J. Composite Odontoma: Diagnosis and Treatment Case Report & Literature Review. *Int. J. Odontostom* **2017**, *11*, 425–430.
23. Vázquez Diego, J.; Gandini Pablo, C.; Carbajal Eduardo, E. Compound odontoma: Radiographic diagnosis and surgical treatment of a clinical case. *Av. Odontoestomatol.* **2008**, *24*, 307–312. Available online: http://scielo.isciii.es/scielo.php?script=sci_arttext&pid=S0213-12852008000500002 (accessed on 2 May 2024).
24. Kadlub, N.; Kreindel, T.; Belle Mbou, V.; Coudert, A.; Ansari, E.; Descroix, V.; Ruhin-Poncet, B.; Coulomb L'hermine, A.; Berdal, A.; Vazquez, M.P.; et al. Specificity of paediatric jawbone lesions: Tumours and pseudotumours. *J. Craniomaxillofac Surg.* **2014**, *42*, 125–131. [CrossRef]
25. El-Mofty, S. Psammomatoid and trabecular juvenile ossifying fibroma of the craniofacial skeleton: Two distinct clinicopathologic entities. *Oral. Surg. Oral. Med. Oral. Pathol. Oral. Radiol. Endod.* **2002**, *93*, 296–304. [CrossRef]
26. Chrcanovic, B.R.; López Alvarenga, R.; Horta, M.C.R.; Freire-Maia, B.; Souza, L.N. Central ossifying fibroma in the maxilla: A case report and review of the literature. *Av. Odontoestomatol.* **2011**, *27*, 33–39. Available online: https://scielo.isciii.es/scielo.php?script=sci_serial&pid=0213-1285&lng=es&nrm=iso (accessed on 2 May 2024). [CrossRef]
27. Lina, Z.; Ting, S.; Haoman, N.; Ning, G.; Yaling, T.; Yu, C. Mandibular ossifying fibroma and compound odontoma: A case report. *Huaxikouqiangyixuezazhi* **2016**, *34*, 100–103. [CrossRef]
28. Amado Cuesta, S.; Gargallo Albiol, J.; Berini Aytés, L.; Gay Escoda, C. Review of 61 cases of odontoma. Presentation of an erupted complex odontoma. *Med. Oral.* **2003**, *8*, 366–373.
29. Khalifa, C.; Omami, M.; Garma, M.; Slim, A.; Sioud, S.; Selmi, J. Compound-complex odontoma: A rare case report. *Clin. Case. Rep.* **2022**, *10*, e05658. [CrossRef]
30. Chang, J.Y.; Wang, J.T.; Wang, Y.P.; Liu, B.Y.; Sun, A.; Chiang, C.P. Odontoma: A clinicopathologic study of 81 cases. *J. Formos. Med. Assoc.* **2003**, *102*, 876–882.

31. Kim, K.S.; Lee, H.G.; Hwang, J.H.; Lee, S.Y. Incidentally detected odontoma within a dentigerous cyst. *Arch. Craniofac Surg.* **2019**, *20*, 62–65. [CrossRef] [PubMed]
32. Soliman, N.; Al-Khanati, N.M.; Alkhen, M. Rare giant complex composite odontoma of mandible in mixed dentition: Case report with 3-year follow-up and literature review. *Ann. Med. Surg.* **2022**, *74*, 103355. [CrossRef] [PubMed]
33. Manfredini, M.; Ferrario, S.; Creminelli, L.; Kuhn, E.; Poli, P.P. Compound odontoma associated with dentigerous cyst incidentally detected in an adult patient: Tomography and histological features. *Case Rep. Dent.* **2022**, *2022*, 6210289. [CrossRef]
34. Neumann, B.L.; Só, B.B.; Santos, L.G.; Silveira, F.M.; Wagner, V.P.; Vargas, P.A.; Dos Santos, J.N.; Mosqueda-Taylor, A.; Fonseca, F.P.; Schuch, L.F.; et al. Synchronous odontogenic tumors: A systematic review. *Oral. Dis.* **2023**, *29*, 2493–2500. [CrossRef]
35. Das, U.M.; Viswanath, D.; Azher, U. A compound composite odontoma associated with unerupted permanent incisor: A case report. *Int. J. Clin. Pediatr. Dent.* **2009**, *2*, 50–55. [CrossRef]
36. Hamada, M.; Okawa, R.; Nishiyama, K.; Nomura, R.; Uzawa, N.; Nakano, K. Compound odontoma removed by endoscopic intraoral approach: Case report. *Dent. J.* **2021**, *9*, 81. [CrossRef]
37. Ćabov, T.; Fuchs, P.N.; Zulijani, A.; Ćabov Ercegović, L.; Marelić, S. Odontomas: Pediatric case report and review of the literature. *Acta Clin. Croat.* **2021**, *60*, 146–152. [CrossRef]
38. Kalra, A.; Pajpani, M.; Webb, R. Ameloblastic Fibro-Odontoma. *J. Dent. Child.* **2018**, *85*, 143–146.
39. Sun, L.; Sun, Z.; Ma, X. Multiple complex odontoma of the maxilla and the mandible. *Oral. Surg. Oral. Med. Oral. Pathol. Oral. Radiol.* **2015**, *120*, e11–e16. [CrossRef]
40. Yassin, O.M.; Hamori, E. Characteristics, clinical features and treatment of supernumerary teeth. *J. Clin. Pediatr. Dent.* **2009**, *33*, 247–250. [CrossRef] [PubMed]
41. Hisatomi, M.; Asaumi, J.I.; Konouchi, H.; Honda, Y.; Wakasa, T.; Kishi, K. A case of complex odontoma associated with an impacted lower deciduous second molar and analysis of the 107 odontomas. *Oral. Dis.* **2002**, *8*, 100–105. [CrossRef] [PubMed]

Disclaimer/Publisher's Note: The statements, opinions and data contained in all publications are solely those of the individual author(s) and contributor(s) and not of MDPI and/or the editor(s). MDPI and/or the editor(s) disclaim responsibility for any injury to people or property resulting from any ideas, methods, instructions or products referred to in the content.

Review

Gallbladder Pancreatic Heterotopia—The Importance of Diagnostic Imaging in Managing Intraoperative Findings

Crenguța Sorina Șerboiu [1,2], Cătălin Aliuș [3,*], Adrian Dumitru [4], Dana Țăpoi [4], Mariana Costache [4], Adriana Elena Nica [5], Mihăilescu Alexandra-Ana [6], Iulian Antoniac [7] and Sebastian Grădinaru [8,9]

[1] Department of Cellular, Molecular Biology and Histology, Carol Davila University of Medicine and Pharmacy, 050474 Bucharest, Romania; crengutas@yahoo.com
[2] Department of Radiology and Medical Imaging, University Emergency Hospital Bucharest, 050098 Bucharest, Romania
[3] Surgical Department IV, University Emergency Hospital Bucharest, 050098 Bucharest, Romania
[4] Pathology Department, University Emergency Hospital Bucharest, 050098 Bucharest, Romania; dr.adriandumitru@yahoo.com (A.D.); dana-antonia.tapoi@drd.umfcd.ro (D.Ț.); m_costache_dermatopat@yahoo.com (M.C.)
[5] Intensive Care Unit, University Emergency Hospital Bucharest, 050098 Bucharest, Romania; adriana.nica@suub.ro
[6] Intensive Care Unit, Foisor Hospital Bucharest, 021382 Bucharest, Romania; mihailescu.alexandra@drd.umfcd.ro
[7] Department of Metallic Materials Sciense and Physical Metallurgy, Faculty of Materials Science and Engineering, University Politehnica of Bucharest, 060042 Bucharest, Romania; antoniac.iulian@gmail.com
[8] Department of General Surgery, County Hospital Ilfov, 050474 Bucharest, Romania; gradinarusebastian@gmail.com
[9] Titu Maiorescu University of Medicine and Pharmacy, 031593 Bucharest, Romania
* Correspondence: alius.catalin@gmail.com; Tel.: +40-769-291-401

Abstract: Pancreatic heterotopy is a rare entity defined as the presence of abnormally located pancreatic tissue without any anatomical or vascular connection to the normal pancreas. Heterotopic pancreatic tissue can be found in various regions of the digestive system, such as the stomach, duodenum, and upper jejunum, with the less commonly reported location being the gallbladder. Gallbladder pancreatic heterotopia can be either an incidental finding or diagnosed in association with cholecystitis. Pancreatitis of the ectopic tissue has also been described. In this context, we report three cases of heterotopic pancreatic tissue in the gallbladder with different types of pancreatic tissue according to the Heinrich classification. One patient was a 24-year-old male who presented with acute pancreatitis symptoms and an ultrasonographical detected mass in the gallbladder, which proved to be heterotopic pancreatic tissue. The other two cases were female patients aged 24 and 32, respectively, incidentally diagnosed on histopathological examination after cholecystectomy for symptomatic cholelithiasis. Both cases displayed chronic cholecystitis lesions; one of them was also associated with low grade dysplasia of the gallbladder. Although a rare occurrence in general, pancreatic heterotopia should be acknowledged as a possible incidental finding in asymptomatic patients as well as a cause for acute cholecystitis or pancreatitis.

Keywords: ectopic; pancreas; heterotopia; gallbladder; pancreatitis; cholecystitis

1. Introduction

A heterotopic pancreas is described as a pancreatic tissue that does not have any anatomical or vascular connections with the pancreas itself. Other terms such as "ectopic pancreas", "accessory pancreatic tissue", "pancreatic choristoma", or "aberrant pancreas" are used in the literature. It is most commonly found in the gastrointestinal tract, with over 90% of the cases reported in its upper part (stomach, duodenum, and upper jejunum). Some rare locations that were reported in association with pancreatic heterotopia include the ileum, Meckel's diverticulum, splenic hilum, common bile duct, and in exceptionally rare cases, the gallbladder [1–3]. Despite being a congenital anomaly pancreatic heterotopia is usually an incidental finding, reported in 13% of cases at autopsy and in only 0.2% after laparotomy [4,5]. Although the majority of these pancreatic remnants are functional, they are usually asymptomatic [6]. When symptoms arise, they are mainly non-specific and consist of abdominal pain or tenderness, dyspepsia, nausea, vomiting, anaemia, or gastrointestinal bleeding [4,7]. Pancreatitis of the ectopic tissue has also been described [8]. In this paper, we report three cases of gallbladder heterotopic pancreas, an entity so rare that there have been fewer than 40 cases reported since 1916 [4]. As highlighted in similar studies reporting uncommon conditions, awareness and dissemination are crucial in helping clinicians ensure early diagnosis and appropriate management. Furthermore, advancements in histopathological analysis, immunohistochemistry techniques, and the introduction of artificial intelligence in specimen readings are expected to increase the number of papers on rare findings.

The first histological classification of pancreatic heterotopia in the gallbladder was published by von Heinrich more than a hundred years ago [9] and was last modified by Gaspar Fuentes et al. in the early 1970s [10]. According to this classification, there are four types of pancreatic heterotopia (Figure 1).

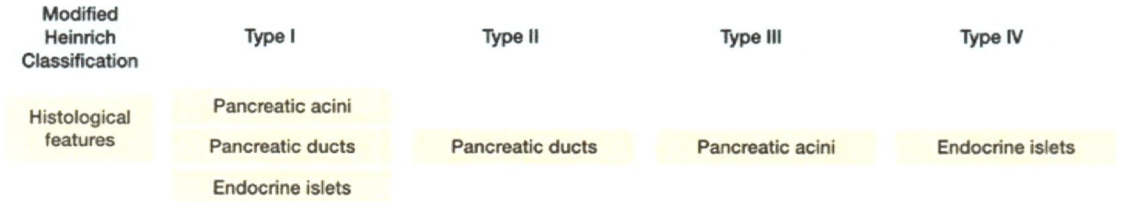

Figure 1. Modified Heinrich Classification for pancreatic heterotopia.

Type I displays pancreatic acini, ducts, and endocrine islets; type II displays pancreatic ducts only; type III displays acini only; and type IV endocrine cells only. Although acini and ducts are visible in conventional HE staining, immunohistochemistry can be employed to identify and confirm the presence of acinar/ductal components using Cytokeratin. The endocrine islets could be identified based on the presence of neuroendocrine markers such as Chromogranin A (non-specific) and Insulin (specific).

2. Types of Pancreatic Heterotopia

2.1. Type 1

A 24-year-old man presented to the hospital with intense upper abdominal pain radiating to the back, nausea, and vomiting. The patient requested medical help after excessive alcohol consumption, so the initial supposition was acute pancreatitis. On physical examination, the abdomen was tender in the right upper quadrant with a positive Murphy's sign. The white cell count was normal but with a left shift of the leukocytes and normal amylase and lipase levels. Ultrasonography revealed a mass initially believed to be an enlarged Mascagni's lymph node, and therefore laparoscopic cholecystectomy was recommended (Figure 2). Upper GI endoscopy revealed no signs of peptic ulcer disease and redirected the diagnosis toward biliary pathology since the only objective findings were a thickened gallbladder wall and an enlarged juxta cystic node. A laparoscopic cholecystectomy was indicated, and intraoperative findings showed a globulous gallbladder with an edematous wall and pericholecystic adhesions. At the time of the operation, a diagnosis of acute cholecystitis was supported by the clinical presentation and the oedematous walls of the gallbladder. The postoperative course of the patient was favorable, with remission of the symptoms and discharge after three days.

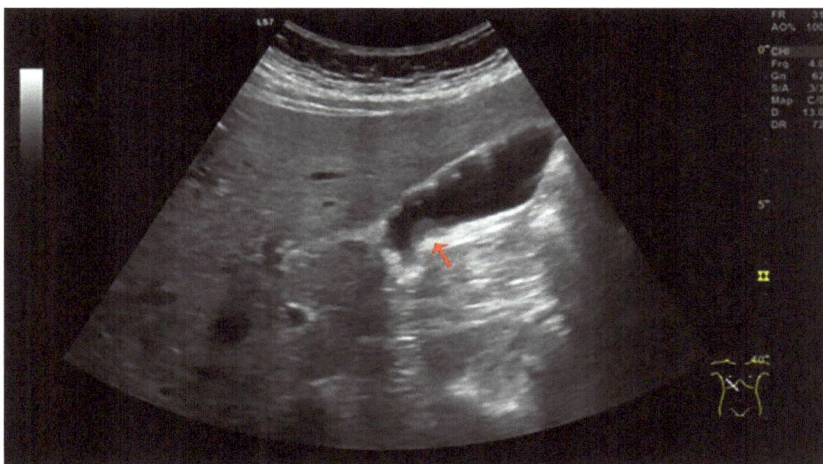

Figure 2. Ultrasonography reveals pancreatic heterotopia Type 1 (red arrow).

After the surgical removal of the gallbladder, the tissue fragments were sent for processing and examination to the Department of Pathology. Gross examination revealed a slightly lobulated white-yellowish pseudo-tumoral mass measuring approximately 1.8/2/1.2 cm (Figure 3). The mass was found in the infundibular area of the gallbladder, adjacent to Mascagni's lymph node. Tissue samples were fixed with 10% buffered Formalin and sent for histopathological processing by conventional methods using Paraffin inclusion and Hematoxylin-Eosin (HE) staining. Also, immunohistochemical tests were performed. The paraffin blocks acquired by histopathological processing were sectioned at the microtome resulting in 2 μm thickness sections mounted on slides covered with poly-L-Lysin. We used the following antibodies from Biocare for ancillary testing: Cytokeratin 8/18, Cytokeratin 19, Chromogranin A, and Insulin. Cytokeratin (Ck) has been used to highlight serous acini and /or pancreatic ducts, while Langerhans cells have been highlighted using either a universal marker for neuroendocrine differentiation (Chromogranin A) or a specific immunomarker: Insulin.

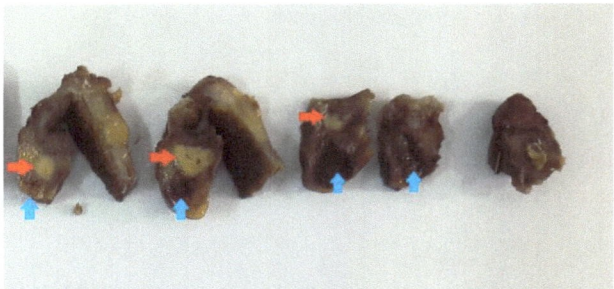

Figure 3. Gross appearance of the heterotopic pancreatic tissue in the wall of the gallbladder (red arrow). Note the Mascagni lymph node in the vicinity (blue arrow).

Microscopic examination showed a well-circumscribed fully developed heterotopic pancreatic tissue in the muscularis layer extending to the subserosa adipose connective tissue. The pancreatic rests were composed of lobules of exocrine pancreatic acini, exocrine ducts and many Langerhans islets. (Figures 4 and 5). The findings were consistent with type I pancreatic heterotopia according to the modified Heinrich classification (Figure 6).

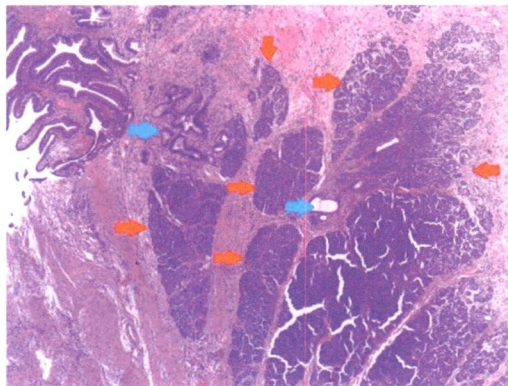

Figure 4. Heterotopic pancreatic tissue of the gallbladder. Hematoxylin and Eosin staining, 4× magnification. It can be observed in serous acini (red arrows) and exocrine ducts (blue arrows).

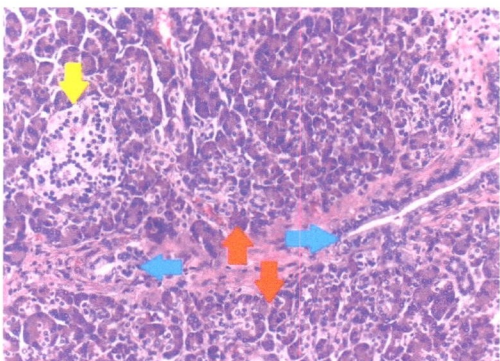

Figure 5. Type 1 gallbladder pancreatic heterotopia according the de modified Heinrich classification. All three histological elements of the pancreas can be observed: serous acini (red arrows), endocrine cells (yellow arrow) and exocrine ducts (blue arrow).

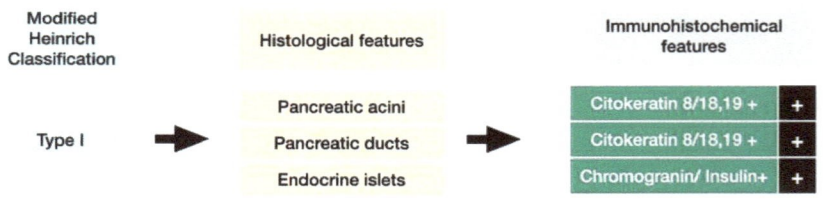

Figure 6. Histological features and IHC (imunohistochemistry) features of type I pancreatic heterotopia.

The islets were strongly and diffusely positive for Chromogranin A and Insulin (Figure 7). The serous acini were positive for Ck8/18. The remaining sections showed features of chronic cholecystitis (Figure 8).

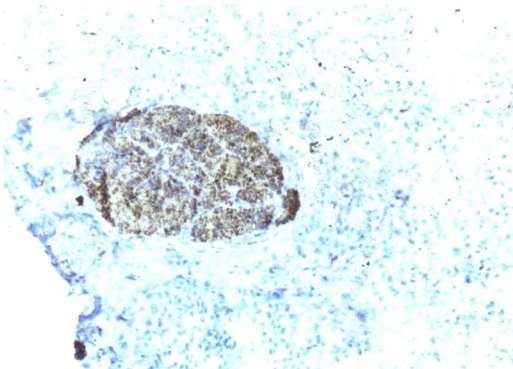

Figure 7. Langerhans islets are strongly positive for Insulin antibodies in heterotopic pancreatic tissue of the gallbladder. IHC staining with DAB chromogen, 20× magnification.

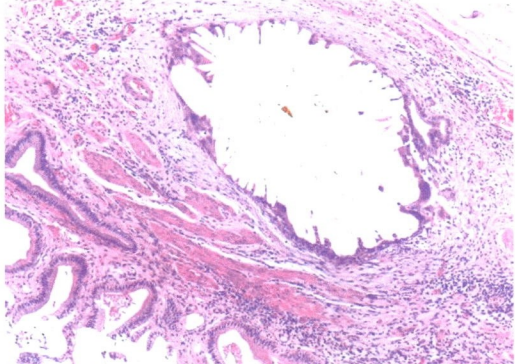

Figure 8. Microscopic aspects suggestive of chronic cholecystitis. Observe a cholesterol calculus included in a Rokitansky-Aschoff sinus. Hematoxylin and Eosin staining, 10× magnification.

The discovery of the heterotopic tissue was incidental, the emergency surgery enabled the removal of the gallbladder with subsequent remission of the symptoms. The patient presented follow-up without any further pathology.

2.2. Type 2

A 24-year-old female presented to the hospital with a history of right hypochondriac pain, nausea, nausea and vomiting. No change in the hematology or biochemistry panels, was noted. On physical examination, there was tenderness in the right upper quadrant of the abdomen. Abdominal ultrasound examination showed cholelithiasis, and the patient underwent laparoscopic cholecystectomy, (Figure 9). The intraoperative findings showed a thickened gallbladder wall and unremarkable neighboring viscera. The postoperative course was uneventful, and the patient was discharged home after two days free of symptoms. Follow-up with the general practitioner was uneventful, and no further visits were requested for this patient. Macroscopic examination did not reveal particular aspects other than those suggestive of chronic cholecystitis. On microscopic examination, ectopic pancreatic tissue was and an incidental finding, being observed within the gallbladder wall.

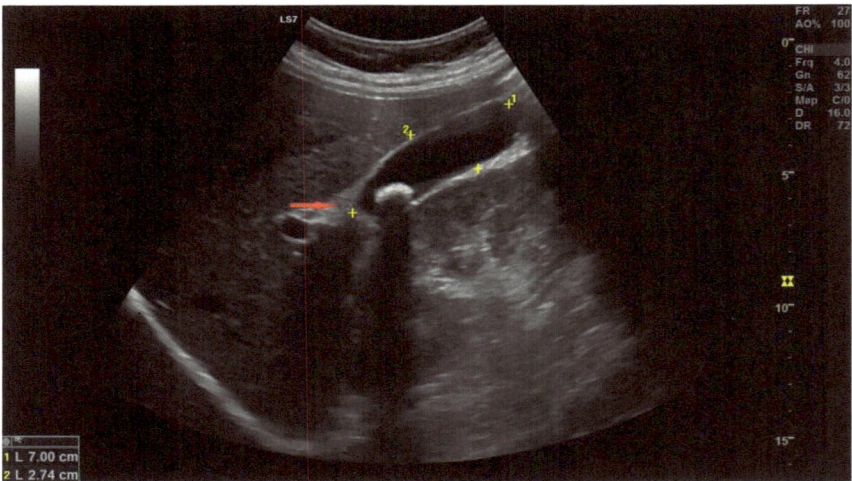

Figure 9. Ultrasonography reveals the site of pancreatic ectopy type 2 (red arrow), opposite the macro calculus with posterior shadow cone.

The ectopic tissue was composed of serous acini and a few exocrine ducts but no endocrine islets, thus this case was classified as type 2 pancreatic heterotopia according to the modified Heinrich's criteria (Figure 10). Pseudo-pyloric metaplasia was observed in the vicinity of the ectopic tissue (Figures 11 and 12).

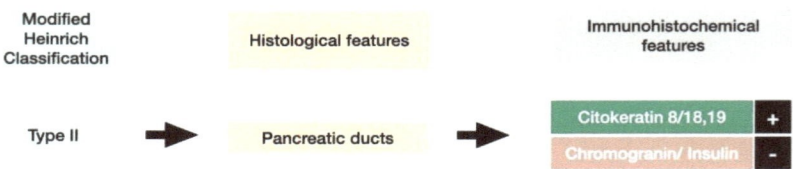

Figure 10. Histological features and IHC features of type II pancreatic heterotopia.

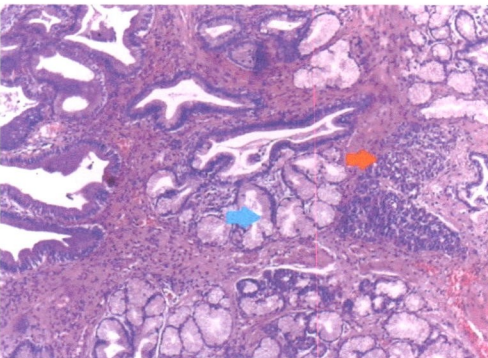

Figure 11. Small foci of heterotopic pancreatic tissue of the gallbladder (red arrow) in the vicinity of pseudo-pyloric metaplasia (blue arrow). Hematoxylin and Eosin staining, 10× magnification.

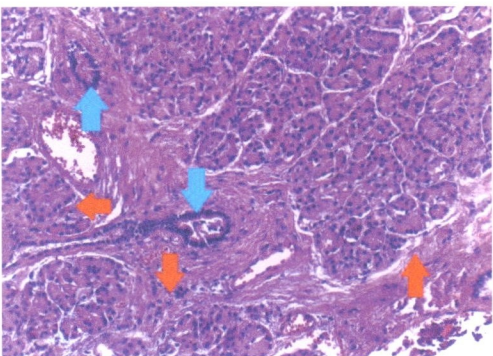

Figure 12. Small foci of heterotopic pancreatic tissue of the gallbladder (red arrow) in the vicinity of pseudo-pyloric metaplasia (blue arrow). High power magnification showing serous acini and exocrine ducts only in the heterotopic pancreatic tissue of the gallbladder (type 2 heterotopic pancreatic tissue according to the Heinrich classification). Hematoxylin and Eosin staining, 40× magnification.

2.3. Type 3

A 32-year-old female presented to the hospital with a history of right upper abdominal pain radiating to the right shoulder, nausea, and vomiting, particularly associated with fatty food intake. The patient had a history of neglected recurrent abdominal pain, and initially used over-the-counter analgesics for self-medication. The right hypochondriac region was tender on physical examination with no change in the CBC (Complete Blood Count) panel. Ultrasonography revealed cholelithiasis and subsequently laparoscopic cholecystectomy was carried out, (Figure 13). On gross examination variable thickening of the gallbladder wall was observed. The wall thickness varied from 0.3 to 0.6 cm. The serosal layer was unremarkable. The mucosa was flattened and focally ulcerated and numerous yellowish-green friable round stones, each measuring up to 0.4 cm in diameter, were noted in the fundus.

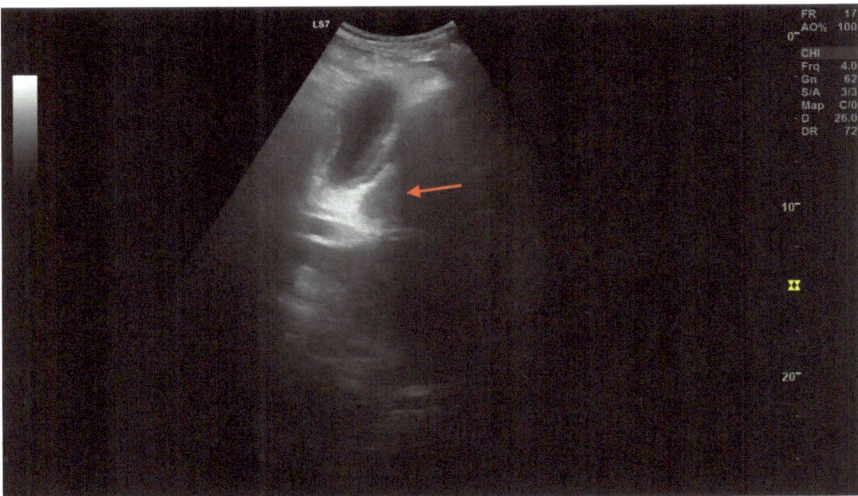

Figure 13. Ultrasonography of a case with type 3 pancreatic heterotopy (red arrow).

A grey-tanned area was seen in the neck region, thought to be the Mascagni's lymph-node, which, instead, on microscopic examination, showed to be a well-circumscribed rest of heterotopic pancreatic tissue, composed of tightly packed lobules of exocrine pancreatic acini (Figure 14). Exocrine ducts or Islets of Langerhans were not seen. The serous acini were strongly positive for Ck 8/18 (Figure 15). This type of heterotopy corresponds to type 3 after Gaspar-Fuentes classification (Figure 16), the original Heinrich classification not having this subtype. The remaining sections showed features of chronic cholecystitis but the incidental findings did not stop here: the mucosa had focal aspects of low -grade biliary intraepithelial dysplasia (Figure 17).

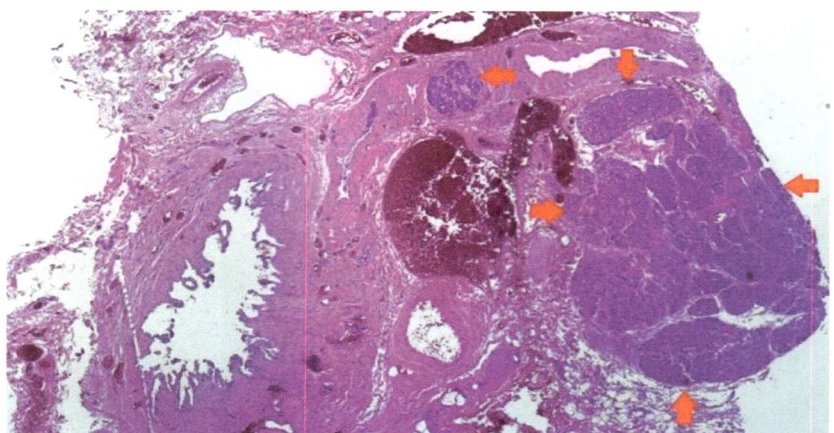

Figure 14. Heterotopic pancreatic tissue (serous acini only-red arrow) in the neck region of the gallbladder. Hematoxylin and Eosin staining, 4× magnification, Leica stitch image software resolution.

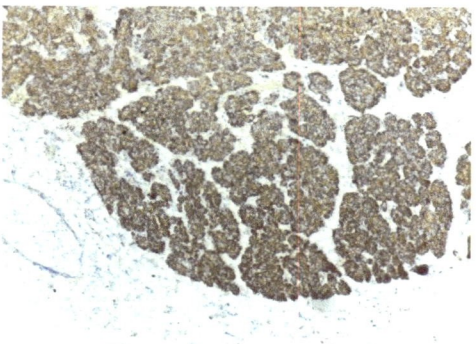

Figure 15. The serous pancreatic acini were strongly positive for Ck8/18 antibody. IHC staining with DAB (Diaminobenzidine) chromogen, 10× magnification.

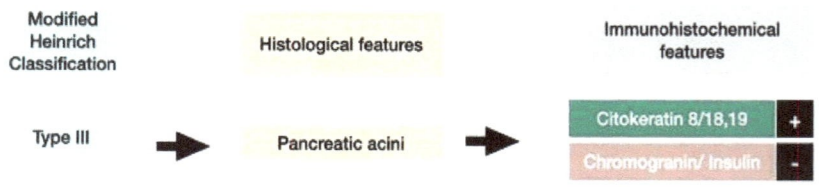

Figure 16. Histological features and IHC features of type I pancreatic heterotopia.

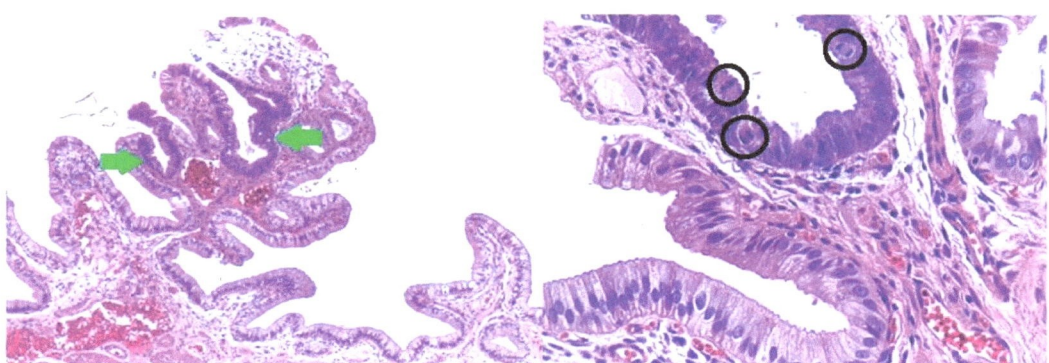

Figure 17. Low grade biliary intraepithelial neoplasia (BilIN1): flat architecture, basal nuclei, pseudostratification within lower two thirds of epithelium (green arrows). Note the mild nuclear abnormalities and frequent mitotic figures (black circles). Hematoxylin and Eosin staining, 10× and 40× magnifications.

3. Discussion

Heterotopic pancreas is a congenital anomaly defined as the presence of pancreatic tissue abnormally located without any connection to the normal pancreas itself [11]. Heterotopic pancreas is usually located in the stomach, small intestine and Meckel's diverticulum [1–3] and it has been rarely encountered in other sites such as the liver or spleen [12]. Gallbladder pancreatic heterotopia was first described by Otschkin in 1916 [13,14] and to this date there are less than 40 cases reported in the literature [15]. It is most frequently located close to the neck of the gallbladder [16]. The overall incidence of pancreatic heterotopia is estimated to be up to 13% on autopsy and 0.2% after laparotomy [4,5]. All these data reflect a low prevalence of heterotopia but suggest ubiquitous potential localizations.

Since the ectopic pancreas is affected by the same pathologies as the orthotopic tissue the clinician should expect pancreatitis, pseudocyst formation, bleeding and malignant transformation hence alterations of the classical clinical patterns would be a natural occurrence. In a young patient such as our first case the presentation with acute upper abdominal pain radiating to the back was suggestive of acute pancreatitis. An elevation of the pancreatic enzymes (although not three to five times higher than the normal value) would fulfil two Atlanta criteria for acute pancreatitis. In the absence of clinical deterioration repeat imaging in pancreatitis is usually performed three days after the onset of the symptoms to allow for mounting of pathological changes visible on USS or CT. On the other hand, the latest Tokyo criteria for the management of acute pancreatitis indicate that for grade I and II acute cholecystitis, early cholecystectomy should be performed within the first 72 h of admission. But this case had only a partially thickened gallbladder wall with no obvious oedematous changes. The USS appearance of the ectopic pancreas is usually an echogenic mass of variable dimensions located mainly near the cystic duct or in the neck of the gallbladder, hence the potential confusion with a lymph node. From acute pancreatitis to dyspepsia and peptic ulcer disease the spectrum of conditions causing similar clinical presentations is large therefore we believe that pancreatic heterotopia, although rare, is a condition that must be considered for differential diagnoses, especially in cases with borderline criteria for acute pancreatitis or lack of correlation between clinical features and imaging findings. The second case presented was a routine case of symptomatic cholelithiasis having atypia diagnosed incidentally on the histology report. There is no data in the literature to suggest a correlation between the presence of pancreatic heterotopia and gallbladder lithiasis. In addition to this, the asymptomatic proportion of patients with both these conditions is quite high. A study performed by Wei on patients with upper gi pancreatic heterotopia suggested that up to 50 per cent of the patients are symptomatic, but because of its low prevalence and the superposable symptoms of more common conditions, underdiagnosis is very likely. The third case was another incidental finding but with importance due to the microscopic changes suggestive of a different type of pancreatic heterotopia. The rarity of these cases coupled with underdiagnosis makes the topic relevant for the clinician who deals with gastrointestinal conditions, especially in acute cases. The occurrence of all three types of pancreatic heterotopia in a single centre while less than 40 cases of gallbladder localisation were reported so far makes the allegation of underdiagnosis even more apt and suggests that perhaps this diagnosis should be sought more frequently.

Since pancreatic heterotopia is a result of abnormal embryological development there are a couple of theories about the mechanisms behind this erratic development. One theory claims that the heterotopic tissue is detached from the primitive pancreas during its rotation, while another theory alleges that during the development of the pancreatic bud, fragments of pancreatic tissue are separated by the longitudinal growth of the intestines [17–19]. Various other studies argue that abnormalities in the Notch signaling pathway may lead to the development of pancreatic heterotopia [20,21]. Hes-1 (Hairy enhancer of split) is a main effector of Notch system and it is involved in region-appropriate differentiation of the pancreas in the developing foregut endoderm. In this respect, the occurrence of pancreatic heterotopia has been noted in Hes-1 knockout mice [22].

Histologically, heterotopic pancreas is composed of endocrine and exocrine tissue in various amounts. The first histological classification on pancreatic heterotopia was published by von Heinrich in 1909 and was lastly modified by Gaspar Fuentes et al. in 1973 [9]. According to this classification, there are 4 types of pancreatic heterotopia: Type I: acini, ducts, and islets of endocrine glands, Type II: canalicular variant with pancreatic ducts, Type III: exocrine pancreas with acinar tissue only. No endocrine tissue is present, Type IV: endocrine pancreas with cellular islets only (no exocrine tissue is present) (Figure 18).

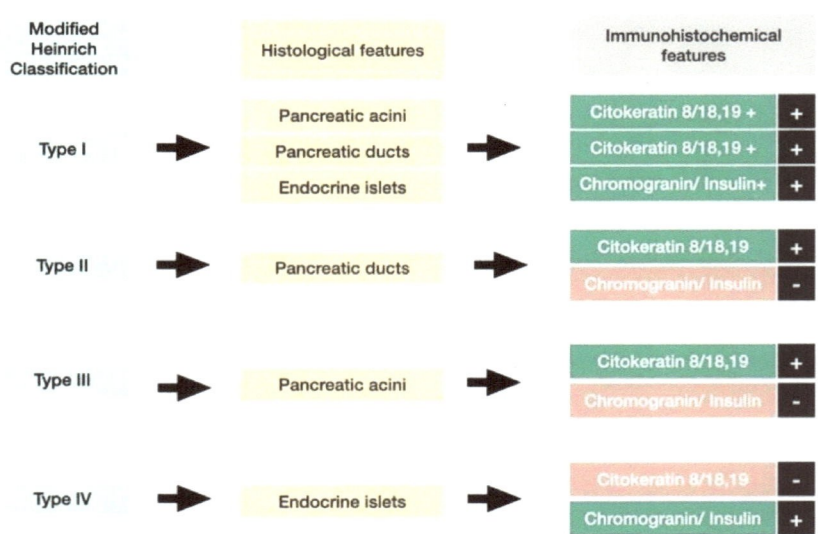

Figure 18. Histological features and IHC features of pancreatic atypia.

In terms of clinical manifestations, pancreatic heterotopia is usually asymptomatic. When symptoms do arise, they are mostly a result of complications such as cholecystitis, bile duct and intestinal obstructions or mucosal ulcers [3], and even gallbladder perforation and peritonitis [18]. There are, however cases, when symptoms are related to the heterotopic pancreas itself. Although rare, pancreatic heterotopia in the stomach can undergo malignant transformation to pancreatic adenocarcinoma [23]. Tumors arising from heterotopic endocrine pancreatic tissue have also been described [24]. In addition to this, heterotopic pancreatic tissue can also cause acute and chronic pancreatitis [25]. Symptoms related to gallbladder pancreatic heterotopia most often resemble acute or chronic cholecystitis. Histopathological examination confirms both the existence of heterotopic pancreatic tissue and lesions of acute and chronic cholecystitis [4,6] It has been demonstrated that pancreatic enzymes levels are elevated in gallbladder bile and as a consequence could be a trigger for gallbladder lesion and therefore lead to acalculous cholecystitis and even gallbladder carcinoma [15,20]. Gallbladder pancreatic heterotopia with chronic cholecystitis was also found in association with pseudo-pyloric metaplasia, and adenomyomatous hyperplasia of the gallbladder [26].

In one of our own cases, the gallbladder mucosa displayed low grade dysplasia. Gallbladder surgery is the most common intervention worldwide with an increasing prevalence due to lifestyle modifications and the growth of obesity. Since every specimen must be sent for histology it is expected that the prevalence of pancreatic heterotopia to rise in correlation with the total number of cholecystectomies which approaches a million cases per year only in Europe. Despite these numbers, very few cases of heterotopia were reported so far. It is true that diagnosing and categorizing it requires the employment of immunohistochemistry techniques which are not universally available and are for some institutions too expensive for routine use.

Since rare diseases affect only a small number of people compared to the general population, this field suffers from a deficit of scientific and medical knowledge input. Hence scientific publications such as case reports and clinical trial studies represent a valuable resource helping to overcome the current imitations [27]. The complexity of this disease requires strong collaboration between the surgeon, radiologist and pathologist to be diagnosed and treated properly. Beside the disease complications, the intraoperative events are not to be neglected either [28].

4. Conclusions

In conclusion, despite being an exceptional encounter, gallbladder pancreatic heterotopia should be considered in the etiology of cholecystitis and as an explanation for incidental ultrasonographic findings such as gallbladder polyps, pseudo-tumoral masses, and other peculiar imaging features. In any case, the definitive diagnosis is made only by histopathological examination. Only strong cooperation between the imaging specialist, the surgical team, and the pathologist can ensure a good outcome and a proper staging of the type of pancreatic heterotopia at the level of the gallbladder. An extensive literature review concerning this entity uncovered a paucity of case reports on this matter, and the authors emphasize the importance of further data collection.

Author Contributions: Conceptualization, C.S.Ș. and S.G.; methodology, C.A.; software, A.D.; validation, D.Ț., M.C. and A.E.N.; formal analysis, M.A.-A.; investigation, I.A.; resources, C.A.; data curation, A.D.; writing—original draft preparation, C.S.Ș.; writing—review and editing, S.G.; visualization, D.Ț.; supervision, M.C.; project administration, A.E.N.; funding acquisition, M.A.-A. and I.A. All authors have read and agreed to the published version of the manuscript.

Funding: This research received no external funding.

Institutional Review Board Statement: Not applicable.

Informed Consent Statement: Informed consent was obtained from all subjects involved in the study.

Data Availability Statement: Not applicable.

Acknowledgments: The authors thank Cristina Veronica Andreescu from the Medical English Department at Carol Davila University of Medicine and Pharmacy, Bucharest, Romania. She kindly agreed to proofread the manuscript.

Conflicts of Interest: The authors declare no conflict of interest.

References

1. Ormarsson, O.T.; Gudmundsdottir, I.; Mårvik, R. Diagnosis and treatment of gastric heterotopic pancreas. *World J. Surg.* **2006**, *30*, 1682–1689. [CrossRef] [PubMed]
2. Pang, L.C. Pancreatic heterotopia: A reappraisal and clinicopathologic analysis of 32 cases. *South. Med. J.* **1988**, *81*, 1264–1275. [CrossRef]
3. Elhence, P.; Bansal, R.; Agrawal, N. Heterotopic pancreas in gall bladder associated with chronic cholecystolithiasis. *Int. J. Appl. Basic Med. Res.* **2012**, *2*, 142–143. [CrossRef]
4. Wilde, G.E.; Gakhal, M.; Sartip, K.A.; Corso, M.J.; Butt, W.G. Pancreatitis in initially occult gastric heterotopic pancreas. *Clin. Imaging* **2007**, *31*, 356–359. [CrossRef]
5. Jovanovic, I.; Knezevic, S.; Micev, M.; Krstic, M. EUS mini probes in diagnosis of cystic dystrophy of duodenal wall in heterotopic pancreas: A case report. *World J. Gastroenterol.* **2004**, *10*, 2609–2612. [CrossRef]
6. Elpek, G.O.; Bozova, S.; Küpesiz, G.Y.; Oğüş, M. An unusual cause of cholecystitis: Heterotopic pancreatic tissue in the gallbladder. *World J. Gastroenterol.* **2007**, *13*, 313–315. [CrossRef] [PubMed]
7. Ferhatoglu, M.F.; Kivilcim, T.; Kartal, A.; Filiz, A.I. A Rare Pathology Mimicking the Gallstone: Heterotopic Pancreas in the Gallbladder. *Cureus* **2018**, *10*, e2659. [CrossRef]
8. Beltrán, M.A.; Barría, C. Heterotopic pancreas in the gallbladder: The importance of an uncommon condition. *Pancreas.* **2007**, *34*, 488–491. [CrossRef]
9. Gaspar Fuentes, A.; Campos Tarrech, J.M.; Fernández Burgui, J.L.; Castells Tejón, E.; Ruíz Rossello, J.; Gómez Pérez, J.; Armengol Miró, J. Ectopias pancreáticas [Pancreatic ectopias]. *Rev. Esp. Enferm. Apar. Dig.* **1973**, *39*, 255–268. (In Spanish) [PubMed]
10. Hickman, D.M.; Frey, C.F.; Carson, J.W. Adenocarcinoma arising in gastric heterotopic pancreas. *West. J. Med.* **1981**, *135*, 57–62.
11. Terada, T.; Nakanuma, Y.; Kakita, A. Pathologic observations of intrahepatic peribiliary glands in 1000 consecutive autopsy livers: Heterotopic pancreas in the liver. *Gastroenterology* **1990**, *98*, 1333–1337. [CrossRef] [PubMed]
12. Poppi, A. Sui pancreas aberranti. *Arch. Ital. Delle Mal. Appar. Dig.* **1935**, *4*, 534–579.
13. Neupert, G.; Appel, P.; Braun, S.; Tonus, C. Heterotopic pancreas in the gallbladder: Diagnosis, therapy, and course of a rare developmental anomaly of the pancreas. *Chirurg* **2007**, *78*, 261–264. [CrossRef]
14. Pendharkar, D.; Khetrapal, S.; Jairajpuri, Z.S.; Rana, S.; Jetley, S. Pancreatic and Gastric Heterotopia in the Gallbladder: A Rare Incidental Finding. *Int. J. Appl. Basic Med. Res.* **2019**, *9*, 115–117. [CrossRef] [PubMed]
15. Kondi-Paphiti, A.; Antoniou, A.G.; Kotsis, T.; Polimeneas, G. Aberrant pancreas in the gallbladder wall. *Eur. Radiol* **1997**, *7*, 1064–1066. [CrossRef]
16. Sharma, S.P.; Sohail, S.K.; Makkawi, S.; Abdalla, E. Heterotopic pancreatic tissue in the gallbladder. *Saudi Med. J.* **2018**, *39*, 834–837. [CrossRef]
17. Ben-Baruch, D.; Sandbank, Y.; Wolloch, Y. Heterotopic pancreatic tissue in the gallbladder. *Acta Chir. Scand.* **1986**, *152*, 557–558. [PubMed]
18. Inceoglu, R.; Dosluoglu, H.H.; Kullu, S.; Ahiskali, R.; Doslu, F.A. An unusual cause of hydropic gallbladder and biliary colic-heterotopic pancreatic tissue in the cystic duct: Report of a case and review of the literature. *Surg. Today* **1993**, *23*, 532–534. [CrossRef] [PubMed]
19. Sato, A.; Hashimoto, M.; Sasaki, K.; Matsuda, M.; Watanabe, G. Elevation of pancreatic enzymes in gallbladder bile associated with heterotopic pancreas. A case report and review of the literature. *JOP* **2012**, *13*, 235–238.
20. Murtaugh, L.C.; Stanger, B.Z.; Kwan, K.M.; Melton, D.A. Notch signaling controls multiple steps of pancreatic differentiation. *Proc. Natl. Acad. Sci. USA* **2003**, *100*, 14920–14925. [CrossRef]
21. Sumazaki, R.; Shiojiri, N.; Isoyama, S.; Masu, M.; Keino-Masu, K.; Osawa, M.; Nakauchi, H.; Kageyama, R.; Matsui, A. Conversion of biliary system to pancreatic tissue in Hes1-deficient mice. *Nat. Genet.* **2004**, *36*, 83–87. [CrossRef]
22. Fukuda, A.; Kawaguchi, Y.; Furuyama, K.; Kodama, S.; Horiguchi, M.; Kuhara, T.; Koizumi, M.; Boyer, D.F.; Fujimoto, K.; Doi, R.; et al. Ectopic pancreas formation in Hes1 -knockout mice reveals plasticity of endodermal progenitors of the gut, bile duct, and pancreas. *J. Clin. Investig.* **2006**, *116*, 1484–1493. [CrossRef]
23. Ogata, M.; Chihara, N.; Matsunobu, T.; Koizumi, M.; Yoshino, M.; Shioya, T.; Watanabe, M.; Tokunaga, A.; Tajiri, T.; Matsumoto, K. A Case of Intra-abdominal Endocrine Tumor Possibly Arising from an Ectopic Pancreas. *J. Nippon. Med. Sch.* **2007**, *74*, 168–172. [CrossRef] [PubMed]
24. Wawrzynski, J.; De Leon, L.; Shah, S.A.; Adrain, A.; Goldstein, L.J.; Feller, E. Gastric Heterotopic Pancreas Presenting as Abdominal Pain with Acute and Chronic Pancreatitis in the Resected Specimen. *Case Rep. Gastrointest. Med.* **2019**, *2019*, 2021712. [CrossRef] [PubMed]
25. Kaur, N.; Chander, B.; Kaur, H.; Kaul, R. Cholecystitis Associated with Heterotopic Pancreas, Pseudopyloric Metaplasia, and Adenomyomatous Hyperplasia: A Rare Combination. *J. Lab. Physicians* **2016**, *8*, 126–128. [CrossRef] [PubMed]
26. Sanchiz-Cárdenas, E.M.; Soler Humanes, R.; Lavado-Fernández, A.I.; Díaz-Nieto, R.; Suárez-Muñoz, M.A. Ectopic pancreas in gallbladder. Clinical significance, diagnostic and therapeutic implications. *Rev. Esp. Enferm. Dig.* **2015**, *107*, 701–703. [CrossRef]

27. Totolici, B.D.; Neamțu, C.; Bodog, F.D.; Bungau, S.; Goldiș, D.S.; Matei, M.; Andercou, O.A.; Amza, O.L.; Gyori, Z.; Coldea, L. Hemobilia by idiopathic aneurysm of cystic artery, fistulized in the biliary ways—Clinical case. *Rom. J. Morphol. Embryol.* **2017**, *58*, 267–270. [PubMed]
28. Dumitru, M.; Berghi, O.N.; Taciuc, I.-A.; Vrinceanu, D.; Manole, F.; Costache, A. Could Artificial Intelligence Prevent Intraoperative Anaphylaxis? Reference Review and Proof of Concept. *Medicina* **2022**, *58*, 1530. [CrossRef]

Disclaimer/Publisher's Note: The statements, opinions and data contained in all publications are solely those of the individual author(s) and contributor(s) and not of MDPI and/or the editor(s). MDPI and/or the editor(s) disclaim responsibility for any injury to people or property resulting from any ideas, methods, instructions or products referred to in the content.

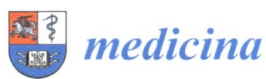 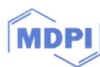

Article

Can MRI Accurately Diagnose and Stage Endometrial Adenocarcinoma?

Ramona-Andreea Rizescu [1], Iulia Alecsandra Sălcianu [2,3,*], Alexandru Șerbănoiu [2,4,5,*], Radu Tudor Ion [2,4,5], Lucian Mihai Florescu [6], Ioana-Andreea Gheonea [6], Gheorghe Iana [2] and Ana Magdalena Bratu [2,3]

1. Doctoral School of the University of Medicine and Pharmacy Craiova, 200349 Craiova, Romania; ramona.rizescu11@gmail.com
2. Department of Radiology and Medical Imaging, University of Medicine and Pharmacy Carol Davila, 050474 Bucharest, Romania; radu.ion@drd.umfcd.ro (R.T.I.); george_iana@yahoo.com (G.I.); ana.bratu@umfcd.ro (A.M.B.)
3. Department of Radiology and Medical Imaging, Colțea Hospital, 030171 Bucharest, Romania
4. Department of Radiology and Medical Imaging, University Emergency Hospital Bucharest, 050098 Bucharest, Romania
5. Doctoral School of "Carol Davila", University of Medicine and Pharmacy, 700115 Bucharest, Romania
6. Department of Radiology and Medical Imaging, University of Medicine and Pharmacy Craiova, 200349 Craiova, Romania; lucian.florescu@umfcv.ro (L.M.F.); ioana.gheonea@umfcv.ro (I.-A.G.)
* Correspondence: iulia.salcianu@umfcd.ro (I.A.S.); alexandru.serbanoiu@drd.umfcd.ro (A.Ș.); Tel.: +40-766524703 (I.A.S.)

Abstract: *Background and Objectives*: Endometrial carcinoma is one of the most common gynecological cancers, and benign lesions such as endometrial hyperplasia, polyps, adenomyosis and leiomyomas should be included in the differential diagnosis. Magnetic resonance imaging has an important role in evaluating endometrial cancer and assessing the depth of myometrial invasion, and it closely correlates with the prognosis of the patient. The purpose of this study is to evaluate the MRI semiology of the endometrial carcinomas that mimic benign lesions, the main factors that may affect the correct diagnosis and the feasibility of magnetic resonance imaging to evaluate the depth of the myometrial invasion of endometrial cancer. *Materials and Methods*: This is a retrospective analysis of 45 patients that underwent MRI examinations and the lesions were pathologically diagnosed as endometrial carcinoma after surgical resection. This study evaluated the staging accuracy of T2-weighted imaging, diffusion-weighted imaging (DWI), ADC mapping and T1-weighted imaging with fat saturation before and after gadolinium injection. *Results*: In 36 of the 45 cases, the MRI of the lesion showed the characteristics of endometrial cancer and the diagnosis was certain. Nine lesions (20%) were described as unequivocal and had unspecific MR appearance. In eight of the nine cases (89%), the histopathologic report revealed the presence of leiomyomas and two of these cases (22%) were also associated with adenomyosis. The cause of underestimation in these patients was coexisting lesions exhibiting heterogenous intensity and contrast enhancement, which made it difficult to detect the margins of the lesions. The depth of the myometrial invasion was underestimated in nine cases and overestimated in three cases. The staging accuracy with MRI was 74%. There was a significant correlation between MR imaging and histopathologic finding in the assessment of myometrial invasion ($p < 0.001$). Cervical extension was noted in eight cases (18%), but was missed on MR imaging in two patients and overstaged in none. Six of them were associated with myometrial invasion in more than 50% of the thickness. There was a significant correlation between MR imaging and histopathologic finding in the assessment of cervical extension ($p < 0.001$). *Conclusions*: Our data confirm the high accuracy of MRI in the diagnosis and local staging of endometrial carcinoma. The information provided by MRI has an important role in planning the treatment and the prognosis of the patients.

Keywords: endometrial cancer; endometroid adenocarcinoma; Federation of Gynecology and Obstetrics staging; magnetic resonance imaging staging

Citation: Rizescu, R.-A.; Sălcianu, I.A.; Șerbănoiu, A.; Ion, R.T.; Florescu, L.M.; Gheonea, I.-A.; Iana, G.; Bratu, A.M. Can MRI Accurately Diagnose and Stage Endometrial Adenocarcinoma? *Medicina* 2024, 60, 512. https://doi.org/10.3390/medicina60030512

Academic Editors: Romica Cergan, Adrian Costache and Mihai Dumitru

Received: 12 February 2024
Revised: 13 March 2024
Accepted: 19 March 2024
Published: 21 March 2024

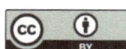

Copyright: © 2024 by the authors. Licensee MDPI, Basel, Switzerland. This article is an open access article distributed under the terms and conditions of the Creative Commons Attribution (CC BY) license (https:// creativecommons.org/licenses/by/ 4.0/).

1. Introduction

Endometrial carcinoma has an incidence rate that accounts for more than 50% malignant tumors in female patients, being one of the most common gynecological cancers [1]. The histological type, tumor grade and the International Federation of Obstetrics and Gynecology (FIGO 2023) staging have a great impact on the prognosis and treatment of endometrial cancer.

Magnetic resonance imaging (MRI) is widely applied in the diagnosing and staging of endometrial cancer [2]. MRI is the best tool for assessing myometrial invasion depth and cervical extension, which correspond with the grade of the tumor, the presence of lymph node invasion and prognosis [3–5]. Conventional MRI is based on the radiologist's perception and experience and sometimes presents interobserver variations [6,7].

This study attempts to comprehensively explore the information derived from T2-weighted imaging, diffusion-weighted imaging (DWI), ADC mapping and T1-weighted imaging with fat saturation before and after gadolinium injection in order to preoperatively distinguish endometrial carcinoma from benign mimics.

Local staging of endometrial cancer requires evaluating the tumor extension in the thickness of the myometrium. Observing an intact junctional zone, with low signal intensity on T2-weighted images and a thin band of early subendometrial enhancement excludes almost completely myometrial invasion [4,5]. The disruption of the subendometrial band indicates myometrial invasion. If there is an invasion of less than 50% of the myometrial thickness, the staging of the tumor is IA, while invasion greater than or equal to 50% of the myometrial thickness indicates a stage IB tumor [8].

There are some possible pitfalls that can result in underestimation and overestimation of myometrial invasion: (1) the tumor may present as a small or isointense lesion; (2) there may be poor visualization of the endometrium or the endometrial–myometrial interface contrast due to the presence of leiomyomas, adenomyosis, myometrium thinning in postmenopausal patients or endometrial thinning in older patients or endometrial cavity distension [4,5].

The purpose of this study is to evaluate the accuracy of MR imaging in diagnosing and staging endometrial carcinoma based on histopathological findings. Another aim is to identify the benign lesions that may affect the correct staging of the tumor.

2. Materials and Methods

2.1. Patient Selection

A retrospective review of the oncologic database from our institution, from January 2019 to November 2023, included 45 women, aged 34 to 81 years (age mean 60 years), who presented with abnormal vaginal bleeding and had undergone MRI examinations. Thirty-five of the patients (78%) attained menopause at the time of presentation. All lesions were pathologically diagnosed with endometrial carcinoma after surgical resection. Four patients were excluded from this study based on the definitive histologic diagnosis that differed from adenocarcinoma: carcinosarcoma in one patient and leiomyosarcoma in three patients.

Our institutional review board does not require approval for this type of retrospective study.

The clinical, pathologic and imaging parameters were collected from electronic medical records.

Patient data are compiled and stored in a anonymized and centralized Microsoft Excel© spreadsheet. Data analysis and graphical representations were performed using SPSS Statistics software (version 29.0 IBM Corporation, Armonk, NY, USA) and Microsoft Excel© (version 16.83, Microsoft, Redmond, WA, USA). The analysis of the correlation between MRI findings and histopathological results was performed using the independent-samples t-test. The statistical significance for the test was chosen to be $p < 0.05$.

2.2. MRI Protocol

The MRI scan was performed with patients in supine position, with free breathing during acquisition on 1.5 T scanners with phased-array abdominal coils.

The protocol included high-resolution sagittal T2-weighted fast spin-echo imaging, T2-weighted scans coronally and axially to the longitudinal axis of the uterine body, diffusion-weighted imaging (DWI) with b = 0 and 800 s/mm^2 (the ADC map is automatically calculated based on DWI by the embedded software of the MRI equipment), T1-weighted images with fat suppression before and after intravenous administration of 10 mL of gadolinium followed by flushing with 20 mL saline.

2.3. Image Analysis

There are several signal characteristics of endometrial cancer on MRI that are commonly recognized. In T2-weighted images, the lesion appears as a well-delineated (regular or irregular) or diffuse mass and is located within the endometrial cavity, showing heterogenous intermediate signal intensity relative to the hyperintense endometrium and hypointense myometrium. In diffusion-weighted images, the tumor appears hyperintense at the high B value, with a corresponding hypointense signal on the ADC map. On the postcontrast images, tumors may show early uptake in comparison with the normal endometrium and slower uptake than the myometrium. The proper timing for evaluating myometrial invasion is 2.5 min after contrast injection. Images obtained at 4 min after contrast injection are useful in detecting cervical invasion [3–5,9,10].

3. Results

Of the patients, 22 (49%) were in the age group between 41 and 60 years, followed by 21 patients (47%) who were more than 60 years old and 2 patients who were less than 40 years old (4%) (Figure 1). The most common symptom was postmenopausal vaginal bleeding, observed in 35 patients (78%). Patients in the perimenopausal age group had irregular and abundant vaginal bleeding (7 patients, 15%), but also intermittent spotting (3 patients, 7%) (Figure 2).

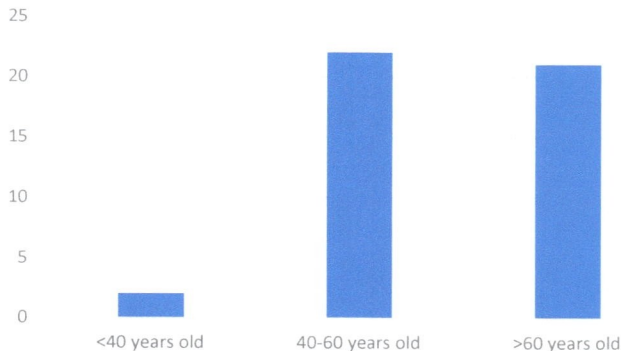

Figure 1. Age distribution of patients included in this study.

On T2-weighted images, endometrial carcinoma appeared hypointense to the adjacent myometrium in 16 patients (35%), isointense in 22 patients (49%) and hyperintense in 7 patients (16%). Forty of the tumors showed high signal intensity on DWI (89%). The contrast enhancement of the tumors was assessed as low in 30 cases (67%), intermediate in 3 cases (7%) and heterogenous in 12 cases (26%). The endometrium appeared thickened in 21 cases (46%).

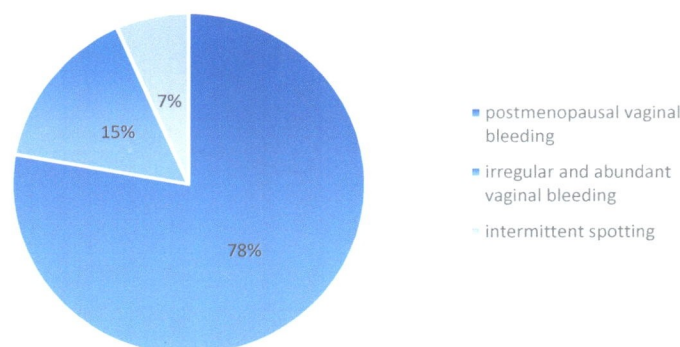

Figure 2. Presenting symptoms of the patients included in this study.

The maximum diameter of the tumor was evaluated; in 7 cases (16%) it measured maximum 20 mm, 21 to 40 mm in 24 cases (53%), 41 to 60 mm in 10 cases (22%), and over 60 mm in 4 cases (9%).

Of these 45 cases of endometrial cancer, 38 patients had endometrioid adenocarcinomas (15 were well differentiated: grade G1; 18 had moderate differentiation: grade G2; 5 were poorly differentiated: grade G3), 4 women had serous adenocarcinoma, 1 had clear cell adenocarcinoma, and 2 cancers were mixed adenocarcinoma (clear cell and serous adenocarcinoma). All of the patients with endometrial carcinoma underwent standard surgical procedure, total abdominal hysterectomy with bilateral salphingo-oophorectomy with pelvic lymph node dissection, and the staging accuracies of the T2, DWI and gadolinium-enhanced T1-weighted images in the assessment of myometrial invasion were evaluated.

The findings on MR imaging were compared with surgical and pathological findings.

Histological examination of the 45 endometrial cancers revealed that tumors were confined to the endometrium in 3 cases, invaded less than 50% of the myometrial thickness in 21 cases, and invaded 50% or more of the myometrial thickness in 21 cases. The depth of the myometrial invasion was underestimated in nine cases and overestimated in three cases. The staging accuracy with MRI was 74% (33/45 lesions). There was a significant correlation between MR imaging and histopathologic finding in the assessment of myometrial invasion ($p < 0.001$) (Table 1).

According to FIGO staging, 31% patients had stage IA disease, 16% had stage IB disease, 15% had stage II disease. Stage IIIa and IIIc were seen in 7% and 20% patients, respectively. 11% of the patients had IVC disease (Table 2).

In 13 cases (29%), distension of the uterine cavity was present.

The histological grade and disease staging (the depth of myometrial invasion, cervical extension) are predictive of the occurrence of extrauterine spread, pelvic nodal metastases, and impact the prognosis and treatment. Based on the stage of the disease, the treatment options include surgery, radiation therapy and chemotherapy [11–14].

Cervical extension was noted in eight cases (18%), but was missed on MR imaging in two patients and overstaged in none. Six of them were associated with myometrial invasion in more than 50% of the thickness. There was a significant correlation between MR imaging and histopathologic finding in the assessment of cervical extension ($p < 0.001$) (Table 3).

Table 1. MRI and histopathologic correlation of myometrial invasion.

			HP_Invasion <50%	HP_Invasion >50%	without	Total
MRI_invasion	<50%	Count	12	1	0	13
		Expected Count	6.1	6.1	0.9	13.0
		% within HP_invasion	57.1%	4.8%	0.0%	28.9%
	>50%	Count	3	18	0	21
		Expected Count	9.8	9.8	1.4	21.0
		% within HP_invasion	14.3%	85.7%	0.0%	46.7%
	without	Count	6	2	3	11
		Expected Count	5.1	5.1	0.7	11.0
		% within HP_invasion	28.6%	9.5%	100.0%	24.4%
Total		Count	21	21	3	45
		Expected Count	21.0	21.0	3.0	45.0
		% within HP_invasion	100.0%	100.0%	100.0%	100.0%

Chi-Square Tests	Value	df	p value
Pearson Chi-Square	32.946	4	<0.001
Likelihood Ratio	34.104	4	<0.001
N of Valid Cases	45		

Table 2. FIGO staging of the patients included in this study.

Figo Staging	Number of Patients	Percentage
IA	14	31
IB	7	16
IC	0	0
IIA	0	0
IIB	2	4
IIC	5	11
IIIA	3	7
IIIB	0	0
IIIC	9	20
IVA	0	0
IVB	0	0
IVC	5	11

Regional lymph node invasion was noted in 11 cases (24%). In these patients, the depth of myometrial invasion was bigger than 50% of the thickness in eight cases (73%). In two cases, the myometrial invasion was absent and less than 50% of the thickness, but the histopathology analysis revealed an aggressive histological type of endometrial carcinoma (serous adenocarcinoma and poorly differentiated endometrioid adenocarcinoma G3). One case with reported lymph node invasion and less than 50% myometrial thickness invaded was histologically described as moderately differentiated endometrioid adenocarcinoma G2.

In 36 of the 45 cases, MRI of the lesion showed the characteristics of endometrial cancer and the diagnosis was certain. The main goal of this study is to evaluate the semiology of the endometrial carcinomas that mimic benign lesions and the main factors that may affect the correct diagnosis.

Table 3. MRI and histopathologic correlation of cervical extension.

			HP Cervix Invasion 0	HP Cervix Invasion 1	Total
MRI cervix invasion	0	Count	37	2	39
		Expected Count	32.1	6.9	39.0
		% within HP cervix invasion	100.0%	25.0%	86.7%
	1	Count	0	6	6
		Expected Count	4.9	1.1	6.0
		% within HP cervix invasion	0.0%	75.0%	13.3%
Total		Count	37	8	45
		Expected Count	37.0	8.0	45.0
		% within HP cervix invasion	100.0%	100.0%	100.0%

Chi-Square Tests					
	Value	df	Asymptotic Significance (2 sided)	Exact Sig. (2 sided)	Exact Sig. (1 sided)
Pearson Chi-Square	32.019	1	<0.001		
Continuity Correction	25.858	1	<0.001		
Likelihood Ratio	26.343	1	<0.001		
Fisher's Exact Test				<0.001	<0.001
Linear-by-Linear Association	31.308	1	<0.001		
N of Valid Cases	45				

Nine lesions (20%) were described as unequivocal and had unspecific MR appearance.

On T2-weighted images, the tumors appeared hypointense to the adjacent myometrium in six patients (67%), isointense in two patients (22%) and hyperintense in one patient (11%). Four of the tumors showed high signal intensity on DWI (44%), while six of the tumors showed low signal on the ADC map. The contrast enhancement of the tumors was assessed as low in two cases (22%), intermediate in one case (11%) and heterogenous in six cases (26%). Endometrial thickness was noted in six cases (66%). None of the cases presented distension of the uterine cavity or cervical extension.

The maximum diameter of the tumor measured maximum 20 mm in three cases (33%), 21 to 40 mm in four cases (45%) 41 to 60 mm in one case (11%) and over 60 mm in one case (11%).

The histopathologic analysis of these nine cases reported eight cancers as endometrioid adenocarcinomas (four were well differentiated: grade G1; three were moderately differentiated: grade G2; one was poorly differentiated: grade G3) and one cancer as serous adenocarcinoma. All nine patients underwent the classical surgical procedure and the myometrial invasion could be evaluated. On the MR images, eight lesions showed no myometrial invasion, while one lesion invaded more than 50% of the myometrial thickness. The histological examination revealed no myometrial invasion in one case, invasion of less than 50% of the myometrial thickness in five cases and invasion of 50% or more of the myometrial thickness in three cases. The depth of the myometrial invasion was underestimated in seven cases. In eight of the nine cases (89%), the histopathologic report revealed the presence of leiomyomas and two of these cases (22%) were also associated with adenomyosis. The cause of underestimation in these patients was coexisting lesions exhibiting heterogenous intensity and contrast enhancement, which made it difficult to detect the margins of the lesions.

In one of these cases, the MRI examination showed invasion of more than 50% of the myometrial thickness with serous extension, high signal intensity on DWI and low signal on the ADC map, heterogenous structure that suggested and infectious etiology. The result of the histopathological report showed poorly differentiated endometrioid adenocarcinoma G3.

4. Discussion

Patients with noninvasive or locally advanced endometrial carcinoma benefit from surgical treatment. The recent less invasive surgical techniques require an accurate preoperative work-up in order to reduce the risk of understaging the disease and affecting the therapeutic plan.

The age at presentation for endometrial carcinoma has a mean of approximately 63 years, 90% of them present with abnormal vaginal bleeding [15,16].

Compared to other gynecological malignancies, the prognosis of endometrial carcinoma is more favorable, with a 5-year survival rate of 84%. 75% of the patients present with stage I disease [17,18] and the treatment is represented by simple hysterectomy [19].

In our study, 22 (49%) were in the age group between 41 and 60 years, followed by 21 patients (47%) who were more than 60 years old and 2 patients who were less than 40 years old (4%) (27.8%). The most common complaint was postmenopausal vaginal bleeding, seen in 35 patients (78%). The patients in the perimenopausal age group presented with irregular and heavy vaginal bleeding (7 patients, 15%), followed by intermittent spotting (3 patients, 7%).

The most common histopathology of endometrial carcinoma in our patients was endometrioid adenocarcinoma (38 patients, 85%), 40% of which were grade I, 47% were grade II, 13% were grade III. The next histopathology findings were serous adenocarcinoma (9%), clear cell adenocarcinoma (2%), and mixed adenocarcinoma (4%). A study by Shrivastava et al. [20] also stated that the most of the cases presented with endometrioid adenocarcinoma histology (27 patients, 75%), out of which 48% were grade I, 37% were grade II and 15% were grade III. This was followed by papillary adenocarcinoma, i.e., 22% and adenosquamous carcinoma (3%). A study by Yoney et al. [21] also stated that most of the cases had endometrioid adenocarcinoma histology (227 patients, 92.3%) out of which 51 (61.4%) cases had grade 1 disease.

MR imaging was used in preoperative assessment of the depth of myometrial invasion [22–26], cervical extension [27] and identification of enlarged pelvic lymph nodes [28,29]. In this study, we evaluated the accuracy of MR imaging in diagnosing, staging endometrial carcinoma in order to efficiently plan the treatment of the disease. Endometrial carcinoma could be detected on T2-weighted images as it appeared hypointense to the adjacent myometrium in 16 patients (35%), isointense in 22 patients (49%) and hyperintense in 7 patients (16%). Dynamic MR imagining performed after intravenous of gadolinium chelates is useful in evaluating the tumor due to different vascularity comparing to the myometrium and it helps in differentiating it from the fluid filling the endometrial cavity. The contrast enhancement of the tumors was assessed as low in 30 cases (67%), intermediate in 3 cases (7%) and heterogenous in 12 cases (26%).

The presence and depth of myometrial invasion are important factors in predicting lymph nodes metastases. Patients with myometrial invasion greater than 50% of the thickness have a six to sevenfold increased prevalence of pelvic and lumboaortic lymph node metastases compared with patients with absent or less than 50% myometrial invasion [12]. Planning the extent of lymphadenectomy is determined by the preoperative determination of myometrial invasion.

The presence and depth of myometrial invasion are best assessed on T2-weighted images and appears as an interruption of the junctional zone. However, in postmenopausal women, the junctional zone may be less visible and the myometrium may be thinned due to the involution of the uterus, making the evaluation of myometrial invasion more difficult to assess. In our patients, there was a significant correlation between MR imaging and histopathologic finding in the assessment of myometrial invasion ($p < 0.001$).

Preoperative evaluation of cervical extension is an important step in planning the treatment as it affects the prognosis of the patients. Several studies have shown that macroscopic cervical involvement is associated with a worse prognosis than microscopic involvement and may help in planning radical surgery or additional radiation therapy [30,31]. In this study, cervical infiltration was missed in two patients and overstaged in none. We report an 75% accuracy in detecting cervical involvement. In our patients, there was a significant correlation between MR imaging and histopathologic finding in the assessment of cervical invasion ($p < 0.001$).

Pelvic lymph node status is one of the most important prognosis factors in endometrial carcinoma. MRI may directly depict lymph nodes without contrast medium. MR imaging also has limitations in assessing the status of the lymph nodes, the most important one being differentiating between metastatic and non-metastatic lymph nodes. The presence of central necrosis has a 100% positive predictive value in the diagnosis of metastasis, although it usually occurs when the diameter of the lymph nodes is over 2 cm in size [28]. Another aspect in oncologic patients is setting a cut-off value of the minimal diameter of the lymph node of 1 cm for differentiating metastatic lymph nodes.

In this study, regional lymph node invasion was noted in 11 cases (24%). In these patients, the depth of myometrial invasion was bigger than 50% of the thickness in eight cases (73%). In two cases, the myometrial invasion was absent and less than 50% of the thickness, but the histopathology analysis revealed an aggressive histological type of endometrial carcinoma (serous adenocarcinoma and poorly differentiated endometrioid adenocarcinoma G3). One case with reported lymph node invasion and less than 50% myometrial thickness invaded was histologically described as moderately differentiated endometrioid adenocarcinoma G2.

A limit of this study was represented by the fact that we evaluated only the regional staging of endometrial carcinoma, focusing on the local extension of the tumor and not searching for distant metastases.

5. Conclusions

Imaging plays an important role in patients suspected of endometrial cancer, and MRI is considered the imaging method of choice in diagnosing and preoperative staging of endometrial carcinoma.

Our data confirm the high accuracy of MRI in local staging of endometrial carcinoma, combining the characteristics of the tumor on T2-weighted imaging, diffusion-weighted imaging, ADC mapping, and dynamic contrast administration, which may be particularly helpful in cases of tumors that are either iso- or hyperintense relative to the myometrium.

The future of diagnosing and staging endometrial carcinoma will benefit from upgraded MR protocols that will include MR perfusion, MR spectroscopy, blood oxygen level-dependent MRI and improved contrast agents. These additions will increase the accuracy of the differential diagnosis, offer a better assessment of associated benign and malignant lesions and a more specific characterization of the tumor type in order to aid the surgical protocol and decrease the morbidity and mortality of this neoplasia.

Author Contributions: All authors have an equal contribution to this study. All authors have read and agreed to the published version of this manuscript.

Funding: This research received no external funding.

Institutional Review Board Statement: Ethical review and approval were waived for this study because this study is retrospective.

Informed Consent Statement: Patient consent was waived because this study is retrospective.

Data Availability Statement: Data are available upon request from the corresponding authors.

Acknowledgments: Publication of this paper was supported by the University of Medicine and Pharmacy Carol Davila, through the institutional program Publish not Perish.

Conflicts of Interest: The authors declare no conflict of interest.

References

1. Siegel, R.L.; Miller, K.D.; Jemal, A. Cancer statistics, 2020. *CA Cancer J. Clin.* **2020**, *70*, 7–30. [CrossRef]
2. Frei, K.A.; Kinkel, K. Staging endometrial cancer: Role of magnetic resonance imaging. *J. Magn. Reson. Imaging* **2001**, *13*, 850–855. [CrossRef]
3. Meissnitzer, M.; Forstner, R. MRI of endometrium cancer—How we do it. *Cancer Imaging* **2016**, *16*, 11. [CrossRef]
4. Nougaret, S. From Staging to Prognostication. *Magn. Reason. Imaging Clin. N. Am.* **2017**, *25*, 611–633. [CrossRef] [PubMed]
5. Nougaret, S. Endometrial Cancer MRI staging: Updated Guidelines of the European Society of Urogenital Radiology. *Eur. Radiol.* **2019**, *29*, 792–805. [CrossRef] [PubMed]
6. Stanzione, A. Deep Myometrial Infiltration of Endometrial Cancer on MRI: A Radiomics-Powered Machine Learning Pilot Study. *Acad. Raidol.* **2021**, *28*, 737–744. [CrossRef]
7. Woo, S.; Kim, S.Y.; Cho, J.Y.; Kim, S.H. Assessment of deep myometrial invasion of endometrial cancer on MRI: Added value of second-opinion interpretations by radiologists subspecialized in gynaecologic oncology. *Eur. Radiol.* **2017**, *27*, 1877–1882. [CrossRef] [PubMed]
8. Berek, J.S. FIGO staging of endometrial cancer: 2023. *Int. J. Gynecol. Obstet.* **2023**, *162*, 383–394. [CrossRef] [PubMed]
9. Park, S.B.; Moon, M.H.; Sung, C.K.; Oh, S.; Lee, Y.H. Dynamic Contrast-Enhanced MR Imaging of Endometrial Cancer: Optimizing the Imaging Delay for Tumour-Myometrium Contrast. *Eur. Radiol.* **2014**, *24*, 2795–2799. [CrossRef] [PubMed]
10. Manfredi, R. Local-Regional Staging of Endometrial Carcinoma: Role of MR Imaging in Surgical Planning. *Radiology* **2004**, *231*, 372–378. [CrossRef] [PubMed]
11. Akin, O.; Mironov, S.; Pandit-Taskar, N.; Hann, L.E. Imaging of Uterine Cancer. *Radiol. Clin. N. Am.* **2007**, *45*, 167–182. [CrossRef] [PubMed]
12. Creasman, W.T.; Morrow, C.P.; Bundy, B.N.; Homesley, H.D.; Graham, J.E.; Heller, P.B. Surgical pathologic spread patterns of endometrial cancer. A Gynecologic Oncology Group Study. *Cancer* **1987**, *60*, 2035–2041. [CrossRef] [PubMed]
13. Scoutt, L.M. Clinical stage I endometrial carcinoma: Pitfalls in preoperative assessment with MR imaging. Work in progress. *Radiology* **1995**, *194*, 567–572. [CrossRef]
14. Nasi, F.; Fiocchi, F.; Pecchi, A.; Rivasi, F.; Torricelli, P. MRI evaluation of myometrial invasion by endometrial carcinoma. Comparison between fast-spin-echo T2w and coronal-FMPSPGR Gadolinium-Dota-enhanced sequences. *Radiol. Med.* **2005**, *110*, 199–210. [PubMed]
15. Manfredi, R.; Gui, B.; Maresca, G.; Fanfani, F.; Vonomo, L. Endometrial cancer: Magnetic resonance imaging. *Abdom. Imaging* **2005**, *30*, 626–636. [CrossRef]
16. Andersen, J.; Shanbhag, S.; Cruikshank, D. Use and accuracy of magnetic resonance imaging (MRI) staging of network treated endometrial cancer (EC): An audit and comparison to best evidence. *Sri Lanka J. Obstet. Gynaecol.* **2010**, *31*, 104. [CrossRef]
17. La Fianza, A.; Alberici, E.; Generoso, P.; Preda, L.; Campani, R. Correlation between pretreatment prognostic factors and lymph node metastases in endometrial adenocarcinoma. Clinical application. *Radiol. Med.* **2000**, *100*, 363–366.
18. Smith, R.C.; McCarthy, S. Magnetic resonance staging of neoplasms of the uterus. *Radiol. Clin. N. Am.* **1994**, *32*, 109–131. [CrossRef] [PubMed]
19. Ascher, S.M.; Reinhold, C. Imaging of cancer of the endometrium. *Radiol. Clin. N. Am.* **2002**, *40*, 563–576. [CrossRef]
20. Shrivastava, S. Magnetic resonance imaging in pre-operative staging of endometrial cancer. *Indian J. Cancer* **2016**, *53*, 181. [CrossRef] [PubMed]
21. Yoney, A.; Yildirim, C.; Bati, Y.; Unsal, M. Low risk stage I endometrial carcinoma: Prognostic factors and out-comes. *Indian J. Cancer* **2011**, *48*, 204. [CrossRef]
22. Takahashi, S. Preoperative staging of endometrial carcinoma: Diagnostic effect of T2-weighted fast spin-echo MR imaging. *Radiology* **1998**, *206*, 539–547. [CrossRef]
23. Sironi, S. Myometrial invasion by endometrial carcinoma: Assessment with plain and gadolinium-enhanced MR imaging. *Radiology* **1992**, *185*, 207–212. [CrossRef]
24. Sironi, S.; Taccagni, G.; Garancini, P.; Belloni, C.; DelMaschi, A. Myometrial invasion by endometrial carcinoma: Assessment by MR imaging. *Am. J. Roentgenol.* **1992**, *158*, 565–569. [CrossRef]
25. Hricak, H.; Rubinstein, L.; Gherman, G.M.; Karstaedt, N. MR imaging evaluation of endometrial carcinoma: Results of an NCI cooperative study. *Radiology* **1991**, *179*, 829–832. [CrossRef]
26. Hardesty, L.A. Use of Preoperative MR Imaging in the Management of Endometrial Carcinoma: Cost Analysis. *Radiology* **2000**, *215*, 45–49. [CrossRef]
27. Toki, T.; Oka, K.; Nakayama, K.; Oguchi, O.; Fujii, S. A comparative study of pre-operative procedures to assess cervical invasion by endometrial carcinoma. *Br. J. Obstet. Gynaecol.* **1998**, *105*, 512–516. [CrossRef]
28. Yang, W.T.; Lam, W.W.M.; Yu, M.Y.; Cheung, T.H.; Metreweli, C. Comparison of Dynamic Helical CT and Dynamic MR Imaging in the Evaluation of Pelvic Lymph Nodes in Cervical Carcinoma. *Am. J. Roentgenol.* **2000**, *175*, 759–766. [CrossRef] [PubMed]

29. Kim, S.H.; Kim, S.C.; Choi, B.I.; Han, M.C. Uterine cervical carcinoma: Evaluation of pelvic lymph node metastasis with MR imaging. *Radiology* **1994**, *190*, 807–811. [CrossRef] [PubMed]
30. Menczer, J. Management of endometrial carcinoma with cervical involvement. An unsettled issue. *Eur. J. Gynaecol. Oncol.* **2005**, *26*, 245–255. [PubMed]
31. Elia, G.; Garfinkel, D.A.; Goldberg, G.L.; Davidson, S.; Runowicz, C.D. Surgical management of patients with endometrial cancer and cervical involvement. *Eur. J. Gynaecol. Oncol.* **1995**, *16*, 169–173. [CrossRef] [PubMed]

Disclaimer/Publisher's Note: The statements, opinions and data contained in all publications are solely those of the individual author(s) and contributor(s) and not of MDPI and/or the editor(s). MDPI and/or the editor(s) disclaim responsibility for any injury to people or property resulting from any ideas, methods, instructions or products referred to in the content.

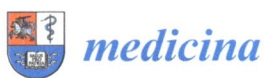 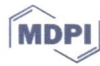

Review

Recent Advances and Adaptive Strategies in Image Guidance for Cervical Cancer Radiotherapy

Beatrice Anghel [1,2,†], Crenguta Serboiu [3,*], Andreea Marinescu [4,*], Iulian-Alexandru Taciuc [1,5], Florin Bobirca [1,6,†] and Anca Daniela Stanescu [1,7]

1. Faculty of Medicine, "Carol Davila" University of Medicine and Pharmacy, 020021 Bucharest, Romania; beatrice.anghel86@gmail.com (B.A.); alexandertaciuc@gmail.com (I.-A.T.); florin.bobirca@umfcd.ro (F.B.); stanescuancadaniela@yahoo.com (A.D.S.)
2. Department of Radiation Oncology, Sanador Oncology Centre, 010991 Bucharest, Romania
3. Department of Histology, Carol Davila University of Medicine and Pharmacy, 020021 Bucharest, Romania
4. Radiology and Imaging Department, Carol Davila University of Medicine and Pharmacy, 020021 Bucharest, Romania
5. Nuclear Medicine Department, Oncological Institute "Prof. Dr. Alexandru Trestioreanu", 022328 Bucharest, Romania
6. General Surgery Department, Cantacuzino Clinical Hospital, 73206 Bucharest, Romania
7. Department of Obstetrics and Gynecology, St. John Emergency Hospital, Bucur Maternity, 040292 Bucharest, Romania
* Correspondence: crengutas@yahoo.com (C.S.); andreea_marinescu2003@yahoo.com (A.M.)
† These authors contributed equally to this work.

Abstract: The standard of care for locally advanced cervical cancer is external beam radiotherapy (EBRT) with simultaneous chemotherapy followed by an internal radiation boost. New imaging methods such as positron-emission tomography and magnetic resonance imaging have been implemented into daily practice for better tumor delineation in radiotherapy planning. The method of delivering radiation has changed with technical advances in qualitative imaging and treatment delivery. Image-guided radiotherapy (IGRT) plays an important role in minimizing treatment toxicity of pelvic radiation and provides a superior conformality for sparing the organs at risk (OARs) such as bone marrow, bowel, rectum, and bladder. Similarly, three-dimensional image-guided adaptive brachytherapy (3D-IGABT) with computed tomography (CT) or magnetic resonance imaging (MRI) has been reported to improve target coverage and reduce the dose to normal tissues. Brachytherapy is a complementary part of radiotherapy treatment for cervical cancer and, over the past 20 years, 3D-image-based brachytherapy has rapidly evolved and established itself as the gold standard. With new techniques and adaptive treatment in cervical cancer, the concept of personalized medicine is introduced with an enhanced comprehension of the therapeutic index not only in terms of volume (three-dimensional) but during treatment too (four-dimensional). Current data show promising results with integrated IGRT and IGABT in clinical practice and, therefore, better local control and overall survival while reducing treatment-related morbidity. This review gives an overview of the substantial impact that occurred in the progress of image-guided adaptive external beam radiotherapy and brachytherapy.

Keywords: cervix cancer; image-guided brachytherapy; ART; external beam radiotherapy; IGRT

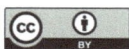

1. Introduction

Cervical cancer is one of the most common malignancies in women worldwide and one of the deadliest forms of cancer with a high burden of disease in developing nations [1,2]. Infection with high-risk subtypes of the human papillomavirus is one of the most important risk factors involved in carcinogenesis [3,4]. Programs and health policies have influenced access to different levels of prevention. The research and development of a vaccine has been proven to significantly reduce the risk of developing cervical cancer in young women [5] but, when diagnosed in advanced stages, the outcomes for cervical cancer remain concerning. The 5-year OS for patients with regional disease is approximately 55% [6,7].

Chemoradiation (CRT) followed by brachytherapy (BT) is the main treatment for locally advanced cervical cancer (LACC) [8]. The addition of concurrent chemotherapy to external beam radiotherapy (EBRT) has improved the prognosis but treatment-related toxicity and distant recurrence remain a challenge [9]. Since 1999, CRT has been recognized as the standard of care in LACC with the results of five randomized controlled phase III trials showing a benefit of 30% to 50% survival advantage by using cisplatin-based chemotherapy to radiation (GOG 85, GOG 120, SWOG 8797/ Intergroup 0107, RTOG 9001) [10–14]. Conventional radiotherapy for cervical cancer is based on cervical examination, 3D conformal radiotherapy, and 2D intracavitary brachytherapy. Definitive CRT for early-stage cervical cancer has shown excellent local control. Compared with 2D or 3D EBRT, intensity-modulated radiation therapy (IMRT) refers to delivering clinical targeted doses using multiple beam angles and field shapes while protecting normal organs such as marrow-containing pelvic bones, bowel, rectum, and bladder [15–18]. With advances in imaging modalities, 3D-IGABT with CT or MRI has been frequently used to refine target coverage and decrease the dose to normal structures [19].

With this review, we would like to emphasize the role of recent imaging tools such as PET–CT, and MRI introduced in the treatment of LACC and technological advances in IGRT and IGABT.

2. Imaging Modalities in Radiotherapy Planning
2.1. The Role of MRI

The FIGO staging is driven by clinical examination, proctoscopy, cystoscopy, and colposcopy in relation to imaging. The old system (FIGO 1999, 2009, 2014) was incorrect, with nearly one-third of stages IB-IIIB cancer being under-staged and more than half of the cases with stage IIIB cancer being over-staged [20]. Limitations have been described regarding size, level of involvement for surrounding structure, and nodal status [21]. After pelvic examination and biopsy +/− colposcopy, to obtain a better initial assessment of pelvic tumor extent, a pelvic MRI is mandatory to guide treatment options. MRI is a noninvasive investigation that can determine an accurate estimation of tumor characteristics (size, parametrial, and pelvic sidewall involvement) as well as lymph node status (pelvic and abdominal lymph nodes), with findings pointing to an accurate staging, prognosis, and treatment planning. This imaging study is vital for diagnosis, monitoring, and follow-up [22].

MRI is indispensable for radiotherapy planning for its accuracy to detect soft tissue tumor involvement and to keep tumor regression under surveillance [23]. Residual disease following EBRT is outlined on MRI for adaptive brachytherapy planning [24].

T2-weighted provides superior resolution to describe primary tumor and soft tissue invasion and for proper imaging of at least two planes (sagittal, coronal, and axial) with detection of extension into the uterus, parametria, and adjacent organs [25]. For a reliable volumetric definition of the target volume, it is relevant to visualize the cervical tumor in multiple planes. An example of collaborative work with the MRI department and Radiotherapy department, for the best interest of our patients, is reviewed in Figures 1 and 2.

In the past, the treatment plan for cervical cancer was developed based on bony landmarks using 2D planning. Analysis of previous studies with MR imaging has looked at tumor coverage with standard pelvic fields and alignment to bony anatomy resulting in geographical miss in up to 66%. MRI is crucial to ensure that the target is satisfactorily covered. When planning the treatment, an MRI should be conducted in the same position as the planned treatment with two options: MR simulation or image registration to a CT simulation. Images should be obtained with 1.5–3 T scanners with body coils. To prevent peristaltic motion, glucagon could be given intravenously prior to or during the exam. To define better, target and OARs multiplanar T2-weighted images are helpful. Improved reproducibility has been noted among experts, particularly in delimitating the parametrium once guidelines are published for delineation targets and OARs on T2-weighted MRI. With this information, MRI in a treatment position represents a standard imaging procedure for 3D conformal and IMRT planning. The large inter- and intrafraction anatomic changes of pelvic organs have an impact on both target volume coverage and dose to normal OARs. This is a factor that strongly influences EBRT precision and considerable motion can be observed between fractions due to bladder filling, rectal filling, and internal motion [26]. Great results have been achieved with the availability of MRI in brachytherapy and superior visualization of the residual tumor dimensions at the time of brachytherapy together with developments of new applicators with interstitial needles to cover laterally the parametrial involvement that would have been underdosed with classical applicator models [27].

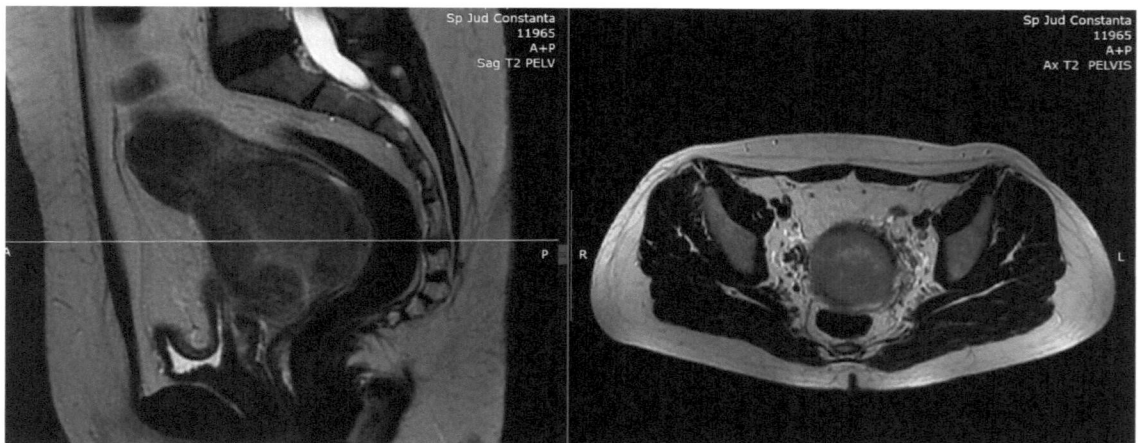

Figure 1. Patient 1 with FIGO stage IIIC2 was treated with EBRT and 3 fractions of HDR CT-based brachytherapy. T2-weighted pretreatment MRI with 6.8 × 6 × 6.2 cm hypointense vaginal wall tumor and superior 1/3 vaginal invasion, bilateral parametrial involvement—sagittal view and axial view.

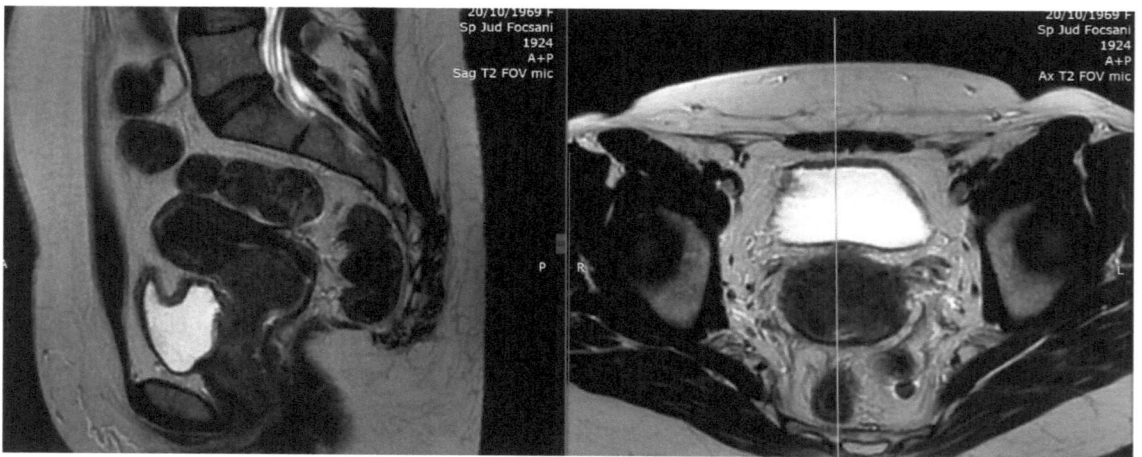

Figure 2. Patient 2 with FIGO stage IVA was treated with EBRT and 3 fractions of HDR CT-based brachytherapy. T2-weighted pretreatment MRI: 4.5 × 5 × 4.6 cm tumor indicating complete vaginal invasion up to urethral meatus and posterior bladder wall involvement—sagittal view and axial view.

Examples of residual large tumors diagnosed and treated in our institutions with MRI performed for planning brachytherapy are available in Figures 3 and 4.

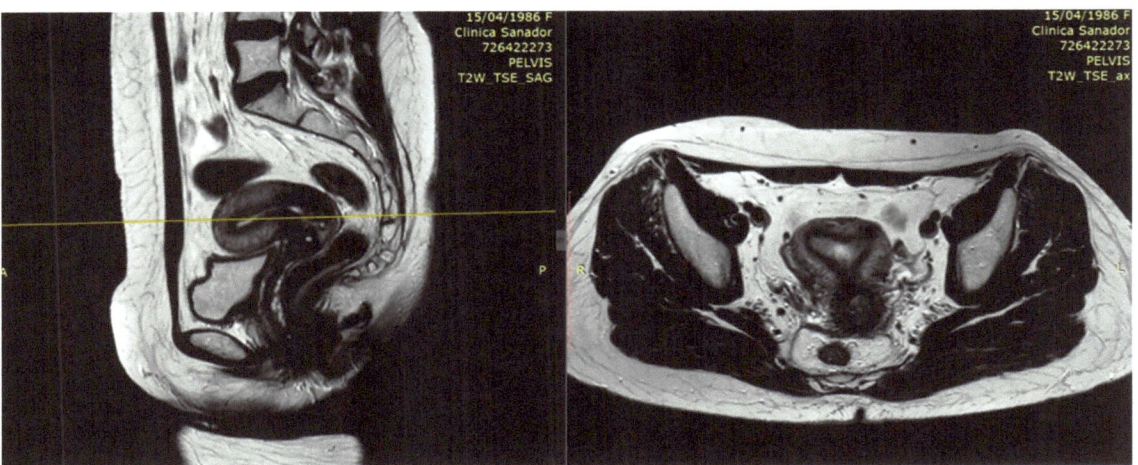

Figure 3. Patient 1 T2-weighted pre-brachytherapy MRI (5th week of CRT): 1.7 × 1.7 × 2.8 cm residual posterior cervix tumor and irregular tumor signal extending to left parametrium (parametrial invasion)—sagittal view and axial view.

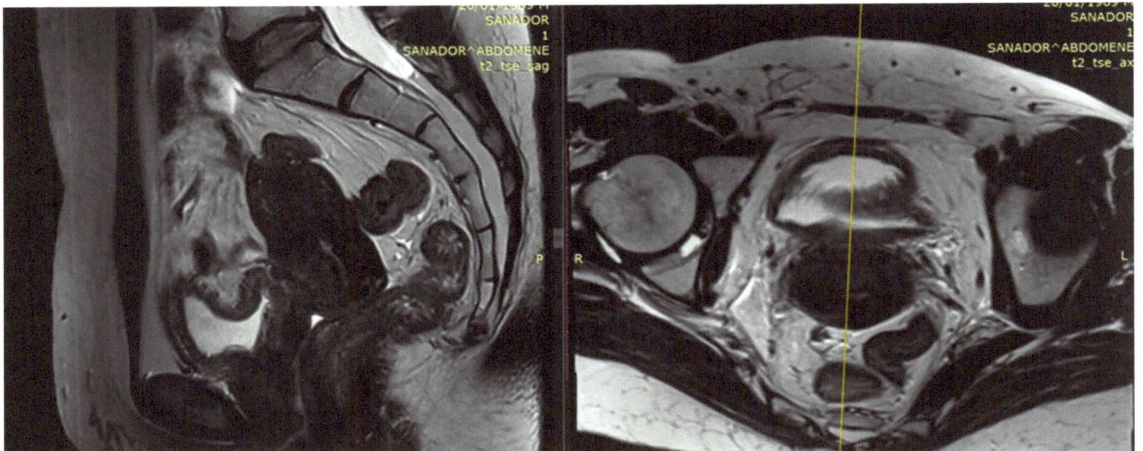

Figure 4. Patient 2 T2-weighted pre-brachytherapy MRI (5th week of CRT): residual tumor and irregular tumor signal extending to parametrium, bladder, and vaginal wall—sagittal view and axial view.

MRI has excellent accuracy to determine remaining tumor early after radiation therapy as well as disease recurrence during follow-up imaging [28]. An important challenge is to identify tumor recurrence versus post-therapy sequelae on MRI (treatment-related fibrosis, inflammation, and necrosis) in view of reducing the high false positive rates when MRI is performed within 3–8 weeks post-treatment. Correctly identifying tumor recurrence is necessary for more than 6 months between treatment and post-therapy assessment [29]. With functional MRI, such as diffusion-weighted imaging (DWI), a potential noninvasive biomarker for tumors, it has been observed that the tumor shrinks with treatment, and water mobility increases. Another indicator of tumor response that may increase and be reliable is the apparent diffusion coefficient (ADC). In more recent data, DWI-MRI is considered an early biomarker of tumor response to chemoradiation with promising results in preliminary studies, and further work is needed in this direction [30]. The availability of MRI in the diagnostic area has brought accurate information for our patients, although, due to the lack of preplanning for infrastructure and qualified personnel, it is hard to implement in radiotherapy departments after department development.

2.2. The Role of PET–CT

In cervical cancer, one of the unfavorable prognostic factors is the presence of lymph node (LN) metastasis. Compared to CT and MRI, FDG PET is more reliable for detecting pelvic and paraaortic (PA) LN metastasis [31,32]. At diagnosis, a study showed that FDG PET detected nearly half of the patients (47%) with positive LN metastasis [33]. In PET-positive LN scans, all had pelvic nodes, 35% PA, and 12% supraclavicular LN metastasis. LN detection via PET–CT could upstage the clinical staging and, therefore, modify the treatment decision and integrate the extended field for the inclusion of metastatic LN into the radiotherapy volume. Excellent local control and acceptable morbidity are offered with IMRT when the PA region is included in the radiotherapy plan [34].

In a randomized trial, 129 patients (I-IVA stages) with positive and negative PA LNs on MRI staging were randomized to have additional FDG–PET for staging or not. Patients with PA LNs FDG avid had an extended field to include LN metastasis. Seven patients had extra pelvic metastases on the PET scan, mainly paraaortic LNs. The conclusions of the study reveal the importance of two imaging modalities, such as pretreatment FDG–PET together with MRI, which can improve the detection of extra pelvic metastasis, particularly PA LNs, and facilitate the selection of cases with extended-field RT. Adding FDG–PET into the staging process has not provided a survival advantage, although the number of PA LN relapses was lower [35]. On the other hand, a more recent study by Su et al. suggests that pretreatment [18] FDG PET–CT might be linked with longer survival in patients with stage IB-IVA treated with CRT, especially in the IGRT and IGABT era [36].

A French analysis highlights the existence of false negative results in 12% of patients staged with negative PA involvement on PET–CT and found positive on laparoscopic PA lymphadenectomy [37]. There is a debate about exposing patients to potential surgical morbidity for those with a negative PET scan. There is a real potential for PET–CT to be integrated into treatment planning to increase the dose to positive LNs with a simultaneous integrated boost (SIB) technique with a perspective to improve regional control [38].

The most recent ESGO/ESTRO/ESP guidelines for the management of patients with cervical cancer—update 2023 Davida Cibula et al.—recommend that nodal status in LACC (T1b3 and higher—except T2a1) and in early-stage disease with highly suspicious LN on imaging should be investigated with a positron emission tomography–computed tomography (PET–CT) [39].

2-deoxy-2 [^{18}F] fluor-D-glucose PET–CT appears to be the best imaging modality for all stages of lymph node involvement with sensitivity and specificity of 82% and 95%, respectively [40,41], and is generally being used for radiation treatment planning in LACC. PA region is essential to be assessed, as 4–30% of patients with LACC have LN metastasis at this level, while 11% have local nodal failure after CRT, from which almost 70% are in PA LNs, as shown by the retroEMBRACE study [41,42].

PET–CT is an important diagnostic tool in LACC management and should be incorporated into the planning process to appreciate and assess the risk for lymph nodes and distant metastasis. In Figures 5 and 6, we provide images with the current role of PET–CT from our database for two different settings: pretreatment work-up and post-treatment follow-up for patients treated with EBRT and image-guided brachytherapy.

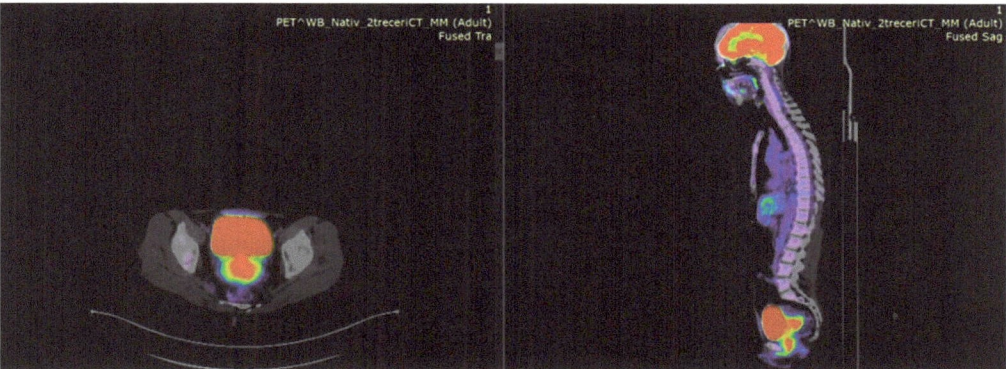

Figure 5. An example of pretreatment [^{18}F] FDG PET–CT showing a locally advanced cervical tumor with complete vaginal invasion and bladder involvement up to urethral meatus—axial view and sagittal view.

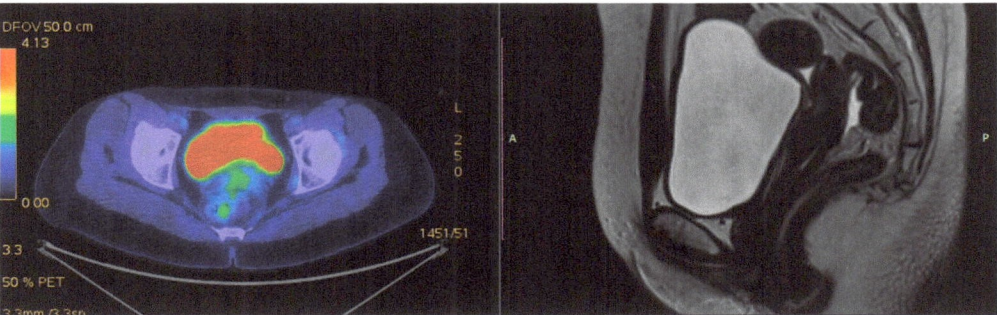

Figure 6. Post IGRT/CRT and IGABT treatment modalities in a FIGO IIIC1 case—left (axial view)—^{18}FDG PET–CT low FDG uptake (SUV max 4) and right (sagittal view)—T2-weighted MR images—no mass in the cervix with low cervical signal intensity. Colposcopy with biopsy was negative for malignancy.

3. Advances in External Beam Radiotherapy

3.1. From 2D to 3D Conformal Radiotherapy

In the past, the treatment of LACC with RT has been implemented with 2D EBRT using anatomical landmarks on X-rays to be able to encompass the primary disease and the potential spread. Two parallel opposed fields (AP–PA) were the basic techniques of EBRT. Later, the "four-field box" technique was introduced to achieve better conformality with four large treatment fields, with the upper border at the level of the aortic bifurcation (L3–L5 vertebral body levels; T12 level in case of extended field in case of paraaortic nodes being involved), the anterior border placed anteriorly to the pubic symphysis, and another border posteriorly outlining the sacrum at the S3/S4 level.

The lateral borders are 1.5–2cm lateral to the pelvic brim and the inferior border is the bottom of the obturator foramen. Although easy to implement in practice, geographical misses have led to reduced LC [43]. CT invention was brought into RT planning after the 1990s, marking the evolution from 2D to 3D conformal RT. Based on the information obtained from a CT scan of the patient imaged in the same position for treatment and in a reproducible way has helped clinicians, physicists, and radiation therapists to understand concepts related to target delineation—gross tumor volume (GTV), clinical target volume (CTV), and planning target volume (PTV)—published in ICRU Report 50 and ICRU Report

62 [44,45]. This technique utilizes anatomical landmarks to better shape the dose distribution of the PTV with the protection of OARs with multileaf collimators (MLCs) [46]. Three-dimensional conformal RT provides volumetric dosimetry and has the advantage of quantifying and correlating treatment outcomes and toxicities.

3.2. Intensity-Modulated Radiotherapy (IMRT) Volumetric Intensity-Modulated Arcs (VMAT)

IMRT is a radiotherapy technique that warrants rigorous conformation of the radiation dose to the target volume. Through IMRT, there is potential to significantly reduce long-term morbidity and improve local control. Compared with conventional EBRT, IMRT uses small beamlets with variable intensity and better conformality to 3D target volumes while minimizing the dose to critical adjacent structures. In 2002, excellent results have been reported with the initial implementation of IMRT for women with gynecological cancers.

TIME-C, Uterus-11, PARCER, INTERTECC-2, Huang et al., and Ghandi et al. are numerous major studies involving advances in radiation therapy techniques with significant lower bowel and bladder toxicity [47–50]. Emerging evidence has shifted the balance increasingly in favor of the ordinary use of IMRT. IMRT can be given via multiple static fields or in arcs, a newer radiation technique known as volumetric intensity-modulated arc radiation therapy (VMAT). Conformality, faster treatment time, and fewer monitor units are some of the main advantages offered by VMAT.

IGRT can deliver a higher dose to the primary tumor and areas at high risk for recurrence with the SIB technique without exposing adjacent normal organs to radiation.

IMRT on a routine basis faces issues such as organ movement during RT (intrafraction) and during treatment (interfraction). Jadon et al. [51] reported that organ motion in EBRT for cervical cancer is present and the degree of movement during radiation therapy should be considered. Bladder and rectal filling influence uterine and cervical motion [52].

As pelvic organ motion seems to be patient-specific, personalized PTV margins and adaptive image-guided radiotherapy (IGRT) have been proposed to cover accurately the target volume while enlarging the normal tissues' protection. As IMRT planning can spare normal OARs, IMRT plans and SIB of LNs are a great strategy to reduce radiation-induced normal tissue complication probability while improving outcomes in a shorter overall treatment time.

3.3. Adaptive External Beam Radiotherapy

IGRT is a dynamic complex process of performing imaging before daily radiotherapy with the intent of achieving target accuracy and precision by correcting geometric and anatomic variations. IGRT techniques consist of planar or volumetric imaging to obtain tighter treatment margins. Highly conformal techniques such as IMRT and stereotactic body radiotherapy (SBRT) demand a high level of setup reproducibility to ensure that the planned dose is delivered to the interest area. Planar IGRT techniques compare 2D radiographs in the same treatment position with digitally reconstructed radiographs (DRR), images obtained from simulation. This allows accurate matching of the radiograph from simulation on bony anatomy with the radiograph from treatment. Volumetric IGRT techniques provide 3D imaging comparable with the initial simulation imaging to check position. This allows for soft tissue and bony anatomy as well (volumetric IGRT: cone-beam CT, CT on rails, and megavoltage CT imaging) [53].

IGRT plays a central role in modern radiotherapy, especially for hypofractionation and stereotactic treatments. It can boost confidence that radiotherapy treatment is in the desired size and margins can be tailored when appropriate. Many factors can determine anatomic deformations to the tumor and OARs throughout a course of treatment:

Firstly, anatomic motion is caused by the system (e.g., musculoskeletal, gastrointestinal, genito-urinary, cardiac, and respiratory).

Secondly, the treatment-induced changes such as tumor reduction, regrowth resulting from accelerated repopulation, weight gain or loss, concomitant chemotherapy, and fibrosis of normal structures.

It can happen at three levels: offline between sessions, online immediately prior to treatment, and real-time during radiotherapy. Based on a predetermined set of scenarios, simple forms of adaptive radiotherapy apply correct measures and will define the concept of a multiadaptive image-guided radiation therapy (IGRT) plan.

In LACC, the uterus and cervix change position during treatment delivery due to variations in rectal and bladder filling and tumor shrinkage during RT [53]. Deformable image registration for transferring anatomic contours and dose between images are described in recent practice advances for forms of adaptive radiotherapy and software tools to analyze automatic treatment planning and deformable dose summation [54].

Adaptive radiotherapy is defined as a temporal adjustment of the treatment plan delivery to a patient, according to objective anatomic changes caused by weight loss, tumor shrinkage, or internal motion (Figures 7 and 8).

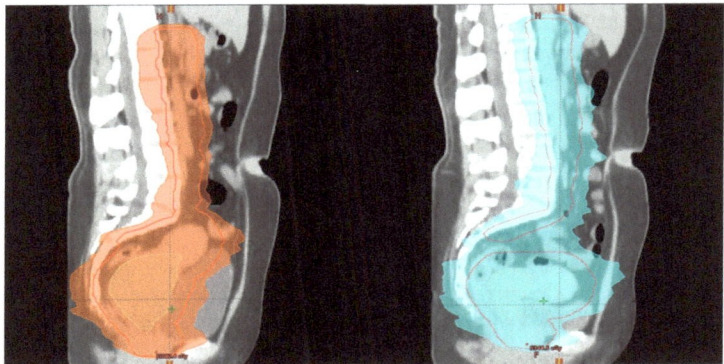

Figure 7. Patient 1 with FIGO stage IIIC2 LACC: **left** image (week 1)—initial plan of EBRT and **right** image (week 3) during EBRT—adaptive planning (sagittal view) for tumor shrinkage.

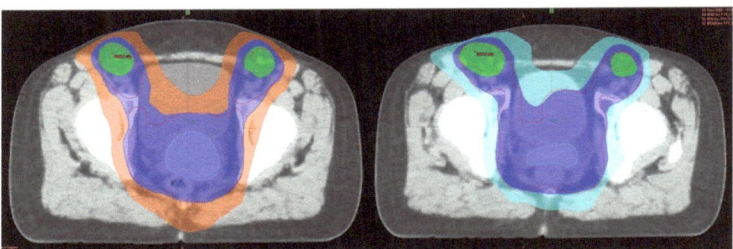

Figure 8. Patient 1 with FIGO stage IIIC2 LACC: **left** image (week 1)—initial plan of EBRT and **right** image (week 3) during EBRT—adaptive planning (axial view) for tumor shrinkage.

A new concept of internal target volume (ITV) is generated to account for various treatment positions for LACC by performing a simulation with a full and an empty bladder and then combining the CTV to be taken into consideration for every move between these two bladder filling extremes [55]. A margin between 3 and 7 mm (PTV) is added to the ITV to fully encompass setup and position errors. Then, volumetric IGRT is applied with cone beam CT (CBCT) to verify the position of the CTV and PTV daily prior to RT delivery. More advanced adaptive strategies have made space for a highly advanced work for treatment delivery called "plan of the day" or "online adaptive RT". These approaches include same-day replanning and recently published review articles are available in the literature [56].

In special scenarios, after paraaortic exploration or hernia repairs, open or laparoscopic, it is vital to use IGRT techniques to protect the wound and prevent complications or even delays in starting radiotherapy for LACC [57].

4. Advances in Brachytherapy

4.1. From 2D Brachytherapy (2D-BT) to 3D Image-Guided Adaptive Brachytherapy (3D-IGABT)

Brachytherapy is an essential component of the treatment of LACC in addition to concurrent CRT. Internal radiation therapy allows an important dose escalation to the gross tumor with the advantage of rapid dose fall-off. This dosimetry analysis shows effective dose coverage of the target while protecting the OARs through technical adjustments of implants (hybrid implants with intracavitary and interstitial needles) and multi-parametric 3D treatment planning [58]. Intracavitary brachytherapy (IC BT) can be accomplished using low dose rate (LDR), pulsed dose rate (PDR), or high dose rate (HDR) sources. HDR has the advantage of exposing the patient care team to less radiation than LDR and there is a need for fewer logistic measures dedicated to source storage and fewer radiation safety measures compared to LDR.

There is an increased risk of exposure, for example, by selecting the inappropriate source strength when retrieving source capsules from storage or incorrect order when implanting sources. For these reasons, IC BT has changed to HDR delivery using remote after-loaders. HDR with a treatment planning process by a computer could optimize the dose to target critical structures. HDR treatments are evaluated using conversion to radio-biologically equivalent doses (EQD2) integrated into clinical practice with caution that comes with model-based conversion (see American Brachytherapy Society Excel worksheet to convert HDR doses to 2Gy equivalent doses). The Manchester system, first introduced in 1938 and then modified in 1953, has established the brachytherapy dose prescription to a specific point; point A was defined as a point 2 cm lateral to the center of the uterine canal and 2 cm superior to the mucosa of the lateral fornix. Later, this system was modified to be relative to the brachytherapy applicator itself to be better visualized on X-ray, which was defined as 2 cm superior to the external cervical ostium and 2 cm lateral to the tandem portion of the applicator [59,60]. Personalization of treatment planning and target-based dose prescription are concepts described in modern BT.

Several options are available: ring and tandem or tandem and ovoid devices, both with the possibility of increasing the complexity of the implant, from an IC one to a hybrid approach (IC plus interstitial needles). The rationale for this mixed approach depends on tumor location, size, and degree of vaginal extent. IC device is recommended for small tumors (<3 cm), with minimal extension into the vagina and no parametrial disease.

When a tumor is large, irregular in shape, and has parametrial involvement, then a hybrid IC/IS can be a better solution with superior dosimetry. In the scenario where a tumor is very large, with extensive vaginal and parametrial involvement and sometimes adjacent organ involvement (e.g., bladder or rectum), interstitial therapy is recommended. For IGABT treatment planning, MRI or CT can be used with significant advantages over point-based planning and there are consensus guidelines for IGBT target delineation [61].

MRI near the time of brachytherapy is an asset and can be used for the identification of GTV. The dose prescribed is to the contouring volume formed by high-risk CTV, which includes GTV, the entire cervix, and macroscopic extension or parametrial involvement. After 45 Gy in 25 treatments to the pelvis (common dose), fractionation schemes to achieve more than 80 Gy Eqd2, including 7 Gy × 4 fractions, 8 Gy × 3 fractions, and 5.5–6 Gy × 5 fractions. Numerous institutional series have showed great results with limited toxicity. In 2008, a prospective observational study was initiated, called EMBRACE, to analyze outcomes from the application of MRI-based IGBT in a multicenter, international population according to Gynecological Groupe Européen de Curiethérapie and the European Society for Radiotherapy & Oncology (Gyn GEC—ESTRO) standards [62,63].

As we know, numerous studies show that IMRT/3D–IGABT is linked to improved survival and reduced gastrointestinal and genitourinary toxicity in patients with LACC compared with those who received 2D EBRT/BT [64,65]. The RetroEMBRACE cohort, an international observational cohort, enrolled 852 patients treated with IGBT prior to participation in EMBRACE [66].

Institutions' MRI-based IGRT users apply GEC—ESTRO recommendations [62] and institutions using CT IGRT are instructed to contour only high-risk CTV [66]. The MRI-based IGBT cohort has a 95% local control at 3 years for < 5 cm tumors, while 85% for tumors > 5 cm. The 3- and 5-year OS rates were 74% and 65%; it is notable that 70% of the overall deaths were due to recurrent disease. Within the Embrace I study, excellent outcomes have been reported, with 51 months being the median follow-up and actuarial 5-year local control was 92% (95% CI 90–93%), with similar local control across all FIGO stages [67]. Local failures in lymph nodes or distant failures occur about half of the time and most local failures have been exposed within the high-risk CTV or intermediate-risk CTV, correlating a dose-dependent relationship [68].

The primary target dosimetry goal was an EQD2 of 85 Gy, assuming an α/β ratio of 10. EMBRACE I early results support the use of combined IC/IS BT, particularly for larger tumors, to reach the target dose with an acceptable toxicity profile [69].

Results from a cancer center in Romania with high addressability of patients with cervical cancer discuss the need to implement the hybrid IC/IS IGABT approach to fulfill the requirements for dose targets and respect surrounding normal tissue constraints [70]. A prospective French STIC trial [71] randomized patients between 2D and 3D BT planning and showed that 3D IGABT is recommended, effective, and safe, with better local control and grade 3–4 toxicity reduced to half, favoring IGABT. In the EMBRACE II cohort, dosimetry and planning advanced features were implemented for patients with FIGO IB-IVA disease with EBRT and IG-IMRT to 45 Gy/25 treatments with MRI-based IGABT with concurrent cisplatin.

Figures 9 and 10 show sample images from a patient treated with a combined IC/IS approach (Figure 9) and then with an intracavitary BT technique (Figure 10) with CT-based image guidance. This is an image-based HDR BT plan for a 64-year-old woman with FIGO IIIC2 cervical cancer (FIGO 2018). After EBRT with concurrent cisplatin, the plan was to receive a brachytherapy boost of 24 Gy in three fractions. She underwent first and second fractions with a combined technique (Figure 9), consisting of a ring and tandem applicator supplemented by the placement of four interstitial needles. The legend shows the isodose curves (colored lines) with a dose-expressed color wash. Not to prolong her OTT while recovering from her low platelet count, she received her last treatment, an IC BT implant (Figure 10).

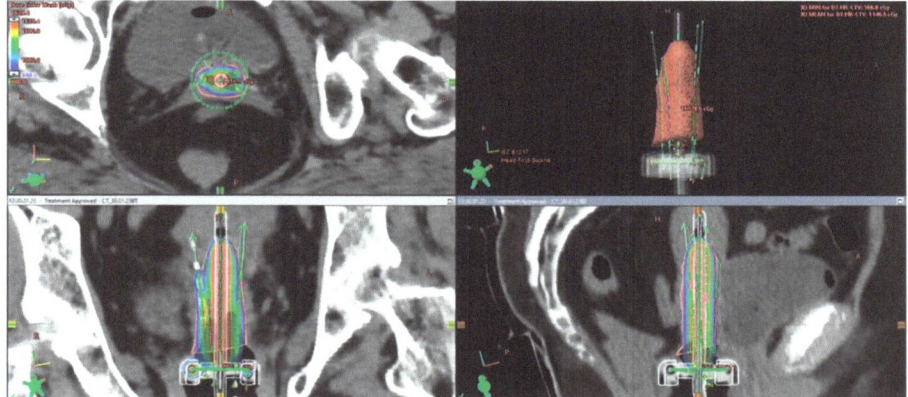

Figure 9. Combined approach (IC + IS). In this example of FIGO IIIC2, a large cervical tumor at presentation with bilateral parametrial involvement and lower uterine segment infiltration and partial response to treatment pre-brachytherapy with residual tumor to the inner third of parametria bilaterally led to the decision to choose a combined approach (implant representation ring and uterine tandem with 4 needles).

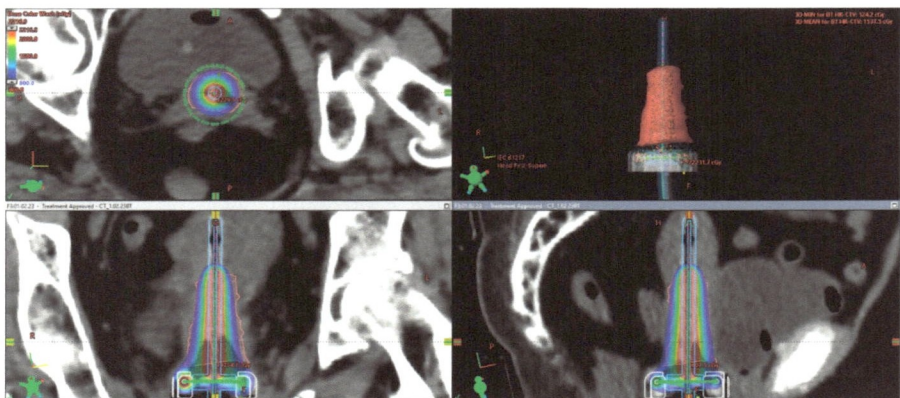

Figure 10. IC approach. The rationale for intracavitary application for the same patient as described in Figure 9: for the last procedure, due to poor blood results (severe thrombocytopenia), the decision was made for an intracavitary approach in order not to prolong overall treatment time (implant representation ring and uterine tandem).

4.2. Adaptive Brachytherapy

The initial implementation of BT in cervical cancer has started with point A dose prescription 2D X-ray dose planning together with standard dose distributions. Unfortunately, point A is a poor substitute for evaluating the dose to a 4-dimensional (4D) target. GEC–ESTRO recommendations introduced image-based target assessment and possibilities to improve prescription, optimization, and dose reporting in a reproducible way. IGABT is conducted in the last 2–3 weeks of an overall treatment time of 7 weeks (50–56 days considered a time constraint) to make the most of the advantage of tumor regression. Tumor regression is more limited in the last weeks, and it may lead to underestimated tumor dose in case the same dose planning concept is applied for all fractions of BT because of the potential reduction of tumors in the high-risk volume. The concepts of "high risk" CTV and "intermediate risk" CTV are implemented in modern BT and are residual gross disease at BT time and, respectively, potential microscopic residual disease. For each BT fraction, there is potential through image-guided dose optimization to spare OARs by tailoring the dose to the target. Significant OAR movement has been observed and it has been highlighted in dosimetry analysis to adjust a repeat adaptive planning for each BT treatment [72,73].

The report released in 2018 by the EMBRACE II study reviewed the outcome and prospect of two decades of progress within the GEC—ESTRO Gyn working group. MRI-guided adaptive BT with combined IC/IS techniques is incorporated within the study and specific dose-volume constraints are recommended for adaptive targets and OARs, for EBRT image guidance for specific targets and techniques (IMRT, IGRT, and SIB for nodal disease), and concurrent CRT. The new concept described is IGABT for its precise delivery of the dose target and excellent protection of OARs. Taking into consideration the time-consuming procedure and the resources needed, IGABT contributes to a reduction in OTT by increasing the fraction size. Another measure adopted is to finish the treatment of EBRT and BT in 7 weeks [74,75].

MRI is the preferred image modality and gold standard for superior soft tissue contrast. The concept of IGABT is based on two main topics: imaging at the time of BT with the applicator in situ and then the same dose planning on the anatomy as the dose delivered.

An adaptive approach results in two major steps: (1) the right applicator to the anatomy and (2) 3D dose optimization with the advantage of having the applicator in situ. Inserting the suitable applicator results in a direct relation between the radioactive source and the topography. For example, in a small tumor, IC BT could be the right choice but, in large tumors with poor response, IC applicator and interstitial component are suitable [76,77]. Another fundamental change with IGABT is the improvement in dose for high-risk CTV, especially for large tumors, with suboptimal dose coverage by 85 Gy EQD2 with standard nonoptimized IC BT (Figures 10 and 11).

3D-IGABT compared with 2D-BT techniques shows a superior safety profile and efficacy in terms of LC. The up-to-date standard for BT is MR image guidance. The major advantage is the dose conformality given by BT regarding both the volume (3D) and the time (4D) [78]. Before each implant, repetitive imaging gives the possibility to adapt the dose to the tumor volume in regression.

A recent systematic review and meta-analysis by Kim et al. have highlighted the important data in the EMBRACE II study stating that 3D-IGABT is a cost-effective option supporting routine use in the treatment of LACC [79–82]. A multidisciplinary team is involved and includes a radiation oncologist, physicists, anesthesiologist, radiation therapists, and nurses. This holistic approach can integrate artificial intelligence (AI) systems to develop algorithms to perform a safe and efficient procedure. Due to current developments, it is important to bring AI as a possible guardship against intraoperative anaphylaxis [83].

Based on the large application of 3D-IGABT for cervical cancer, the ICRU/GEC—ESTRO launched Report 89, with a focus on adaptive brachytherapy. The concept of 4D (four-dimensional) image-guided adaptive brachytherapy (4D-IGABT) is a new approach with great clinical results and has included the 4D concept, which is formed by three spatial dimensions and time. The four-dimensional IGABT design improves the efficacy-to-toxicity ratio by exploiting the tumor-volume reduction commonly seen in cervical cancer after the first part of treatment. Numerous factors should be considered in real-life practice, such as tumor regression, internal organ motion, and organ filling. The main objective of this concept is a more precise treatment through adaptive contouring, imaging, and replanning, replacement of the applicator, and the addition of the interstitial needles while quality assurance procedures are checked simultaneously.

In Figures 11 and 12, we would like to emphasize our work on an HDR CT-based BT plan for a 14-year-old girl with FIGO IIIC2 cervical cancer (FIGO 2018). After EBRT with simultaneous cisplatin, she underwent a brachytherapy boost of 24 Gy in three fractions with a combined technique (Figure 11), consisting of a ring and tandem applicator supplemented by the placement of eight interstitial needles. The legend shows the isodose curves (colored lines) with dose-expressed color wash (see Figure 12).

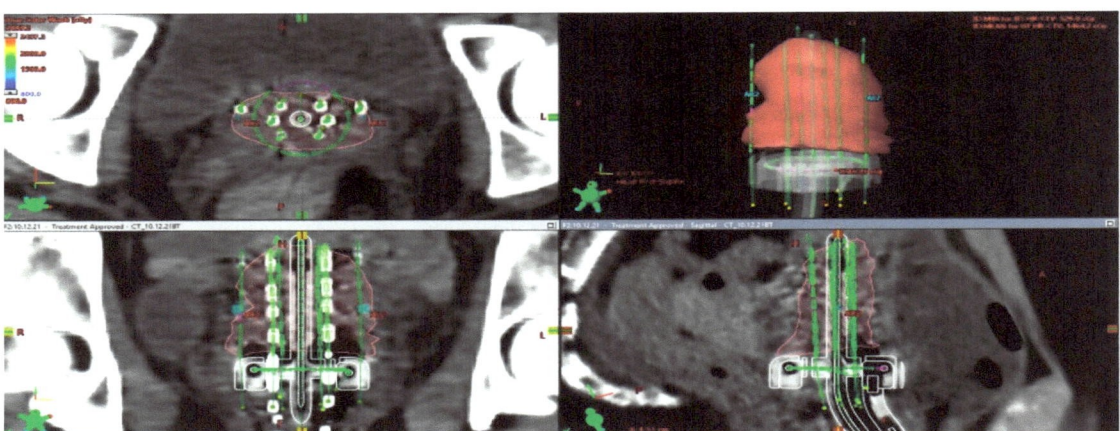

Figure 11. Rationale for interstitial application. In this example, bilateral parametrial involvement at the time of diagnosis and residual tumor to the inner third of parametria bilaterally led to a decision to choose a hybrid approach (implant representation ring and uterine tandem with 8 needles).

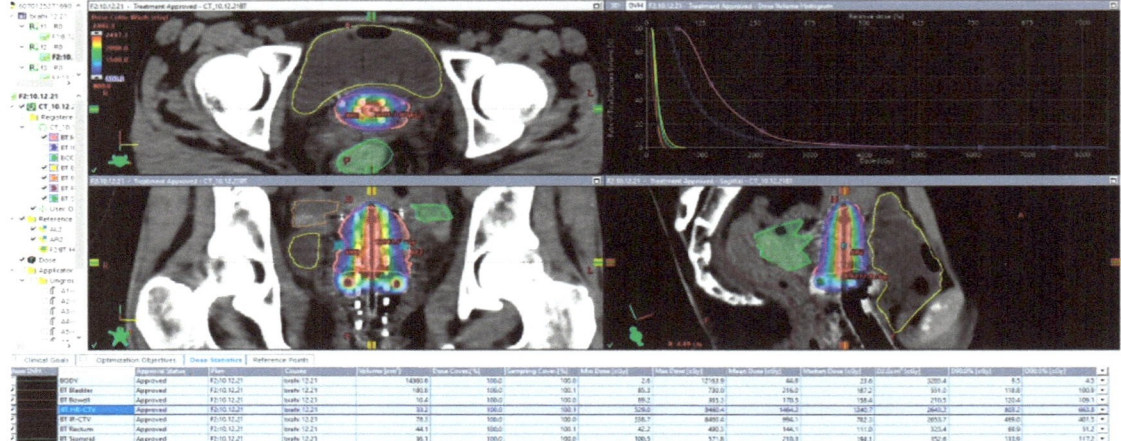

Figure 12. Implant representation ring and uterine tandem with 8 needles with isodose curves–tumor coverage and OARs representation.

5. New Modalities of Radiation Techniques

5.1. MRI-LINAC Using Adaptive Radiotherapy

The MR-LINAC is a ground-breaking system with an extensive care path that has the potential to revolutionize cancer treatment, refine treatment, and enable radiotherapy for hard-to-treat cancers [84]. Magnetic resonance imaging-guided radiotherapy (MRgRT) outlines the greatest potential to achieve the therapeutic gains of image-guided delivery of planned radiation dose. Major advances are noticed with the agility of the MRI LINAC to capture tumors and OARs with on-table MRI, to ensure motion management and delivery of the dose prescribed in real-time, and then to adapt the plan on the same day of the treatment while the patient is on the machine table [85,86]. Imaging for therapy guidance, real-time imaging, and gating for intrafractional management are the main topics analyzed. A brand-new concept is adaptive treatment planning for interfractional management.

This increased eligibility for RT or opportunity for reirradiation leads to improved quality of life for more patients. Dynamic real-time adaptation provides the ability to tailor each MRI-guided radiation therapy based on anatomical changes in size, shape, and position of the tumor or near organs. Diagnostic quality MRI with precise radiation delivery allows treatment dose to be escalated and the tumor to be visualized at every moment, leading to increased protection of normal organs, and providing opportunities for better outcomes and fewer side effects [87].

5.2. 3D Printing in Cervical Cancer Brachytherapy

To perform brachytherapy, an applicator is needed, a medical device that decreases the radiation received by medical personnel. Interstitial brachytherapy can utilize a transperineal template, which has several hollows, allowing guiding tubes to be inserted directly into the tumor or nearby. After-loading and interstitial brachytherapy are appropriate for cervical cancer due to anatomy and the location in the proximity of the cervical tumor. The basic concept remains to deliver a high dose to the cervical target tumor area while protecting OARs. CT and MRI are frequent imaging tools in cervical cancer brachytherapy and significant progress has been made with technology, software, and image guidance. 3D image guidance in cervical cancer brachytherapy can improve local control and minimize radiation effects in OARs. However, 3D-IGABT needs to be implemented by an experienced physician to manipulate the right applicator, insert it at the right position, and revisit all different patient tumor characteristic scenarios, such as size and location. Occasionally, it can be quite difficult to achieve individual treatment by conventional after-loading or interstitial brachytherapy.

Recent gynecological brachytherapy groups are offering high expectations with the application of 3D printing technology in order to solve this issue and ensure personalized treatment with the potential to improve survival rates. With respect to accurate radiotherapy, personalized RT products can be created for each patient by using 3D printing technology. Personalized products can be designed using this technology to perform preoperative planning. The major objective would be to display tumor shape in an anatomic relationship between the tumor and surrounding structures. The next step will be manufacturing a personalized guidance template. Getting the right optimization from needle positions will translate into favorable target dose distributions. Current advances are upgrading the common applicator to an individual design applicator to fit the patient's anatomy and achieve optimal accuracy in dose distribution. A few challenges are described in Huo et al.'s review: 3D-printing materials, 3D-printing model construction, and dose distribution calculation [88,89]. The application of a 3D-printing individualized applicator and template could have enormous potential to improve accuracy in brachytherapy in clinical practice.

6. Future Directions

Based on clinical evidence and guidelines in the literature, real data are available for clinical implementation in gynecological cancers in the era of pelvic IGRT for routine practice. General recommendations are made for the implementation of an institutional pelvic IGRT protocol. Specific features include consistency between treatment intent and the IGRT approach with consideration for minimum national and international IGRT guidance when daily volumetric IGRT is applied. It is important that appointed appropriate health professionals (RTTs) lead on undertaking IGRT with continuous professional development. An IGRT workflow procedure must be clear and, when difficult cases are encountered, the process can be escalated with transparency and strategic directions. Before implementing advanced adaptive strategies, it is mandatory to ensure a robust IGRT service is already in place [90].

Overall, IGABT has significant improvements in local control for all stages in LACC, particularly with 3D and 4D adaptive measures. However, there is potential for further advances in IGABT with hybrid approaches at the time of BT. Unfortunately, cervical cancer is diagnosed in large numbers and with a significant burden of disease in low- and middle-income countries. The need for brachytherapy equipment, imaging modalities, access to treatment, and state-of-the-art options remains a problem and different approaches and workflows must be adopted for these patients. A few ongoing studies mention the use of concurrent CRT plus BT in combination with immune checkpoint inhibitors in patients with LACC, but limited data are available on the sequence of treatments and overall efficacy and safety.

There are promising ways to refine adaptive radiotherapy in both limited and LACC, tailoring the treatment to the individual patient, tumor burden, and response. Furthermore, it is known that there are important changes in the tumor microenvironment and biological factors are investigated for response to radiation. Radiomics has shown promise in precision medicine and advances are reported that will become a valuable tool for the clinical arena. Additional progress in this direction will offer a possibility to provide, in the future, an assessment of tumor characteristics with personalized biological dose planning and dose painting. Cone beam CT quality and the integration of MR-guided EBRT and BT will need technological developments.

7. Conclusions

Imaging modalities are rapidly integrated into current practice in modern radiotherapy for cervical cancer, in work-up radiological investigations, and in treatment delineation, planning, and delivery of radiation. FDG–PET is a valuable imaging tool in LN status definition for cervical cancer. Regarding treatment planning in radiotherapy, PET offers advantages in tumor delineation and defines the real impact of this imaging modality in radiation treatment planning and further treatment decision-making.

MRI remains an important diagnostic tool in pretreatment work-up and its role is obtaining exceptional results in tumor delineation for EBRT and in IGABT, providing higher spatial soft tissue resolution. The general tumoral description and extension depicted by MRI include a more accurate assessment of tumor size (due to multiplanar evaluation), which could reduce staging morbidity, and, therefore, superior results in terms of toxicity post-treatment.

IGRT and IGABT are promising technique tools that can achieve greater local control while reducing complication rates in LACC patients. These modalities are complementary and should be implemented in prospective trials with a move towards a more personalized line of action. Technology advances with superior imaging together with magnetic-resonance-guided radiation therapy and 3D printing in IGABT may hold the greatest potential to improve treatment and reduce potential side effects.

Although there is a possibility to introduce adaptive strategies with clinical benefit, several improvements in automated planning, quality assurance, and imaging quality need to be developed.

Author Contributions: Conceptualization, B.A. and C.S.; methodology, A.M.; software, I.-A.T.; validation, B.A., F.B. and A.D.S.; formal analysis, C.S.; investigation, A.M.; resources, I.-A.T.; data curation, F.B.; writing—original draft preparation, B.A.; writing—review and editing, A.D.S.; visualization, C.S.; supervision, A.M.; project administration, F.B.; funding acquisition, A.D.S. All authors have read and agreed to the published version of the manuscript.

Funding: This research received no external funding.

Institutional Review Board Statement: Not applicable because it is a review.

Informed Consent Statement: Informed consent was obtained from all subjects used to illustrate the review. Written informed consent has been obtained from the patient(s) to publish this review.

Data Availability Statement: Data are available upon request from the corresponding authors.

Conflicts of Interest: The authors declare no conflict of interest.

Abbreviations

ADC	apparent diffusion coefficients
BT	brachytherapy
CBCT	cone beam computed tomography
CI	confidence interval
CRT	chemo-radiotherapy
CT	computed tomography
CTV	clinical target volume
DCE MRI	dynamic contrast-enhanced MRI
DW-MRI	diffusion-weighted MRI
DFS	disease free survival
DRR	digitally reconstructed radiograph
EBRT	external beam radiotherapy
EMBRACE	European study on MRI-guided brachytherapy in locally advanced cervical cancer
EQD2	biologically equivalent dose in 2 Gy fractions
FDG	fluorodeoxyglucose
FIGO	International Federation of Gynaecology and Obstetrics
GEC-	The Groupe Européen de Curiethérapie and the European society for ESTRO radiotherapy & oncology
GOG	Gynecologic Oncology Group
GTV	gross tumor volume
HDR	high dose rate
HR CTV	high risk clinical target volume

ICRU	International Comission on Radiation Units and Measurements
IGABT	image-guided adaptive brachytherapy
IGRT	image-guided radiotherapy
IMRT	intensity modulated radiation therapy
IR CTV	intermediate risk clinical target volume
ITV	internal target volume
LACC	locally advanced cervical cancer
LC	local control
LDR	low dose rate
LINAC	linear accelerator
LN	lymph node
MLC	multileaf collimator
MRI	magnetic resonance imaging
OARs	organs at risk
OS	overall survival
OTT	overall treatment time
PA	paraaortic
PDR	pulsed dose rate
PET	positron emission tomography
PTV	planning target volume
RTOG	Radiation Therapy Oncology Group
SIB	simultaneous integrated boost
SWOG	Southwest Oncology Group
T	Tesla

References

1. Arbyn, M.; Weiderpass, E.; Bruni, L.; de Sanjosé, S.; Saraiya, M.; Ferlay, J.; Bray, F. Estimates of incidence and mortality of cervical cancer in 2018: A worldwide analysis. *Lancet Glob. Health* **2020**, *8*, E191–E203. [CrossRef] [PubMed]
2. Brenner, D.R.; Weir, H.K.; Demers, A.A.; Ellison, L.F.; Louzado, C.; Shaw, A.; Turner, D.; Woods, R.R.; Smith, L.M. Canadian Cancer Statistics Advisory Committee. *CMAJ* **2020**, *192*, E199–E205. [CrossRef] [PubMed]
3. Otter, S.; Whitaker, S.; Chatterjee, J.; Stewart, A. The human papillomavirus as a common pathogen in oropharyngeal, anal, and cervical cancers. *Clin. Oncol.* **2019**, *31*, 81–90. [CrossRef] [PubMed]
4. Walboomers, J.M.M.; Jacobs, M.V.; Manos, M.M.; Bosch, F.X.; Kummer, J.A.; Shah, K.V.; Snijders, P.J.; Peto, J.; Meijer, C.J.; Muñoz, N. Human papillomavirus is a necessary cause of invasive cervical cancer worldwide. *J. Pathol.* **1999**, *189*, 12–19. [CrossRef]
5. Lei, J.; Ploner, A.; Elfström, K.M.; Wang, J.; Roth, A.; Fang, F.; Sundström, K.; Dillner, J.; Sparén, P. HPV Vaccination and the Risk of Invasive Cervical Cancer. *N. Engl. J. Med.* **2020**, *383*, 1340–1348. [CrossRef] [PubMed]
6. Benard, V.B.; Watson, M.; Saraiya, M.; Harewood, R.; Townsend, J.S.; Stroup, A.M.; Weir, H.K.; Allemani, C. Cervical cancer survival in the United States by race and stage (2001–2009): Findings from the CONCORD-2 study. *Cancer* **2017**, *123* (Suppl. 24), 5119–5137. [CrossRef]
7. Han, K.; Milosevic, M.; Fyles, A.; Pintilie, M.; Viswanathan, A.N. Trends in the utilization of brachytherapy in cervical cancer in the United States. *Int. J. Radiat. Oncol. Biol. Phys.* **2013**, *87*, 111–119. [CrossRef]
8. Cervical Cancer Version 1.2024. Available online: https://www.nccn.org/professionals/physician_gls/pdf/cervical.pdf (accessed on 22 August 2023).
9. Vale, C.; Tierney, J.F.; Stewart, L.A.; Brady, M.; Dinshaw, K.; Jakobsen, A. Chemoradiotherapy for Cervical Cancer Meta-Analysis Collaboration. Reducing uncertainties about the effects of chemoradiotherapy for cervical cancer: A systematic review and meta-analysis of individual patient data from 18 randomized trials. *J. Clin. Oncol.* **2008**, *26*, 5802–5812.
10. Morris, M.; Eifel, P.J.; Lu, J.; Grigsby, P.W.; Levenback, C.; Stevens, R.E.; Rotman, M.; Gershenson, D.M.; Mutch, D.G. Pelvic radiation with concurrent chemotherapy compared with pelvic and para-aortic radiation for high-risk cervical cancer. *N. Engl. J. Med.* **1999**, *340*, 1137–1143. [CrossRef]
11. Keys, H.M.; Bundy, B.N.; Stehman, F.B.; Muderspach, L.I.; Chafe, W.E.; Suggs, C.L.; Walker, J.L.; Gersell, D. Cisplatin, radiation, and adjuvant hysterectomy compared with radiation and adjuvant hysterectomy for bulky stage IB cervical carcinoma. *N. Engl. J. Med.* **1999**, *340*, 1154–1161. [CrossRef]
12. Whitney, C.W.; Sause, W.; Bundy, B.N.; Malfetano, J.H.; Hannigan, E.V.; Fowler, W.C.; Clarke-Pearson, D.L.; Liao, S.Y. Randomized comparison of fluorouracil plus cisplatin versus hydroxyurea as an adjunct to radiation therapy in stage IIB-IVA carcinoma of the cervix with negative para-aortic lymph nodes: A Gynecologic Oncology Group and Southwest Oncology Group study. *J. Clin. Oncol.* **1999**, *17*, 1339–1348. [CrossRef] [PubMed]
13. Peters, W.A., III; Liu, P.Y.; Barrett, R.J.; Stock, R.J.; Monk, B.J.; Berek, J.S.; Souhami, L.; Grigsby, P.; Gordon, W., Jr.; Alberts, D.S. Concurrent chemotherapy and pelvic radiation therapy compared with pelvic radiation therapy alone as adjuvant therapy after radical surgery in high-risk early-stage cancer of the cervix. *J. Clin. Oncol.* **2000**, *18*, 1606–1613. [CrossRef] [PubMed]

14. Rose, P.G.; Bundy, B.N.; Watkins, E.B.; Thigpen, J.T.; Deppe, G.; Maiman, M.A.; Clarke-Pearson, D.L.; Insalaco, S. Concurrent cisplatin-based radiotherapy and chemotherapy for locally advanced cervical cancer. *N. Engl. J. Med.* **1999**, *340*, 1144–1153. [CrossRef] [PubMed]
15. Mundt, A.J.; Lujan, A.E.; Rotmensch, J.; Waggoner, S.E.; Yamada, S.D.; Fleming, G.; Roeske, J.C. Intensity-modulated whole pelvic radiotherapy in women with gynecologic malignancies. *Int. J. Radiat. Oncol. Biol. Phys.* **2002**, *52*, 1330–1337. [CrossRef]
16. Mundt, A.J.; Mell, L.K.; Roeske, J.C. Preliminary analysis of chronic gastrointestinal toxicity in gynecology patients treated with intensity-modulated whole pelvic radiation therapy. *Int. J. Radiat. Oncol. Biol. Phys.* **2003**, *56*, 1354–1360. [CrossRef]
17. Chen, M.F.; Tseng, C.J.; Tseng, C.C.; Kuo, Y.C.; Yu, C.Y.; Chen, W.C. Clinical outcome in posthysterectomy cervical cancer patients treated with concurrent cisplatin and intensity-modulated pelvic radiotherapy: Comparison with conventional radiotherapy. *Int. J. Radiat. Oncol. Biol. Phys.* **2007**, *67*, 1438–1444. [CrossRef]
18. Beriwal, S.; Gan, G.N.; Heron, D.E.; Selvaraj, R.N.; Kim, H.; Lalonde, R.; Kelley, J.L.; Edwards, R.P. Early clinical outcome with concurrent chemotherapy and extended-field, intensity-modulated radiotherapy for cervical cancer. *Int. J. Radiat. Oncol. Biol. Phys.* **2007**, *68*, 166–171. [CrossRef]
19. Pötter, R.; Tanderup, K.; Kirisits, C.; de Leeuw, A.; Kirchheiner, K.; Nout, R.; Tan, L.T.; Haie-Meder, C.; Mahantshetty, U.; Segedin, B.; et al. The EMBRACE II study: The outcome and prospect of two decades of evolution within the GEC—ESTRO GYN working group and the EMBRACE studies. *Clin. Transl. Radiat. Oncol.* **2018**, *9*, 48–60. [CrossRef]
20. Lee, S.I.; Atri, M. 2018 FIGO staging system for uterine cervical cancer: Enter cross-sectional imaging. *Radiology* **2019**, *292*, 15–24. [CrossRef]
21. Dhoot, N.M.; Kumar, V.; Shinagare, A.; Kataki, A.C.; Barmon, D.; Bhuyan, U. Evaluation of carcinoma cervix using magnetic resonance imaging: Correlation with clinical FIGO staging and impact on management. *J. Med. Imaging Radiat. Oncol.* **2012**, *56*, 58–65. [CrossRef]
22. Bipat, S.; Glas, A.S.; van der Velden, J.; Zwinderman, A.H.; Bossuyt, P.M.; Stoker, J. Computed tomography and magnetic resonance imaging in staging of uterine cervical carcinoma. *Gynecol. Oncol.* **2003**, *91*, 59–66. [CrossRef] [PubMed]
23. Kerkhof, E.M.; Raaymakers, B.W.; van der Heide, U.A.; van de Bunt, L.; JurgenliemkSchulz, I.M.; Lagendijk, J.J. On line MRI guidance for healthy tissue sparing in patients with cervical cancer. *Radiother. Oncol.* **2008**, *88*, 241–249. [CrossRef] [PubMed]
24. Dimopoulos, J.C.; Lang, S.; Kirisits, C.; Fidarova, E.F.; Berger, D.; Georg, P.; Dörr, W.; Pötter, R. Dosevolume histogram parameters and local tumor control in magnetic resonance image-guided cervical cancer brachytherapy. *Int. J. Radiat. Oncol. Biol. Phys.* **2009**, *75*, 56–63. [CrossRef] [PubMed]
25. Balleyguier, C.; Sala, E.; Da Cunha, T.; Bergman, A.; Brkljacic, B.; Danza, F.; Forstner, R.; Hamm, B.; Kubik-Huch, R.; Lopez, C.; et al. Staging of uterine cervical cancer with MRI: Guidelines of the European Society of Urogenital Radiology. *Eur. Radiol.* **2011**, *21*, 1102–1110. [CrossRef] [PubMed]
26. Fields, E.C.; Weiss, E. A practical review of magnetic resonance imaging for the evaluation and management of cervical cancer. *Radiat. Oncol.* **2016**, *11*, 15. [CrossRef] [PubMed]
27. Hatano, K.; Sekiya, Y.; Araki, H.; Sakai, M.; Togawa, T.; Narita, Y.; Akiyama, Y.; Kimura, S.; Ito, H. Evaluation of the therapeutic effect of radiotherapy on cervical cancer using magnetic resonance imaging. *Int. J. Radiat. Oncol. Biol. Phys.* **1999**, *45*, 639–644. [CrossRef]
28. Vincens, E.; Balleyguier, C.; Rey, A.; Uzan, C.; Zareski, E.; Gouy, S.; Pautier, P.; Duvillard, P.; Haie-Meder, C.; Morice, P. Accuracy of magnetic resonance imaging in predicting residual disease in patients treated for stage IB2/II cervical carcinoma with chemoradiation therapy: Correlation of radiologic findings with surgico-pathologic results. *Cancer* **2008**, *113*, 2158–2165. [CrossRef]
29. Park, J.J.; Kim, C.K.; Park, S.Y.; Simonetti, A.W.; Kim, E.; Park, B.K.; Huh, S.J. Assessment of early response to concurrent chemoradiotherapy in cervical cancer: Value of diffusion-weighted and dynamic contrast-enhanced MR imaging. *Magn. Reson. Imaging* **2014**, *32*, 993–1000. [CrossRef]
30. Havrilesky, L.J.; Kulasingam, S.L.; Matchar, D.B.; Myers, E.R. FDG—PET for management of cervical and ovarian cancer. *Gynecol. Oncol.* **2005**, *97*, 183–191. [CrossRef]
31. Akkas, B.E.; Demirel, B.B.; Vural, G.E. Clinical impact of 18F-FDG PET/CT in the pretreatment evaluation of patients with locally advanced cervical carcinoma. *Nucl. Med. Commun.* **2012**, *33*, 1081–1088. [CrossRef]
32. Kidd, E.A.; Siegel, B.A.; Dehdashti, F.; Rader, J.S.; Mutch, D.G.; Powell, M.A.; Grigsby, P.W. Lymph node staging by positron emission tomography in cervical cancer. *J. Clin. Oncol.* **2010**, *28*, 2108–2113. [CrossRef] [PubMed]
33. Lee, J.; Lin, J.B.; Sun, F.J.; Chen, Y.J.; Chang, C.L.; Jan, Y.T.; Wu, M.H. Safety and efficacy of semi-extended field intensity-modulated radiation therapy and concurrent cisplatin in locally advanced cervical cancer patients: An observational study of 10-year experience. *Medicine* **2017**, *96*, e6158. [CrossRef] [PubMed]
34. Tsai, C.S.; Lai, C.H.; Chang, T.C.; Yen, T.C.; Ng, K.K.; Hsueh, S.; Lee, S.P.; Hong, J.-H. A prospective randomized trial to study the impact of pretreatment FDG—PET for cervical cancer patients with MRI-detected positive pelvic but negative paraaortic lymphadenopathy. *Int. J. Radiat. Oncol. Biol. Phys.* **2010**, *76*, 477–484. [CrossRef] [PubMed]
35. Su, C.H.; Chen, W.M.; Chen, M.; Shia, B.C.; Wu, S.Y. Survival effect of pre-RT PET—CT on cervical cancer: Image-guided intensity-modulated radiation therapy era. *Front. Oncol.* **2023**, *13*, 1012491. [CrossRef]
36. Gouy, S.; Morice, P.; Narducci, F.; Uzan, C.; Martinez, A.; Rey, A.; Bentivegna, E.; Pautier, P.; Deandreis, D.; Querleu, D.; et al. Prospective multicenter study evaluating the survival of patients with locally advanced cervical cancer undergoing laparoscopic

37. Lazzari, R.; Cecconi, A.; Jereczek-Fossa, B.A.; Travaini, L.L.; Dell'Acqua, V.; Cattani, F.; Rizzo, S.; Fodor, C.; Landoni, F.; Orecchia, R. The role of [(18)F]FDG—PET/CT in staging and treatment planning for volumetric modulated RapidArc radiotherapy in cervical cancer: Experience of the European Institute of Oncology, Milan, Italy. *Ecancermedicalscience* **2014**, *8*, 405. [CrossRef]
38. Cibula, D.; Raspollini, M.R.; Planchamp, F.; Centeno, C.; Chargari, C.; Felix, A.; Fischerová, D.; Jahnn-Kuch, D.; Joly, F.; Kohler, C.; et al. ESGO/ESTRO/ESP Guidelines for the management of patients with cervical cancer—Update 2023. *Int. J. Gynecol. Cancer* **2023**, *33*, 649–666. [CrossRef]
39. Choi, H.J.; Ju, W.; Myung, S.K.; Kim, Y. Diagnostic performance of computer tomography, magnetic resonance imaging, and positron emission tomography or positron emission tomography/computer tomography for detection of metastatic lymph nodes in patients with cervical cancer: Meta-analysis. *Cancer Sci.* **2010**, *101*, 1471–1479. [CrossRef]
40. Adam, J.A.; van Diepen, P.R.; Mom, C.H.; Stoker, J.; van Eck-Smit, B.L.F.; Bipat, S. [18^F] FDG—PET or PET/CT in the evaluation of pelvic and para-aortic lymph nodes in patients with locally advanced cervical cancer: A systematic review of the literature. *Gynecol. Oncol.* **2020**, *159*, 588–596. [CrossRef]
41. Nomden, C.N.; Pötter, R.; de Leeuw, A.A.C.; Tanderup, K.; Lindegaard, J.C.; Schmid, M.P.; Fortin, I.; Haie-Meder, C.; Mahantshetty, U.; Hoskin, P.; et al. EMBRACE Collaborative Group. Nodal failure after chemo-radiation and MRI guided brachytherapy in cervical cancer: Patterns of failure in the EMBRACE study cohort. *Radiother. Oncol.* **2019**, *134*, 185–190. [CrossRef]
42. Ramlov, A.; Kroon, P.S.; Jürgenliemk-Schulz, I.M.; De Leeuw, A.A.; Gormsen, L.C.; Fokdal, L.U.; Tanderup, K.; Lindegaard, J.C. Impact of radiation dose and standardized uptake value of (18)FDG PET on nodal control in locally advanced cervical cancer. *Acta Oncol.* **2015**, *54*, 1567–1573. [CrossRef] [PubMed]
43. Bonin, S.R.; Lanciano, R.M.; Corn, B.W.; Hogan, W.M.; Hartz, W.H.; Hanks, G.E. Bony landmarks are not an adequate substitute for lymphangiography in defining pelvic lymph node location for the treatment of cervical cancer with radiotherapy. *Int. J. Radiat. Oncol. Biol. Phys.* **1996**, *34*, 167–172. [CrossRef] [PubMed]
44. International Commission on Radiation Units and Measurements. *ICRU Report 50 Prescribing, Recording, and Reporting Photon Beam Therapy*; International Commission on Radiation Units and Measurements: Bethesda, MD, USA, 1993; Volume 21.
45. International Commission on Radiation Units and Measurements. *ICRU Report 62 Prescribing, Recording, and Reporting Photon Beam Therapy*; Supplement to ICRU Report 50; International Commission on Radiation Units and Measurements: Bethesda, MD, USA, 1999; Volume 21.
46. Gerstner, N.; Wachter, S.; Knocke, T.H.; Fellner, C.; Wambersie, A.; Pötter, R. The benefit of Beam's eye view-based 3D treatment planning for cervical cancer. *Radiother. Oncol.* **1999**, *51*, 71–78. [CrossRef] [PubMed]
47. Klopp, A.H.; Yeung, A.R.; Deshmukh, S.; Gil, K.M.; Wenzel, L.; Westin, S.N.; Gifford, K.; Gaffney, D.K.; Small Jr, W.; Thompson, S.; et al. Patient-reported toxicity during pelvic intensity-modulated radiation therapy: NRG oncology-RTOG 1203. *J. Clin. Oncol.* **2018**, *36*, 2538–2544. [CrossRef] [PubMed]
48. Marnitz, S.; Tsunoda, A.T.; Martus, P.; Vieira, M.; Affonso Junior, R.J.; Nunes, J.; Budach, V.; Hatel, H.; Mustea, A.; Sehouli, J.; et al. Surgical versus clinical staging prior to primary chemoradiation in patients with cervical cancer FIGO stages IIB-IVA: Oncologic results of a prospective randomized international multicenter (Uterus-11) intergroup study. *Int. J. Gynecol. Cancer* **2020**, *30*, 1855–1861. [CrossRef]
49. Chopra, S.; Dora, T.; Gupta, S.; Kannan, S.; Engineer, R.; Mangaj, A.; Maheshwari, A.; Shylasree, T.S.; Ghosh, J.; Paul, S.N.; et al. Phase III randomized trial of postoperative adjuvant conventional radiation (3DCRT) versus image-guided intensity-modulated radiotherapy (IG-IMRT) in cervical cancer (PARCER): Final analysis. *Int. J. Radiat. Oncol. Biol. Phys.* **2020**, *108*, S1–S2. [CrossRef]
50. Mell, L.K.; Sirák, I.; Wei, L.; Tarnawski, R.; Mahantshetty, U.; Yashar, C.M.; McHale, M.T.; Xu, R.; Honerkamp-Smith, G.; Carmona, R.; et al. Bone marrow-sparing intensity modulated radiation therapy with concurrent cisplatin for stage IB-IVA cervical cancer: An international multicenter phase II clinical trial (INTERTECC-2). *Int. J. Radiat. Oncol. Biol. Phys.* **2017**, *97*, 536–545. [CrossRef]
51. Jadon, R.; Pembroke, C.A.; Hanna, C.L.; Palaniappan, N.; Evans, M.; Cleves, A.E.; Staffurth, J. A systematic review of organ motion and image-guided strategies in external beam radiotherapy for cervical cancer. *Clin. Oncol. R. Coll. Radiol.* **2014**, *26*, 185–196. [CrossRef]
52. Hoppe, R.T.; Phillips, T.L.; Roach, M. Chapter 12: Image-guided Adaptive Radiotherapy. In *Textbook of Radiation Oncology*, 3rd ed.; Keall, P.J., Hsu, A., Xing, L., Eds.; Saunders: Philadelphia, PA, USA, 2004.
53. Verellen, D.; De Ridder, M.; Storme, G. A (short) history of image-guided radiotherapy. *Radiother. Oncol.* **2008**, *86*, 4–13. [CrossRef]
54. Chan, P.; Dinniwell, R.; Haider, M.A.; Cho, Y.B.; Jaffray, D.; Lockwood, G.; Levin, W.; Manchul, L.; Fyles, A.; Milosevic, M. Inter- and intrafractional tumor and organ movement in patients with cervical cancer undergoing radiotherapy: A cinematic-MRI point-of-interest study. *Int. J. Radiat. Oncol. Biol. Phys.* **2008**, *70*, 1507–1515. [CrossRef]
55. Bondar, L.; Hoogeman, M.; Mens, J.W.; Dhawtal, G.; de Pree, I.; Ahmad, R.; Quint, S.; Heijmen, B. Toward an individualized target motion management for IMRT of cervical cancer based on model-predicted cervix-uterus shape and position. *Radiother. Oncol.* **2011**, *99*, 240–245. [CrossRef] [PubMed]
56. Shelley, C.E.; Barraclough, L.H.; Nelder, C.L.; Otter, S.J.; Stewart, A.J. Adaptive Radiotherapy in the Management of Cervical Cancer: Review of Strategies and Clinical Implementation. *Clin. Oncol. R. Coll. Radiol.* **2021**, *33*, 579–590. [CrossRef] [PubMed]

57. Dumitrescu, V.; Serban, D.; Costea, D.; Dumitrescu, D.; Bobirca, F.; Geavlete, B.; Bratu, D.G.; Tribus, L.; Serboiu, C.; Alius, C.; et al. Transabdominal Preperitoneal Versus Lichtenstein Procedure for Inguinal Hernia Repair in Adults: A Comparative Evaluation of the Early Postoperative Pain and Outcomes. *Cureus* **2023**, *15*, e41886. [CrossRef] [PubMed]
58. Smith, G.L.; Eifel, P.J. Comment on Trends in the utilization of brachytherapy in cervical cancer in the United States. *Int. J. Radiat. Oncol. Biol. Phys.* **2014**, *88*, 459–460. [CrossRef] [PubMed]
59. Tod, M.C.; Meredith, W.J. A dosage system for use in the treatment of cancer of the uterine cervix. *Br. J. Radiol.* **1938**, *11*, 809–824. [CrossRef]
60. Tod, M.C.; Meredith, W.J. Treatment of cancer of the cervix uteri, a revised Manchester method. *Br. J. Radiol.* **1953**, *26*, 252–257. [CrossRef]
61. Viswanathan, A.N.; Erickson, B.; Gaffney, D.K.; Beriwal, S.; Bhatia, S.K.; Lee Burnett, O.; D'Souza, D.P.; Patil, N.; Haddock, M.G.; Jhingran, A.; et al. Comparison and consensus guidelines for delineation of clinical target volume for CT- and MR-based brachytherapy in locally advanced cervical cancer. *Int. J. Radiat. Oncol. Biol. Phys.* **2014**, *90*, 320–328. [CrossRef]
62. Haie-Meder, C.; Pötter, R.; Van Limbergen, E.; Briot, E.; De Brabandere, M.; Dimopoulos, J.; Dumas, I.; Hellebust, T.P.; Kirisits, C.; Lang, S.; et al. Recommendations from Gynaecological (GYN) GEC—ESTRO Working Group (I): Concepts and terms in 3D image-based 3D treatment planning in cervix cancer brachytherapy with emphasis on MRI assessment of GTV and CTV. *Radiother. Oncol.* **2005**, *74*, 235–245. [CrossRef]
63. Pötter, R.; Haie-Meder, C.; Van Limbergen, E.; Barillot, I.; De Brabandere, M.; Dimopoulos, J.; Dumas, I.; Erickson, B.; Lang, S.; Nulens, A.; et al. Recommendations from Gynaecological (GYN) GEC ESTRO Working Group (II): Concepts and terms in 3D image-based treatment planning in cervix cancer brachytherapy. *Radiother. Oncol.* **2006**, *78*, 67–77. [CrossRef]
64. Rijkmans, E.C.; Nout, R.A.; Rutten, I.H.; Ketelaars, M.; Neelis, K.J.; Laman, M.S.; Coen, V.L.; Gaarenstroom, K.N.; Kroep, J.R.; Creutzberg, C.L. Improved survival of patients with cervical cancer treated with image-guided brachytherapy compared with conventional brachytherapy. *Gynecol. Oncol.* **2014**, *135*, 231–238. [CrossRef]
65. Lin, A.J.; Kidd, E.; Dehdashti, F.; Siegel, B.A.; Mutic, S.; Thaker, P.H.; Massad, L.S.; Powell, M.A.; Mutch, D.G.; Markovina, S.; et al. Intensity Modulated Radiation Therapy and Image-Guided Adapted Brachytherapy for Cervix Cancer. *Int. J. Radiat. Oncol. Biol. Phys.* **2019**, *103*, 1088–1097. [CrossRef] [PubMed]
66. Viswanathan, A.N.; Dimopoulos, J.; Kirisits, C.; Berger, D.; Pötter, R. Computed tomography versus magnetic resonance imaging-based contouring in cervical cancer brachytherapy: Results of a prospective trial and preliminary guidelines for standardized contours. *Int. J. Radiat. Oncol. Biol. Phys.* **2007**, *68*, 491–498. [CrossRef] [PubMed]
67. Pötter, R.; Tanderup, K.; Schmid, M.P.; Jürgenliemk-Schulz, I.; Haie-Meder, C.; Fokdal, L.U.; Sturdza, A.E.; Hoskin, P.; Mahantshetty, U.; Segedin, B.; et al. MRI-guided adaptive brachytherapy in locally advanced cervical cancer (EMBRACE-I): A multicentre prospective cohort study. *Lancet Oncol.* **2021**, *22*, 538–547. [CrossRef]
68. Schmid, M.; Haie-Meder, C.; Mahanshetty, U.; Jürgenliemk-Schulz, I.M.; Segedin, B.; Hoskin, P.; Pötter, R. OC-0055: Local failures after radiochemotherapy and MR-image-guided brachytherapy in cervical cancer patients. *Radiother. Oncol.* **2017**, *123*, S26. [CrossRef]
69. Fortin, I.; Tanderup, K.; Haie-Meder, C.; Lindegaard, J.C.; Mahantshetty, U.; Segedin, B.; Jürgenliemk-Schulz, I.M.; Hoskin, P.; Kirisits, C.; Potter, R.; et al. Image-guided brachytherapy in cervical cancer: A comparison between intracavitary and combined intracavitary/interstitial brachytherapy in regard to doses to HR CTV, OARs and late morbidity—Early results from the Embrace study in 999 patients. *Brachytherapy* **2016**, *15*, S21. [CrossRef]
70. Anghel, B. PO24: High Dose-Rate Tandem and Ovoid 3D CT Based Brachytherapy in Cervical Cancer: Initial Single Center Experience. *Brachytherapy* **2021**, *20*, S66–S67. [CrossRef]
71. Charra-Brunaud, C.; Harter, V.; Delannes, M.; Haie-Meder, C.; Quetin, P.; Kerr, C.; Castelain, B.; Thomas, L.; Peiffert, D. Impact of 3D image-based PDR brachytherapy on outcome of patients treated for cervix carcinoma in France: Results of the French STIC prospective study. *Radiother. Oncol.* **2012**, *102*, 305–313. [CrossRef]
72. Kirisits, C.; Lang, S.; Dimopoulos, J.; Oechs, K.; Georg, D.; Potter, R. Uncertainties when using only one MRI-based treatment plan for subsequent high-dose-rate tandem and ring applications in brachytherapy of cervix cancer. *Radiother. Oncol.* **2006**, *81*, 269–275. [CrossRef]
73. Beriwal, S.; Kim, H.; Coon, D.; Mogus, R.; Heron, D.E.; Huq, M.S. Single magnetic resonance imaging vs magnetic resonance imaging/computed tomography planning in cervical cancer brachytherapy. *Clin. Oncol. R. Coll. Radiol.* **2009**, *21*, 483–487. [CrossRef]
74. Kim, H.; Rajagopalan, M.S.; Beriwal, S.; Huq, M.S.; Smith, K.J. Cost-effectiveness analysis of 3D image-guided brachytherapy compared with 2D brachytherapy in the treatment of locally advanced cervical cancer. *Brachytherapy* **2015**, *14*, 29–36. [CrossRef]
75. Tan, L.T.; Tanderup, K.; Kirisits, C.; Mahantshetty, U.; Swamidas, J.; Jürgenliemk-Schulz, I.; Lindegaard, J.; de Leeuw, A.; Nesvacil, N.; Assenholt, M.; et al. Education and training for image-guided adaptive brachytherapy for cervix cancer-The (GEC)-ESTRO/EMBRACE perspective. *Brachytherapy* **2020**, *19*, 827–836. [CrossRef] [PubMed]
76. Dimopoulos, J.C.; Kirisits, C.; Petric, P.; Georg, P.; Lang, S.; Berger, D.; Potter, R. The Vienna applicator for combined intracavitary and interstitial brachytherapy of cervical cancer: Clinical feasibility and preliminary results. *Int. J. Radiat. Oncol. Biol. Phys.* **2006**, *66*, 83–90. [CrossRef] [PubMed]
77. De Brabandere, M.; Mousa, A.G.; Nulens, A.; Swinnen, A.; Van Limbergen, E. Potential of dose optimisation in MRI-based PDR brachytherapy of cervix carcinoma. *Radiother. Oncol.* **2008**, *88*, 217–226. [CrossRef] [PubMed]

78. Lindegaard, J.C.; Tanderup, K.; Nielsen, S.K.; Haack, S.; Gelineck, J. MRI-guided 3D optimization significantly improves DVH parameters of pulsed-dose-rate brachytherapy in locally advanced cervical cancer. *Int. J. Radiat. Oncol. Biol. Phys.* **2008**, *71*, 756–764. [CrossRef]
79. Tanderup, K.; Lindegaard, J.C.; Kirisits, C.; Haie-Meder, C.; Kirchheiner, K.; de Leeuw, A.; Jürgenliemk-Schulz, I.; Van Limbergen, E.; Pötter, R. Image Guided Adaptive Brachytherapy in cervix cancer: A new paradigm changing clinical practice and outcome. *Radiother. Oncol.* **2016**, *120*, 365–369. [CrossRef]
80. Sturdza, A.E.; Knoth, J. Image-guided brachytherapy in cervical cancer including fractionation. *Int. J. Gynecol. Cancer: Off. J. Int. Gynecol. Cancer Soc.* **2022**, *32*, 273–280. [CrossRef]
81. Vojtíšek, R. Image guided adaptive brachytherapy of cervical cancer—Practical recommendations. *Klin. Onkol.* **2023**, *36*, 96–103. [CrossRef]
82. Sturdza, A.E.; Pötter, R.; Kossmeier, M.; Kirchheiner, K.; Mahantshetty, U.; Haie-Meder, C.; Lindegaard, J.C.; Jurgenliemk-Schulz, I.; Tan, L.T.; Hoskin, P.; et al. Nomogram predicting overall survival in patients with locally advanced cervical cancer treated with radiochemotherapy including image-guided brachytherapy: A Retro-EMBRACE study. *Int. J. Radiat. Oncol. Biol. Phys.* **2021**, *111*, 168–177. [CrossRef]
83. Dumitru, M.; Berghi, O.N.; Taciuc, I.A.; Vrinceanu, D.; Manole, F.; Costache, A. Could Artificial Intelligence Prevent Intraoperative Anaphylaxis? Reference Review and Proof of Concept. *Medicina* **2022**, *58*, 1530. [CrossRef]
84. Corradini, S.; Alongi, F.; Andratschke, N.; Belka, C.; Boldrini, L.; Cellini, F.; Debus, J.; Guckenberger, M.; Hörner-Rieber, J.; Lagerwaard, F.J.; et al. MR-guidance in clinical reality: Current treatment challenges and future perspectives. *Radiat. Oncol.* **2019**, *14*, 92. [CrossRef]
85. Ng, J.; Gregucci, F.; Pennell, R.T.; Nagar, H.; Golden, E.B.; Knisely, J.P.S.; Sanfilippo, N.J.; Formenti, S.C. MRI-LINAC: A transformative technology in radiation oncology. *Front. Oncol.* **2023**, *13*, 1117874. [CrossRef] [PubMed]
86. Randall, J.W.; Rammohan, N.; Das, I.J.; Yadav, P. Towards Accurate and Precise Image-Guided Radiotherapy: Clinical Applications of the MR-Linac. *J. Clin. Med.* **2022**, *11*, 4044. [CrossRef] [PubMed]
87. Cusumano, D.; Boldrini, L.; Dhont, J.; Fiorino, C.; Green, O.; Güngör, G.; Jornet, N.; Klüter, S.; Landry, G.; Mattiucci, G.C.; et al. Artificial Intelligence in magnetic Resonance guided Radiotherapy: Medical and physical considerations on state of art and future perspectives. *Phys. Med.* **2021**, *85*, 175–191. [CrossRef] [PubMed]
88. Huo, W.; Ding, Y.; Sheng, C.; Pi, Y.; Guo, Y.; Wu, A.; Zhang, Z. Application of 3D printing in cervical cancer brachytherapy. *J. Radiat. Res. Appl. Sci.* **2022**, *15*, 18–24. [CrossRef]
89. Marar, M.; Simiele, E.; Niedermayr, T.; Kidd, E.A. Applying 3D-Printed Templates in High-Dose-Rate Brachytherapy for Cervix Cancer: Simplified Needle Insertion for Optimized Dosimetry. *Int. J. Radiat. Oncol. Biol. Phys.* **2022**, *114*, 111–119. [CrossRef]
90. Webster, A.; Appelt, A.L.; Eminowicz, G. Image-Guided Radiotherapy for Pelvic Cancers: A Review of Current Evidence and Clinical Utilisation. *Clin. Oncol. R. Coll. Radiol.* **2020**, *32*, 805–816. [CrossRef]

Disclaimer/Publisher's Note: The statements, opinions and data contained in all publications are solely those of the individual author(s) and contributor(s) and not of MDPI and/or the editor(s). MDPI and/or the editor(s) disclaim responsibility for any injury to people or property resulting from any ideas, methods, instructions or products referred to in the content.

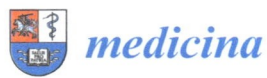

Article

Prostatic Artery Origin Variability: Five Steps to Improve Identification during Percutaneous Embolization

Alexandru Șerbănoiu [1,2,3], Rareș Nechifor [4], Andreea Nicoleta Marinescu [1,2,*], Gheorghe Iana [1], Ana Magdalena Bratu [1,5], Iulia Alecsandra Sălcianu [1,5], Radu Tudor Ion [1,2,3,*] and Florin Mihail Filipoiu [1]

1. Department of Radiology and Medical Imaging, University of Medicine and Pharmacy Carol Davila, 050474 Bucharest, Romania; alexandru.serbanoiu@drd.umfcd.ro (A.Ș.)
2. Department of Radiology and Medical Imaging, University Emergency Hospital Bucharest, 050098 Bucharest, Romania
3. Doctoral School of "Carol Davila", University of Medicine and Pharmacy, 700115 Bucharest, Romania
4. Endovascular Network Bucharest, 075100, Bucharest, Romania
5. Department of Radiology and Medical Imaging, Colțea Hospital, 030171 Bucharest, Romania
* Correspondence: andreea_marinescu2003@yahoo.com (A.N.M.); iradutudor@gmail.com (R.T.I.); Tel.: +40-723257619 (A.N.M.)

Abstract: *Background and Objectives*: The purpose of the current paper is to present our study on the variability in the prostatic artery origin, discuss the less frequent origins, and present the challenges of the prostatic artery embolization (PAE) procedure, thus aiding young interventional radiologists. *Materials and Methods*: We studied the origins of the prostatic artery on digital subtraction angiography (DSA) examinations from PAE procedures on 35 male pelvises (70 hemi-pelvises). *Results*: Our study has demonstrated that the most frequent origin of the prostatic artery (PA) is the internal pudendal artery (IPA), 37.1%, followed by the anterior gluteal trunk, 27.1%, and the superior vesical artery (SVA), 21.4%. Less frequent origins are the obturator artery (OBT), 11.4%, and the inferior gluteal artery (IGA), 2.8%. *Conclusions*: Compared to other studies, we notice some differences in the statistical results, but the most frequent origins remain the same. What is more important for young interventional radiologists is to be aware of all the possible origins of the PA in order to be able to offer a proper treatment to their patients. The important aspect that will ensure the success of the procedure without post-procedural complications is represented by the successful embolization of the targeted prostatic parenchyma.

Keywords: prostatic arterial embolization; interventional radiology; benign prostate hyperplasia; anatomy

Citation: Șerbănoiu, A.; Nechifor, R.; Marinescu, A.N.; Iana, G.; Bratu, A.M.; Sălcianu, I.A.; Ion, R.T.; Filipoiu, F.M. Prostatic Artery Origin Variability: Five Steps to Improve Identification during Percutaneous Embolization. *Medicina* 2023, 59, 2122. https://doi.org/10.3390/medicina59122122

Academic Editor: Giuseppe Lucarelli

Received: 9 October 2023
Revised: 30 November 2023
Accepted: 30 November 2023
Published: 5 December 2023

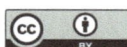

Copyright: © 2023 by the authors. Licensee MDPI, Basel, Switzerland. This article is an open access article distributed under the terms and conditions of the Creative Commons Attribution (CC BY) license (https://creativecommons.org/licenses/by/4.0/).

1. Introduction

Benign prostate hyperplasia (BPH) has been a very common pathology in the male population over the past 50 years (50% incidence) associated with lower urinary tract symptoms (LUTSs) that affect the quality of life [1]. Treatment options for BPH include medication, surgery (transurethral incision of prostate, TUIP, and transurethral resection of the prostate, TURP), and minimally invasive treatments, like prostatic artery embolization (PAE) and prostatic urethral lift. Prostatic artery embolization is a minimally invasive treatment for BPH that consists of the supra-selective embolization of prostatic arteries (PAs), which reduces the volume of the prostate parenchyma and improves the symptomatology of the patients. Described in 2010 as a therapy for BPH by Carnevale, the procedure has been adapted and developed by several interventional radiology centers [2].

Post-procedural outcomes for PAE and TURP are similar regarding LUTSs; however, PAE has advantages such as preservation of the urinary and sexual functions. Studies on the TURP procedure note adverse reactions such as bleeding, infection, and urethral stricture, as well as increased morbidity with retrograde ejaculation and urinary incontinence [3]. Other important advantages of PAE are the minimally invasive nature of the procedure with no need for hospitalization or general anesthesia and the increased quality of life; nevertheless, incidents such as non-targeted embolization (NTE) of the bladder or rectum causing pelvic pain or rectal bleeding can occur; usually, the area of ischemia is small and the adverse reactions are transient and do not need treatment [4,5]. Penile ischemia is possible in the case of NTE due to the vascularization origin from the IIA branches, but at the same time, erectile dysfunction after PAE has not been reported [6]. The high success rate of prostatic artery embolization procedures and the decrease rate of post-procedural incidents is directly related to good knowledge of the prostatic vascularization and its variability [4].

The indication for PAE is considered to be patients with moderate to severe lower urinary tract symptoms in direct relation to a benign prostatic obstruction who do not respond to medication or have a severe adverse reaction to it [7,8].

The main purpose of this paper is to present the procedural protocol in our department and the results of the study on the arterial origin of the PA. We expect this study to serve as a guide for young interventional radiologists who want to perform PAE by presenting the protocol of the procedure from our department and the main challenges we have encountered [9].

2. Materials and Methods

This retrospective study is based on digital subtraction angiography (DSA) examinations of 35 male patients, aged 50–83 with BPH that undergo PAE. The procedures were performed from March 2021 to May 2023 by two interventional radiologists in the Endovascular Network department. All patients have agreed to participate in this study by signing the preprocedural consent and information form.

In our department for PAE, we used the left brachial approach with a 5F introducer (Terumo™, West Collins Avenue Lakewood, CO, USA) with a 5F JR (125 cm) shape catheter (Merit Medical™, South Jordan, UT, USA), a Radiofocus™ guide wire 0.035″ (180 cm) from Terumo™, and a nonionic contrast agent (Omnipaque™ 350 mL 1/mL GE Healthcare™, Chicago, IL, USA). For the supra-selective catheterization of prostatic arteries, we used a Direxion Transend 14™ and pre-loaded torqueable microcatheter from Boston Scientific™ (Marlborough, MA, USA).

We used five steps in the arterial mapping in order to identify the PA and successfully obtain the supra-selective catheterization:

1. Contralateral 45° with 10° cranio-caudal-oriented DSA in order to catheterize the internal iliac artery.
2. Ipsilateral 45° with 10° cranio-caudal-oriented DSA in order to obtain the mapping of the main branches of the iliac artery and include them in one of the Yamaki classifications (Table 1) [10];
3. After we identified the four main branches (superior gluteal artery, inferior gluteal artery, obturator artery, internal pudendal artery), we searched for the PA artery, which usually has a characteristic corkscrew aspect and parallel trajectory with the IPA.
4. The next step is represented by the positioning of the JR catheter in an optimal position near the origin of the PA and catheterization with the Direxion™ microcatheter.
5. Study the aspect of the PA: we can find two branches of the PA, which are represented by the posterior PA (vascularization of the prostatic capsule) and anterior PA (vascularization of the prostatic parenchyma) [2].

This five-step method of mapping the arterial vascularization of the pelvis has the purpose of offering an organized search of the PA and reducing the exposure to radiation while concluding in a proper prostatic embolization.

Table 1. Yamaki classification of internal iliac artery branching patterns.

Group	Branching Pattern
Group A	The internal iliac artery divides into two branches, the superior gluteal artery and the common trunk of the inferior gluteal and internal pudendal arteries.
Group B	The internal iliac artery divides into two branches, the internal pudendal artery and the common trunk of the superior gluteal and inferior gluteal arteries.
Group C	The internal iliac artery simultaneously divides into three major branches.
Group D	The internal iliac artery divides into the common trunk for the superior gluteal and internal pudendal arteries and the inferior gluteal artery.

Variabilities that must be taken into consideration when identifying the PA:

- Type of internal iliac artery (IIA) branching pattern from Yamaki classification which helps to identify possible origins of the PA [3].
- Prostatic arteries realize the vascularization of the prostate, the anterior for the prostatic parenchyma and the posterior prostatic arteries for the prostatic capsule. Depending on the variability, we can frequently find a common trunk and a distal bifurcation near the prostate, but there are also cases of two PAs with different origins (Figure 1) [11].
- There are cases when we can identify IPA and IPA accessories, which must not be confused with the PA. At the level of accessory IPAs, we can find the origin of the middle rectal artery, which has a characteristic pattern of enhancement that cannot be mistaken with the prostatic blush [12] (Figure 2);

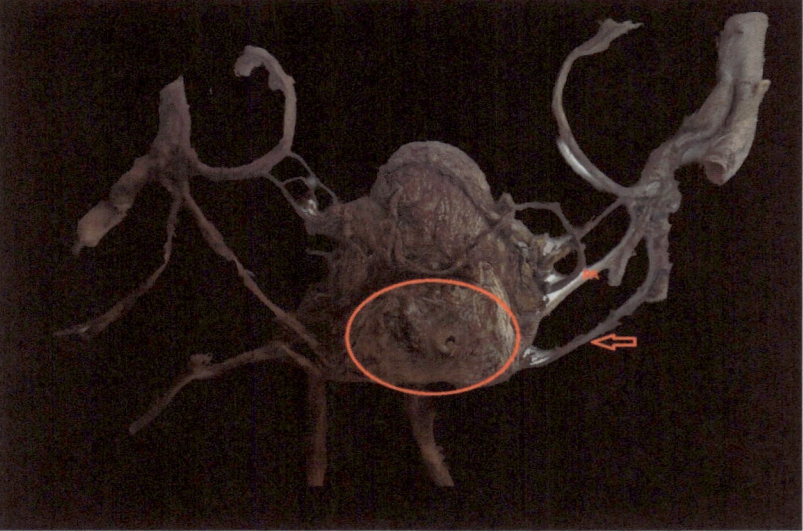

Figure 1. Prostate (red circle) and bladder complex obtained from anatomical dissection also with main branches from the IIA and anatomical variation with two PAs on the left side. Prostatic artery noted with PA and accessory prostate artery (arrow).

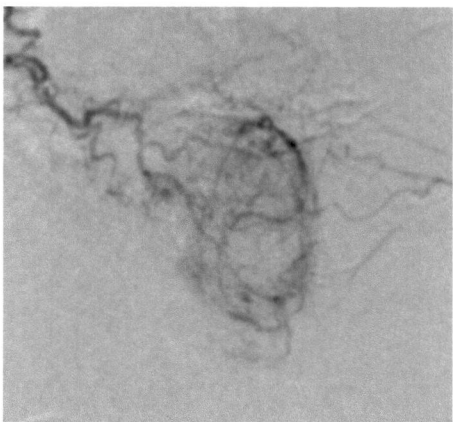

Figure 2. Contrast enhancement at the level of right prostatic lobe with the characteristic "blush" aspect, and we also can see the "cork-screw" aspect of the right PA.

3. Results

We were able to identify the origin of the PA of all patients included in this study with the most common origin found at the level of IPA (37.1% of 70 hemi-pelvises) followed by the anterior gluteal trunk above the bifurcation (27.1% of 70 hemi-pelvises), the superior vesical artery (21.4% of 70 hemi-pelvises), and the obturator artery (11.4% of 70 hemi-pelvises). Less frequent origins were found at the level of the inferior gluteal artery (2.8% of 70 hemi-pelvises). Compared with other studies, the percentage of each origin is slightly different but the main order of frequency is maintained [13–15] (Table 2).

Table 2. Comparison of recent studies results regarding the origin of PA.

Study	IPA (%)	Anterior Gluteal Trunk (%)	SVA (%)	Obturator Artery (%)	IGA (%)
Serbanoiu et al.	26 (37.1%)	19 (27.1%)	15 (21.4%)	8 (11.4%)	2 (2.8%)
Bilhim (2010) [14]	28 (56%)	14 (28%)	-	6 (12%)	2 (4%)
Bilhim (2012) [13]	73 (34%)	38 (17.8%)	42 (20%)	27 (12.6%)	8 (3.7%)
Zhang (2015) [7]	32 (27.9%)	45 (39.5%)	37 (32.6%)	-	-
DeAssis (2015) [11]	45 (31.1%)	-	43 (28.7%)	28 (18.8%)	-
Garcia-Monaco (2015) [15]	8 (17.4%)	26 (56.6%)	-	2 (4.3%)	-

3.1. Prostatic Artery Origin

3.1.1. PA with Origin from IPA

We can consider this example as the ideal patient for PA catheterization from the point of view of the vascular anatomy. Nevertheless, it is mandatory to respect all the steps of the procedure and verify the catheterized artery before embolization(Figure 3).

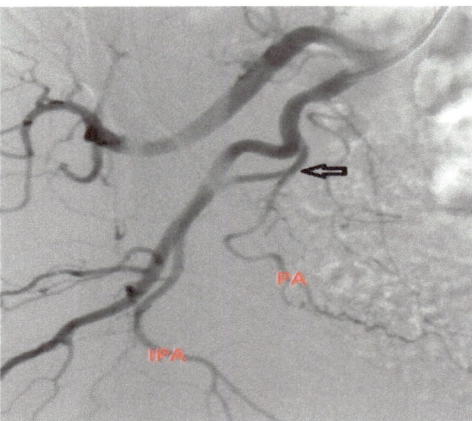

Figure 3. Case of a patient with PA origin (arrow) from the IPA with no significant angulation of the origin and no important collaterals.

3.1.2. PA with Origin from Anterior Gluteal Trunk

The origin at this level is usually accessible for catheterization with the JR catheter due to its particular shape, as it can be placed near the origin of the PA, and it will offer good support and good handling for the Direxion microcatheter (Figure 4).

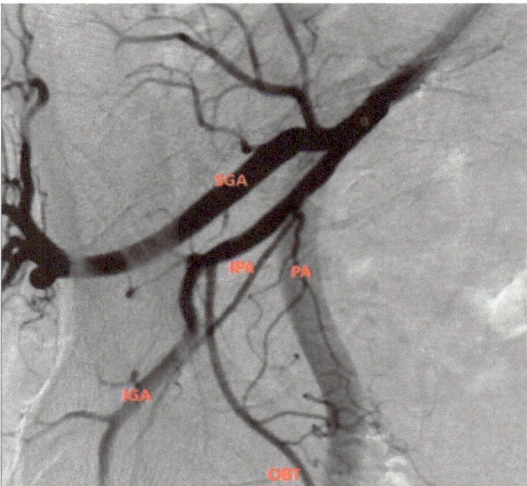

Figure 4. PA with origin from the anterior gluteal trunk. We can identify the obturator artery (OBT) and IPA as branches from the anterior trunk. After the origin of the PA, there are small visible arterial branches that represent inferior vesical arteries.

3.1.3. PA with Origin from SVA

For this anatomic variant, it is important to place the microcatheter distally to the PA origin in order to avoid non-targeted embolization of the bladder (Figure 5).

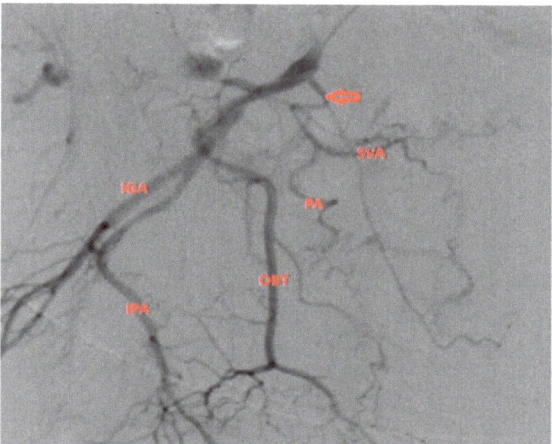

Figure 5. This is the case of PA with an origin from the superior vesical artery (arrow). PA has its origin in the proximal part of SVA.

3.1.4. PA with Distal Origin from Internal Pudendal Artery

The most frequent origin of PA is from IPA, nevertheless distal origin is very rare and may be challenging to catheterize due to its long path and direction of the vessel (Figure 6).

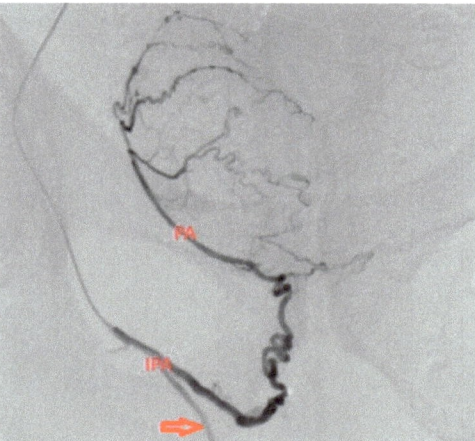

Figure 6. In this figure, we have a particular case of PA originating distally from the IPA with ascendent trajectory. The important aspect in this case is the supra-selective catheterization in order to not accidentally embolize the penile artery (arrow).

3.2. Importance of Supra-Selective Catheterization in Case of PA with Common Trunk or Anastomosis

3.2.1. PA origin with Common Trunk

We can often identify PAs that have a common trunk with the superior or inferior ves-ical artery (Figure 7) that require the microcatheter to be placed after the origin of the vesical arteries in order to manage a targeted embolization.

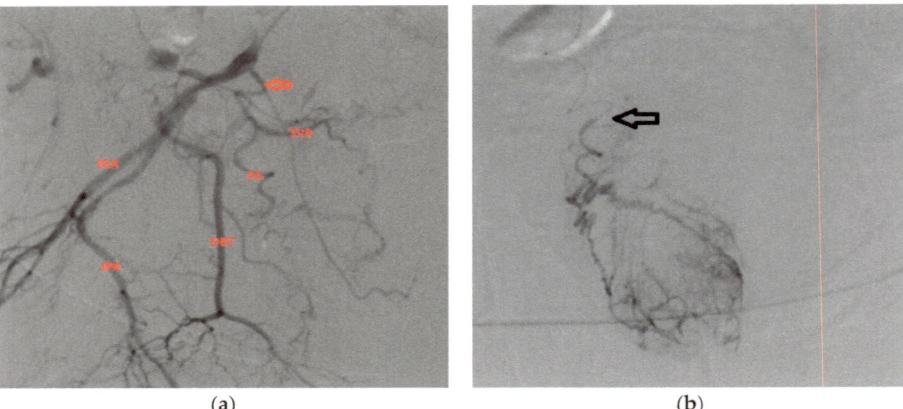

Figure 7. (**a**) Origin of PA from SVA (arrow); (**b**) correct position of microcatheter (arrow) distally from the origin of PA in order to ensure targeted embolization of the prostate, which we can identify by the characteristic blush of contrast enhancement.

3.2.2. Anastomoses of PA with Penile Artery

For arterial anastomosis and collaterals, we have to follow the same rule in order to obtain targeted embolization (Figure 8); otherwise, embolization particles will reach unwanted territories and may cause small areas of necrosis. What are most common and with severe symptoms are the bladder, penis, and rectum, causing urinary and sexual function deficiency and ischemic rectitis with inferior abdominal pain, respectively [2].

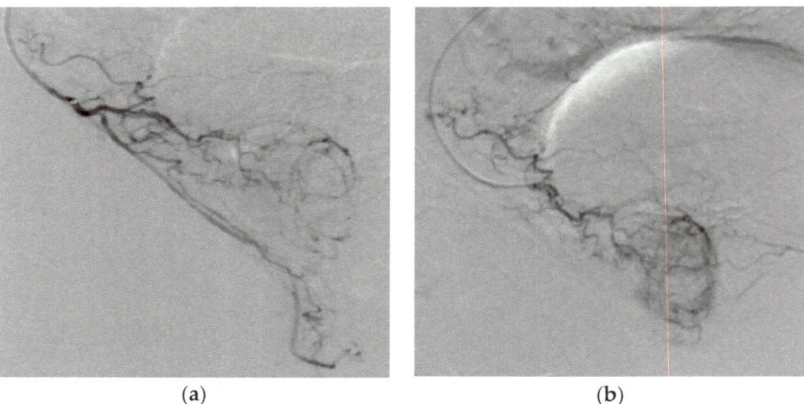

Figure 8. (**a**) Catheter positioned in proximal part of PA; we can identify arterial branches for the penis. Embolization should be made distally from the origin of these branches in order to have a targeted embolization. (**b**) Correct position of the microcatheter, distal from the origin of penile arterial branches, ensures targeted embolization of the prostate.

3.2.3. Middle Rectal Artery with Origin from PA

We can find cases of middle rectal artery with the origin at the level of posterior PA, and as a key finding we can search for the characteristic vertical blush of the rectal arteries. In this case we have to correct the position of the microcatheter at the level of the anterior PA in order to perform the targeted embolization and not damage the rectal tissue [16]. Always before embolization, we have to demonstrate the correct position with DSA acquisition in which we can identify the prostatic blush (Figure 9).

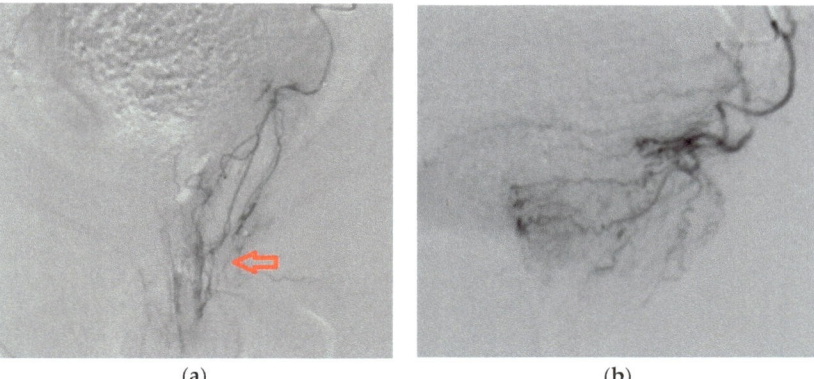

Figure 9. (**a**) Rectal arteries characteristic vertical blush (arrow). (**b**) Correct position of the microcatheter with the characteristic prostatic enhancement pattern.

3.3. Post-Procedural Short-Term Complications

We report no major periprocedural events for any of the patients included in this study such as non-targeted embolization with areas of necrosis at the level of the rectum, bladder, or penis. None of the patients included in this study had vascular complications after the procedure such as pseudoaneurysms or arterial dissection. Minor post-procedural side-effects have been reported such as pelvic pain in the first 24 h at 22 of the patients from the 35 included in this study (62.8%).

4. Discussion

Because the PAE procedure has become increasingly popular in recent years, it is important to discuss in this paper the method and challenges encountered related to the anatomical variability of PA origin. The variability in the male pelvic arterial vascularization is significant; nevertheless, some patterns are identified as recurrent. Compared to the present literature, the results of this study agree with the scientific consensus that there are three most frequent origins, which are the IPA, anterior common trunk, and SVA. However, our paper, as well as the ones which we have cited, found different proportions of the main origins, which might be explained by regional differences. This is fundamental to improvement of the procedure, especially taking the exposure to radiation of both the patient and doctor into consideration.

PAE is a demanding procedure and the outcome is directly related to the skills and the knowledge of the performing doctor, so it is necessary to highlight certain helpful information. The left brachial with a 5F introducer represents a better approach that will make the catheterization of both sides of the pelvis easier and also result in less frequent post-procedural local complications.

The five aforementioned steps of arterial mapping before the embolization represent a coordinated search of the PA that will significantly reduce the time of the procedure and the radiation exposure to both the patient and the doctor, by having the typical anatomical variations in mind. When using the arterial mapping, we can correlate the results of the current study that will help identify the PA based on the most frequent or less frequent origins. The similar results of the current study compared to the cited studies represent a confirmation of the accuracy of our data.

The characteristic "cork-screw" aspect of the PA is helpful in identifying it in the numerous pelvic small vessels.

After the supra-selective catheterization of the PA, it is recommended to use 200–300 μm embolic particles highly diluted with contrast agent and saline solution injected slowly for the embolization. Repeated verification with DSA is needed in order to prevent embolization particle reflux from the PA in other arterial branches.

During the procedure, there are some challenges that can be encountered such as the angulation of the artery from the origin. The path and branches that may have an origin at this level are highly susceptible to variability and may represent a challenge for young interventional radiologists. The solution is represented by performing the end part of the microguide with a similar angle of the artery for a better navigation and catheterization.

BPH is one of the most frequent pathologies in the elderly male population; at the same time, atherosclerotic disease is very common in this age group. In many cases of PAE, it is expected to encounter vascular stenosis and tortuosity that will transform the catheterization of the prostatic artery in the most difficult part of the procedure and increase the radiation exposure to the patient and doctor [17–19]. The position of the JR catheter is important and helpful in these cases because it can ensure the proper support for the microcatheter navigation through the atherosclerotic plaques.

It is required to identify the collaterals or anastomosis of the PA before embolization in order to take proper action to ensure targeted embolization. The most frequent collateral arteries are with middle rectal artery, inferior vesical arteries, and IPA. If supra-selective catheterization is not possible, micro-coil embolization of the branch is recommended in order to ensure a proper embolization [6].

The endovascular navigation technique for the pelvic arterial supply discussed in this paper can find its application also in other special procedures that are intended to solve rare post-surgical complications such as bleeding and pseudoaneurysm that may occur. Cases with a very good outcome have been reported with a low morbidity [20,21]. It is essential to adapt the embolic material (coil, glue, particles) depending on the affected branch of the IIA.

Targeted embolization is one of the most important steps for a successful embolization procedure because it reduces the chances of post-procedural complications [22]. All aspects discussed must be taken into consideration when embolization is performed in order to have an efficient procedure without other post-procedural complications.

5. Conclusions

The PAE procedure is a safe and effective method of treatment for LUTSs in BPH as long as there is proper knowledge of the technique and anatomic variability of the arterial vascularization in the pelvic region. Due to its minimally invasive nature and low rate of complications, the popularity of this procedure has increased in the past years.

Compared to other studies, we noticed a difference in the percentage of the origins, but the most frequent variations are agreed upon in literature. It is important for young interventional radiologists to be aware of all the possible origins of PAs in order to be able to catheterize the PA and offer a proper treatment to their patients with BPH.

Author Contributions: Conceptualization, A.Ș. and R.N.; methodology, G.I.; formal analysis, A.M.B. and I.A.S.; resources, R.N.; writing—original draft preparation, A.Ș. and R.T.I.; writing—review and editing. A.Ș. and A.N.M.; supervision F.M.F. All authors have read and agreed to the published version of the manuscript.

Funding: This research received no external funding.

Institutional Review Board Statement: The study was conducted in accordance with the Declaration of Helsinki and approved by the Ethic Committee of Endovascular Network in March 2021 with registration number 43/2021.

Informed Consent Statement: Informed consent was obtained from all subjects involved in the study.

Data Availability Statement: Data are available upon request from the corresponding authors.

Acknowledgments: Publication of this paper was supported by the University of Medicine and Pharmacy Carol Davila, through the institutional program Publish not Perish.

Conflicts of Interest: The authors declare no conflict of interest.

Abbreviations

BPH	benign prostatic hyperplasia
PAE	prostatic arterial embolization
DSA	digital subtraction angiography
PA	prostatic artery
SGA	superior gluteal artery
IGA	inferior gluteal artery
OBT	obturator artery
IIA	internal iliac artery
SVA	superior vesical artery

References

1. Berry, S.J.; Coffey, D.S.; Walsh, P.C.; Ewing, L.L. The Development of Human Benign Prostatic Hyperplasia with Age. *J. Urol.* **1984**, *132*, 474–479. [CrossRef] [PubMed]
2. Carnevale, F.C.; Antunes, A.A.; da Motta Leal Filho, J.M.; de Oliveira Cerri, L.M.; Baroni, R.H.; Marcelino, A.S.Z.; Freire, G.C.; Moreira, A.M.; Srougi, M.; Cerri, G.G. Prostatic Artery Embolization as a Primary Treatment for Benign Prostatic Hyperplasia: Preliminary Results in Two Patients. *Cardiovasc. Interv. Radiol.* **2010**, *33*, 355–361. [CrossRef]
3. Ahyai, S.A.; Gilling, P.; Kaplan, S.A.; Kuntz, R.M.; Madersbacher, S.; Montorsi, F.; Speakman, M.J.; Stief, C.G. Meta-analysis of Functional Outcomes and Complications Following Transurethral Procedures for Lower Urinary Tract Symptoms Resulting from Benign Prostatic Enlargement. *Eur. Urol.* **2010**, *58*, 384–397. [CrossRef] [PubMed]
4. Moreira, A.M.; de Assis, A.M.; Carnevale, F.C.; Antunes, A.A.; Srougi, M.; Cerri, G.G. A Review of Adverse Events Related to Prostatic Artery Embolization for Treatment of Bladder Outlet Obstruction Due to BPH. *Cardiovasc. Interv. Radiol.* **2017**, *40*, 1490–1500. [CrossRef] [PubMed]
5. Jones, P.; Rai, B.P.; Nair, R.; Somani, B.K. Current Status of Prostate Artery Embolization for Lower Urinary Tract Symptoms: Review of World Literature. *Urology* **2015**, *86*, 676–681. [CrossRef] [PubMed]
6. Kim, S.D.; Huh, J.S.; Kim, Y.-J. Necrosis of the Penis with Multiple Vessel Atherosclerosis. *World J. Mens Health* **2014**, *32*, 66. [CrossRef] [PubMed]
7. Picel, A.C.; Hsieh, T.-C.; Shapiro, R.M.; Vezeridis, A.M.; Isaacson, A.J. Prostatic Artery Embolization for Benign Prostatic Hyperplasia: Patient Evaluation, Anatomy, and Technique for Successful Treatment. *RadioGraphics* **2019**, *39*, 1526–1548. [CrossRef] [PubMed]
8. Pereira, J.; Bilhim, T.; Duarte, M.; Rio Tinto, H.; Fernandes, L.; Martins Pisco, J. Patient Selection and Counseling before Prostatic Arterial Embolization. *Tech. Vasc. Interv. Radiol.* **2012**, *15*, 270–275. [CrossRef]
9. Moulin, B.; di Primio, M.; Vignaux, O.; Sarrazin, J.L.; Angelopoulos, G.; Hakime, A. Prostate Artery Embolization: Challenges, Tips, Tricks, and Perspectives. *J. Pers. Med.* **2022**, *13*, 87. [CrossRef]
10. Yamaki, K.-I.; Saga, T.; Doi, Y.; Aida, K.; Yoshizuka, M. A Statistical Study of the Branching of the Human Internal Iliac Artery. *Kurume Med. J.* **1998**, *45*, 333–340. [CrossRef]
11. de Assis, A.M.; Moreira, A.M.; de Paula Rodrigues, V.C.; Harward, S.H.; Antunes, A.A.; Srougi, M.; Carnevale, F.C. Pelvic Arterial Anatomy Relevant to Prostatic Artery Embolisation and Proposal for Angiographic Classification. *Cardiovasc. Interv. Radiol.* **2015**, *38*, 855–861. [CrossRef]
12. Nguyen Xuan, H.; do Huy, H.; Nguyen Thi Bich, N.; Phan Hoang, G.; le Van, K.; Nguyen Duy, T.; Anh Tran, T.; Thi Nga, V.; Bui Minh, L. Anatomical Characteristics and Variants of Prostatic Artery in Patients of Benign Hyperplasia Prostate by Digital Subtraction Angiography. *Open Access Maced. J. Med. Sci.* **2019**, *7*, 4204–4208. [CrossRef] [PubMed]
13. Bilhim, T.; Pisco, J.M.; Rio Tinto, H.; Fernandes, L.; Pinheiro, L.C.; Furtado, A.; Casal, D.; Duarte, M.; Pereira, J.; Oliveira, A.G.; et al. Prostatic arterial supply: Anatomic and imaging findings relevant for selective arterial embolization. *J. Vasc. Interv. Radiol.* **2012**, *23*, 1403–1415. [CrossRef] [PubMed]
14. Bilhim, T.; Pisco, J.M.; Furtado, A.; Casal, D.; Pais, D.; Pinheiro, L.C.; O'Neill, J.E.G. Prostatic arterial supply: Demonstration by multirow detector Angio CT and Catheter Angiography. *Eur. Radiol.* **2011**, *21*, 1119–1126. [CrossRef] [PubMed]
15. Garcia-Monaco, R.; Garategui, L.; Kizilevsky, N.; Peralta, O.; Rodriguez, P.; Palacios-Jaraquemada, J. Human cadaveric specimen study of the prostatic arterial anatomy: Implications for arterial embolization. *J. Vasc. Interv. Radiol.* **2014**, *25*, 315–322. [CrossRef] [PubMed]
16. Moreira, A.M.; Marques CF, S.; Antunes, A.A.; Nahas, C.S.R.; Nahas, S.C.; de Gregorio Ariza, M.Á.; Carnevale, F.C. Transient Ischemic Rectitis as a Potential Complication after Prostatic Artery Embolization: Case Report and Review of the Literature. *Cardiovasc. Interv. Radiol.* **2013**, *36*, 1690–1694. [CrossRef]
17. Bin Lim, K. Epidemiology of clinical benign prostatic hyperplasia. *Asian J. Urol.* **2017**, *4*, 148–151. [CrossRef]

18. Taylor, B.C.; Wilt, T.J.; Fink, H.A.; Lambert, L.C.; Marshall, L.M.; Hoffman, A.R.; Beer, T.M.; Bauer, D.C.; Zmuda, J.M.; Orwoll, E.S. Prevalence, severity, and health correlates of lower urinary tract symptoms among older men: The MrOS study. *Urology* **2006**, *68*, 804–809. [CrossRef]
19. Jaffer, F.A.; O'Donnell, C.J.; Larson, M.G.; Chan, S.K.; Kissinger, K.B.; Kupka, M.J.; Salton, C.; Botnar, R.M.; Levy, D.; Manning, W.J. Age and Sex Distribution of Subclinical Aortic Atherosclerosis. *Arterioscler. Thromb. Vasc. Biol.* **2002**, *22*, 849–854. [CrossRef]
20. Gonzalez-Araiza, G.; Haddad, L.; Patel, S.; Karageorgiou, J. Percutaneous Embolization of a Postsurgical Prostatic Artery Pseudoaneurysm and Arteriovenous Fistula. *J. Vasc. Interv. Radiol.* **2019**, *30*, 269–271. [CrossRef]
21. della Corte, M.; Amparore, D.; Sica, M.; Clemente, E.; Mazzuca, D.; Manfredi, M.; Fiori, C.; Porpiglia, F. Pseudoaneurysm after Radical Prostatectomy: A Case Report and Narrative Literature Review. *Surgeries* **2022**, *3*, 229–241. [CrossRef]
22. Carnevale, F.C.; Moreira, A.M.; Harward, S.H.; Bhatia, S.; de Assis, A.M.; Srougi, M.; Cerri, G.G.; Antunes, A.A. Recurrence of Lower Urinary Tract Symptoms Following Prostate Artery Embolization for Benign Hyperplasia: Single Center Experience Comparing Two Techniques. *Cardiovasc. Interv. Radiol.* **2017**, *40*, 366–374. [CrossRef] [PubMed]

Disclaimer/Publisher's Note: The statements, opinions and data contained in all publications are solely those of the individual author(s) and contributor(s) and not of MDPI and/or the editor(s). MDPI and/or the editor(s) disclaim responsibility for any injury to people or property resulting from any ideas, methods, instructions or products referred to in the content.

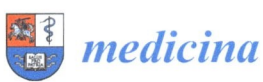

Article

Profile of Newly Diagnosed Patients with HIV Infection in North-Eastern Romania

Isabela Ioana Loghin [1,2], Andrei Vâță [1,2,*], Ioana Florina Mihai [1], George Silvaș [2], Șerban Alin Rusu [2], Cătălina Mihaela Luca [1,2,*] and Carmen Mihaela Dorobăț [2]

[1] Department of Infectious Diseases, "Grigore T. Popa" University of Medicine and Pharmacy, 700115 Iasi, Romania
[2] Department of Infectious Diseases, "St. Parascheva" Clinical Hospital of Infectious Diseases, 700116 Iasi, Romania
* Correspondence: andreiandrei@yahoo.com (A.V.); catalina_luca2006@yahoo.com (C.M.L.)

Abstract: *Background and Objectives*: Human immunodeficiency virus infection and the acquired immunodeficiency syndrome (HIV/AIDS) pandemic are unquestionably the most serious public crisis of our time. Identifying, preventing, and treating HIV-associated comorbidities remains a challenge that must be addressed even in the era of antiretroviral therapy. *Materials and Methods*: In this study, we aimed to characterize the aspects of newly diagnosed patients with HIV/AIDS, during 2021–2022 in Northeastern Romania. We reviewed the frequency and associated comorbidities of these patients in correspondence with national and global results. *Results*: Our study found that of all newly diagnosed HIV cases (167 cases—74 cases in 2021 and 98 cases in 2022), 49.70% were diagnosed with HIV infection and 50.30% had AIDS. Based on sex correlated with the CD4+ T-lymphocyte level, the most affected were males, with a lower CD4+ T-lymphocyte level overall. The average HIV viral load was 944,689.55 copies/mL. Half of males had an abnormal ALT or AST (39.53% and 49.61%); as for the females, less than a quarter had an increased value of ALT or AST, respectively (18% and 26%). The most frequent co-infections were as follows: oral candidiasis (34.73% of patients), hepatitis B (17.37% of patients), and SARS-CoV-2 infection (8.38%), followed by hepatitis C (6.39%), tuberculosis (TB), syphilis, toxoplasmosis, *Cryptococcus*, *Cytomegalovirus* infections. Males were more affected than females, with a higher percentage of co-infections. The prescribed antiretroviral treatment focused on a single-pill regimen (79.04%) to ensure adherence, effectiveness, and safety. Therefore, 20.96% had been prescribed a regimen according to their comorbidities. *Conclusions*: Our study found a concerning rise in the incidence of HIV in 2022 compared to that in 2021 in Northeastern Romania, because of the rise in post-SARS-CoV-2 pandemic addressability. Advanced immunodeficiency and the burden of opportunistic infections characterize newly diagnosed HIV patients. The physicians should keep in mind that these patients may have more than one clinical condition at presentation.

Keywords: HIV/AIDS; opportunistic infections; HBV; HCV; ART; UNAIDS

Citation: Loghin, I.I.; Vâță, A.; Mihai, I.F.; Silvaș, G.; Rusu, Ș.A.; Luca, C.M.; Dorobăț, C.M. Profile of Newly Diagnosed Patients with HIV Infection in North-Eastern Romania. *Medicina* 2023, 59, 440. https://doi.org/10.3390/medicina59030440

Academic Editors: Romica Cergan, Adrian Costache and Mihai Dumitru

Received: 30 January 2023
Revised: 20 February 2023
Accepted: 21 February 2023
Published: 23 February 2023

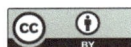

Copyright: © 2023 by the authors. Licensee MDPI, Basel, Switzerland. This article is an open access article distributed under the terms and conditions of the Creative Commons Attribution (CC BY) license (https://creativecommons.org/licenses/by/4.0/).

1. Introduction

Human immunodeficiency virus infection and the acquired immunodeficiency syndrome (HIV/AIDS) pandemic are unquestionably the most serious public crisis of our time despite the international and local efforts to combat this calamity. The life expectancy of HIV-positive individuals who receive efficient antiretroviral therapy (ART) and sustained viral suppression is close to normal. Identifying, preventing, and treating HIV-associated comorbidities remains a challenge that must be addressed even in the era of antiretroviral therapy.

Patients who have recently been diagnosed with HIV infection may be asymptomatic or develop a wide range of symptoms associated with opportunistic infections, acute seroconversion disease, or other disorders [1].

HIV infection can spread through three different routes: parenteral, vertical, and sexual. Among women, heterosexual transmission has decreased substantially in Europe in recent years. While transmission through injected drug use has declined steadily since 2012, it remains high in the East [2].

In addition to traditional risk factors, such as age, dyslipidemia, diabetes, lipodystrophy, high blood pressure, obesity, smoking, and drug use, comorbidities may be caused by HIV infection itself (through microbial translocation, low-grade persistent chronic inflammation, immune system activation, and pro-coagulant mechanisms), co-infections (with hepatitis viruses, herpes viruses), opportunistic infections (*Myco-bacterium tuberculosis, Cryptococcus neoformans, Pneumocystis jiroveci*) and ART (toxicities, drug–drug interactions) [3]. The Joint United Nations Programme on HIV/AIDS (UNAIDS) confirmed that 38.4 million people globally were infected with HIV in 2021 from which 1.5 million people became newly infected with HIV in the year 2021 and 650,000 people died from AIDS-related illnesses in 2021.

New HIV infections have been reduced by 54% since their peak in 1996. In 2021, around 1.5 million people were newly infected with HIV, compared to 3.2 million people in 1996. Women and girls accounted for 49% of all new infections in 2021. Since 2010, new HIV infections have declined by 32%, from 2.2 million to 1.5 million. Since 2010, new HIV infections among children have declined by 52%, from 320,000 in 2010 to 160,000 in 2021.

On World AIDS Day 2014, UNAIDS set targets aimed at ending the AIDS epidemic by 2030. To achieve this, countries are working toward reaching the interim "95-95-95" targets of 95% of people living with HIV knowing their HIV status, 95% of people who know their HIV positive status based on treatment, and 95% of people on treatment with suppressed viral loads—by 2025. Of all people living with HIV, 85% knew their status, 75% were accessing treatment, and 68% were virally suppressed in 2021 [4].

In Romania, The National Institute of Infectious Diseases "Prof. Dr. Matei Balș" published statistics stating that since the beginning of 2022 up until the end of September 2022, 445 new HIV–AIDS patients were identified, from which 126 had passed away due to HIV–AIDS-associated conditions [3]. From 1985 to 2022, Romania recorded 26,791 HIV-infected cases, from which there were 10,053 pediatric cases, 16,738 adult cases, and 8293 patients passed away during this period [5].

In this study, we aimed to characterize the aspects of newly diagnosed patients with HIV/AIDS, during 2021–2022 in Northeastern Romania. We reviewed the frequency and associated comorbidities of the newly diagnosed patients with HIV infection in correspondence with national and global results.

2. Materials and Methods

2.1. Database Description

We conducted a retrospective clinical study, based on hospital medical records of newly diagnosed patients with HIV/AIDS, in Northeastern Romania, hospitalized in the "Sf. Parascheva" Clinical Hospital of Infectious Diseases from Iasi, aiming to highlight the profile and associated comorbidities of the new HIV/AIDS cases, in the context of the SARS CoV-2 pandemic. The studied period was between 1 January 2021 and 31 December 2022.

Inclusion criteria selected patients over 18-years-old with an HIV-positive enzyme-linked immunosorbent assay (ELISA) test and confirmation of HIV/AIDS infection via Western blotting (WB), hospitalized in our Regional HIV/AIDS Center of Northeastern Romania. Patients who tested positive for HIV/AIDS infection were also evaluated based on the HIV plasma viral load and CD4+ T cell levels. Our study group included 74 patients in 2021 and 93 patients in 2022.

The study obtained the approval of the Ethics Committee of the "Sf. Parascheva" Clinical Hospital of Infectious Diseases, Iasi, Romania. (Approval No. 32/5 December 2022). All participants signed informed consent at the time of admission.

The collected data included demographic aspects (age, sex), personal pathological antecedents, clinical characteristics, blood tests (viro-immunological testing), assessment of potential associated opportunistic infections, patient staging, antiretroviral treatment initiated, and the evolution and prognosis after therapy of patients newly diagnosed with HIV/AIDS infection.

The HIV infection stage, based on age-specific CD4+ T-lymphocyte counts or CD4+ T-lymphocyte percentage of total lymphocytes CD4 T cells level, was established according to the Centers for Disease Control and Prevention (CDC) Atlanta Classification—surveillance data on HIV infection and AIDS: stage 1, when the CD4+ T-lymphocyte level is $\geq$500 cells/μL; stage 2, CD4+ T-lymphocytes between 200 and 499 cells/μL; and stage 3, a CD4+ T-lymphocyte level $\leq$200 cells/μL. Stages 1 and 2 represent HIV infection and stage 3 is associated with AIDS [4,6].

The people suspected of having HIV were serologically evaluated through two ELISA tests, and the serological confirmation was achieved by performing the Western blot test. All this was carried out by the epidemiologists within the regional public health management network, and later, the patients were directed to the regional HIV/AIDS center.

All blood tests were performed by the hospital's central laboratory, and the HIV plasmatic viral load and CD4+ T cell level were assessed by the hospital's molecular biology laboratory. The method used for identifying HIV viremia, as well as monitoring the viral load levels, was a measurement based on RT-PCR HIV 1 using Cepheid's GeneXpert® (Headquarters: Sunnyvale, California, U.S, Factory: Solna, Sweden). The viral load was considered undetectable when values were under 40 copies/mL and detectable when values were above 40 copies/mL.

All newly diagnosed PWH (people with HIV) were clinically and biologically evaluated periodically, for metabolic syndrome and liver enzymes. The laboratory reference values were between 5 and 31 UI/l for ALT (alanine transaminase) and for AST (aspartate transaminase), between 7 and 32 UI/l for GGT (gamma-glutamyl transferase), between 122 and 200 mg/dL for COL (cholesterol), between 40 and 66 mg/dL for HDL-COL (high-density lipoprotein cholesterol), 30 and 159 mg/dL for LDL-COL (low-density lipoprotein cholesterol), and 30 and 150 mg/dL for TG (triglycerides), with no differences between sexes.

2.2. Statistical Analysis

The correlation analysis among demographic parameters, clinical data, and outcomes was performed using the Pearson test in XLSTAT version 2019 software (ADDINSOFT, Paris, France) Kendall's Tau correlation coefficients were calculated (11). Statistical analysis was performed using Statistical Software for Excel (XLSTAT) version 2019 (Addinsoft, New York, NY, USA).

3. Results

In the Northeastern part of Romania, in 2022 and 2021, there was a total of 167 cases (93 in 2022, representing 55.69%, and 74 cases in 2021, representing 44.31%), and HIV infection was most frequent in men (129 cases, 77.25%) than in women (38 cases, 22.75%) (Figure 1).

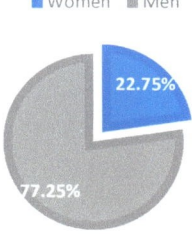

Figure 1. Distribution of new HIV/AIDS cases by sex.

The majority of cases were young adults, aged between 31- and 40-years-old—67 patients (40.12%), followed by the age group 21–30—48 patients (28.74%), 41–50 years—22 patients (13.17%), 51–60-years-old—11 patients (6.59%), over 61-years-old—10 patients (6.99%), and 0–20 years—9 patients (5.39%) (Table 1). The average age in the study group was 35-years-old.

Table 1. Distribution of new HIV/AIDS cases by age.

Age (Years)	n	%
0–20	9	5.39
21–30	48	28.74
31–40	67	40.12
41–50	22	13.17
51–60	11	6.59
over 61	10	5.99

The distribution of our study group based on county showed that almost a third of the patients were from Iasi (48 cases, 28.74%), followed by Bacau (35 cases, 20.96%), Neamt (31 cases, 18.56%), Suceava (31 cases, 18.56%), Botosani (16 cases, 9.58%), and Vaslui (6 cases, 3.59%) (Table 2). From the urban area in Northeast Romania, there were 101 patients (60.48%), and the remaining 66 cases (39.52%) were from rural areas (Figure 2).

Table 2. Distribution of new HIV/AIDS cases by county in Northeast Romania.

County	n	%
Iasi	48	28.74
Neamt	31	18.56
Vaslui	6	3.59
Bacau	35	20.96
Botosani	16	9.58
Suceava	31	18.56

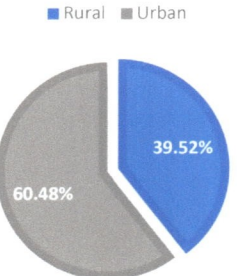

Figure 2. New HIV/AIDS cases, distribution by area.

Considering the route of transmission, only 159 cases (95.21%) reported a possible cause. For the remaining eight cases (4.79%), the route of transmission remains unknown (Table 3).

Table 3. Route of transmission of the study group.

	n	%
Route of transmission	159	95.21
Sexual (heterosexual and MSM)	151	90.42
Intravenous drug-use	5	2.99
Perinatal	3	1.8
Unknown	8	4.79

Regarding the sexual route of transmission (heterosexual and MSM/men having sex with men—90.42% cases), the most affected group was young adult males (aged 21–40) with a medium education level. Intravenous drug use was recorded at 2.99% with three perinatal cases (1.8%).

All of the newly diagnosed patients from the Iasi HIV/AIDS Regional Center between 1 January 2021 and 31 December 2022 were virologically and immunologically evaluated.

It was observed that 43.11% of cases had a CD4+ T-lymphocyte level between 1 and 199 cells/μL, 37.72% of cases had a CD4+ T-lymphocyte value between 200 and 499 cells/μL, and 19.16% had CD4+ T-lymphocyte values over 500 cells/μL, with an average CD4+ T-lymphocyte level of 300.45 cells/μL (Table 4, Figures 3 and 4).

Based on gender correlated with the CD4+ T-lymphocyte level, the most affected were males, with a lower CD4+ T-lymphocyte level overall. The average HIV viral load was 944,689.55 copies/mL.

We used the CDC (Center for Disease Control and Prevention) stages of HIV/AIDS, and the results showed the following: 32 patients were stage 1 HIV infection (19.16%), 51 patients were in the 2nd stage (30.54%), and 84 patients in the 3rd stage (50.3%) (Table 5).

Table 4. Distribution of new HIV/AIDS cases by CD4+ T-lymphocyte level and sex.

CD4+ T-lymphocyte Level $p \geq 0.05$	Male		Female		Total	
	n	%	n	%	N	%
0–199 cells/μL	58	34.73	14	8.38	72	43.11
200–499 cells/μL	52	31.14	11	6.59	63	37.72
>500 cells/μL	19	11.38	13	7.78	32	19.16

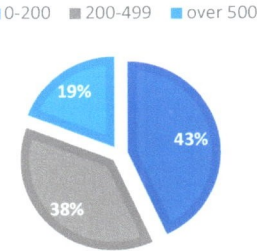

Figure 3. Distribution of cases by CD4+ T-lymphocyte level (cells/μL).

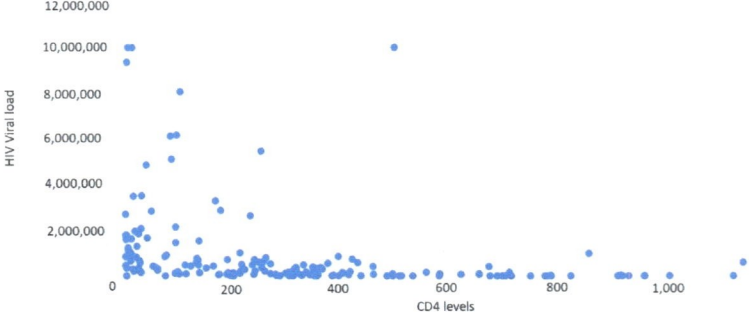

Figure 4. Distribution of new HIV/AIDS cases by CD4+ T-lymphocyte level and HIV viral load.

Table 5. Distribution of study cases by CDC, HIV/AIDS classification.

Classification of the Studied Cases	n	%
Stage 1	32	19.16
Stage 2	51	30.54
Stage 3	84	50.30

In the study group, it was observed that almost half of the males had an abnormal ALT or AST (39.53% and 49.61%); as for the females, less than a quarter had an increased value of ALT or AST, respectively (18% and 26%). Of 39.53% of the males with an abnormal ALT value, 5.43% (7 cases) had hepatitis B, 0.78% (1 case) had hepatitis C, and only 9.3% (12 cases) declared occasional alcohol consumption. Of 49.61% of male patients with abnormal AST, 3.1% (4 cases) had hepatitis B, 1.55% (2 cases) had hepatitis C, and only 12.48% (16 cases) declared occasional alcohol consumption. The rest of the patients did not have an identified cause of elevated transaminase values.

Regarding the metabolic profile, cholesterol levels were increased in a third of the study group, regardless of sex (31.01% males and 34% females); the triglyceride levels were more than a third, affecting almost equally both sexes (44.19% males and 39% females) (Table 6).

Table 6. Distribution of cases based on sex and metabolic syndrome and liver enzymes.

Laboratory Marker	Value	Male		Female		Total	
		n	%	N	%	N	%
ALT	normal	78	60.47	31	82	109	65.27
	abnormal	51	39.53	7	18	58	34.73
AST	normal	65	50.39	28	74	93	55.69
	abnormal	64	49.61	10	26	74	44.31
GGT	normal	65	50.39	32	84	97	58.08
	abnormal	64	49.61	6	16	70	41.92
Cholesterol	normal	89	68.99	25	66	114	68.26
	abnormal	40	31.01	13	34	53	31.74
HDL-COL	normal	123	95.35	35	92	158	94.61
	abnormal	6	4.65	3	8	9	5.39
LDL-COL	normal	103	79.84	31	82	134	80.24
	abnormal	26	20.16	7	18	33	19.76
Triglycerides	normal	72	55.81	23	61	95	56.89
	abnormal	57	44.19	15	39	72	43.11

The study group was screened for the most common co-infections associated with HIV/AIDS. The results showed that two-thirds (65.87%) of the patients admitted to our clinic in the studied period had different opportunistic infections. Many of the opportunistic infections were identified in stages 2 and 3 (25.75%, and 32.34%), when the CD4 T-lymphocyte level was under 500 cells/μL (Table 7).

Table 7. Distribution of opportunistic infections by CDC stage in our study group.

HIV/AIDS Status	Stage 1		Stage 2		Stage 3		Total	
	n	%	n	%	N	%	N	%
No opportunistic infections	18	10.78	15	8.98	24	14.37	57	34.13
Opportunistic infections	13	7.78	43	25.75	54	32.34	110	65.87

The results showed that the most frequent co-infections were oral candidiasis (34.73% of patients), hepatitis B (17.37% of patients), and SARS-CoV-2 infection (8.38%), followed by hepatitis C (6.39%). To a lesser extent, cases of tuberculosis (TB), syphilis, toxoplasmosis, *Cryptococcus*, *Cytomegalic virus* (CMV), *Herpes virus*, and *varicella-zoster virus* (VZV) infections were recorded. Males were more affected than females, with a higher percentage of co-infections (Table 8).

Table 8. Distribution of new HIV/AIDS cases by co-infections.

Co-Infections	Men		Women		Total	
$p < 0.05$	n	%	n	%	n	%
HBV	15	8.98	14	8.38	29	17.37
HCV	6	3.59	5	2.99	11	6.59
TB	8	4.79	1	0.60	9	5.39
Syphilis	1	0.60	2	1.20	3	1.80
Candidiasis	39	23.35	19	11.38	58	34.73
Toxoplasmosis	3	1.80	0	0.00	3	1.80
CMV	1	0.60	1	0.60	2	1.20
VZV	4	2.40	1	0.60	5	2.99
Herpesviruses	3	1.80	1	0.60	4	2.40
Cryptococcus	1	0.60	0	0.00	1	0.60
SARS CoV-2	6	3.59	8	4.79	14	8.38

All of the newly diagnosed patients in the Iasi HIV/AIDS Regional Center were prescribed ART (antiretroviral treatment) with a focus on a single-pill regimen to ensure adherence to treatment. Therefore, 79.04% of cases were prescribed a single-pill regimen, and the remaining 20.96% had been prescribed a regimen that took into account their comorbidities (Table 9). The treatment was initiated as soon as the diagnosis and antiretroviral therapy were established. The period of time between diagnosis and ART initiation ranged between 72 h and 14 days according to the severity of the cases, in order to avoid IRIS (immune reconstruction inflammatory syndrome), also following www.hiv-druginteractions.org.

Table 9. Distribution of new HIV/AIDS cases by ART regimen.

ART Regimen	N	%
BIC/FTC/TAF (Bictegravir/Emtricitabine/Tenofovir alafenamide)	56	33.53
DTG/3TC (Dolutegravir/Lamivudine)	38	22.75
DOR/3TC/TDF (Doravirine/Lamivudine/Tenofovir disoproxil)	33	19.76
DTG/ABC/3TC (Dolutegravir/Abacavir/Lamivudine)	5	2.99
Other	35	20.96

The patients were evaluated after one month, and the viro-immunological status showed, in Table 9, an increased CD4+ T-lymphocyte level and a significant decrease in HIV viremia. As such, 56 patients (33.53%) had a CD4 value between 1 and 199 cells/µL, 74 patients (44.31%) had a value between 200 and 499 cells/µL, and 37 patients (22.16%) had a value above 500 cells/µL. The median CD4 value was 363.52 cells/µL. The average HIV viral load was 57,907.2 copies/mL. In both sexes, most of the cases had a CD4+ T-lymphocyte level between 200 and 499 cells/µL (Table 10, Figure 5).

Table 10. Distribution by CD4+ T-lymphocyte level and sex, one month after ART.

CD4 Levels $p \leq 0.05$	Male		Female		Total	
	n	%	n	%	n	%
0–200 cells/µL	47	28.14	9	5.39	56	33.53
200–499 cells/µL	59	35.33	15	8.98	74	44.31
>500 cells/µL	23	13.77	14	8.38	37	22.16

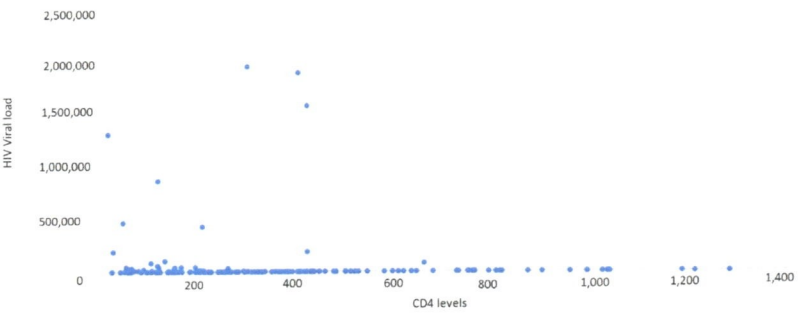

Figure 5. Distribution of HIV/AIDS cases by CD4+ T-lymphocytes level and HIV viral load, one month after ART.

The patients were initially evaluated at diagnosis and then one month after starting ART. The HIV viral load showed a significant decrease after starting antiretroviral therapy, with viral suppression being obtained in 50.9% of cases (85 cases) (Table 11).

Table 11. Distribution by HIV viral load level, at initial assessment, and one month after ART.

HIV Viral Load ($p < 0.05$)	Initial Assessment		One Month after ART	
	n	%	n	%
Undetectable (<40 copies/mL)	9	5.39	85	50.9
Detectable >40 copies/mL	158	94.6	82	49.1

4. Discussion

HIV infection is becoming a chronic disease because of effective ART treatment regimens. More HIV-infected patients are developing additional chronic diseases due to an increase in the quality of life, which is becoming close to normal. HIV-related healthcare requirements will rise, putting more strain on health systems and significantly impacting public health.

Our study found that of all the newly diagnosed HIV cases (167 cases), 49.70% were diagnosed with HIV infection and 50.30% had AIDS-related symptoms. Moreover, we found a concerning rise in the incidence of HIV in 2022 (93 cases) compared to that in 2021 (74 cases) in our region (North-eastern Romania), probably because of the rise in post-SARS-CoV-2 pandemic addressability.

The number of new HIV diagnoses in 2021 in Europe was 16,624 cases, with 40% (6648 cases) of all new HIV diagnoses in 2021 and more than half (55%) of diagnoses with the route of transmission known. MSM continues to be the most common method of HIV transmission recorded in the European Union. More than 60% of new HIV diagnoses, among those with a documented route of HIV transmission, were caused by sexual contact between men. In Europe, heterosexual contact accounted for 29% (4848 cases) of HIV infections, and in 40% of the number of cases, the mode of transmission was known, making it the second most often reported mode of HIV transmission. Nearly 4% of HIV diagnoses in 2021 were attributable to the transmission through injected drugs. Less than 1% of new HIV diagnoses in Europe in 2021 were attributable to vertical transmission, while 27% of new HIV diagnoses did not have a known mode of transmission. In East Europe, in 2020, HIV infection in new cases was transmitted through sex between men 3.1%, heterosexual transmission (men) at 32.7%, heterosexual transmission (women) at 32.6%, injected drug use at 28.1%, mother-to-child transmission at 28.1%, and unknown at 3.0%. In our region, we had similar results; from 159 cases, the most frequent was sexual transmission (heterosexual contact and MSM) (90.42%), with only a few known cases of intravenous drug usage and perinatal cases.

In the WHO European Region, 43 countries reported 8.194 new AIDS cases in 2021, with a diagnosis rate of 1.2 per 100,000 people. Over the past ten years, the number of AIDS cases has steadily decreased in the West, European Union, and the East. Furthermore, in the East, the number of infections stabilized between 2012 and 2018 and even decreased in 2019. The rate continued to fall in 2020–2021, though it is possible that this was because of the COVID-19 pandemic's impact on reporting [2]. In our region, we also found a decreasing rate; in 2021, we had admitted, from a total of 159 cases, 74 patients (44.31%), and in 2022, 93 patients (55.69%).

In a study from South Asia, it was found that the mean age of HIV/AIDS patients was 36.38 ± 10.62 years. The data presented are consistent with those from our study (mean age of our study group—35.35). The most common symptoms were fever (28.89%), weight loss (28.61%), and generalized weakness (22.22%). The overall mean CD4 count was 176.04 ± 163.49 cells/mm^3. Regarding the results from our study group, the mean CD4 count was 300.45 cells/mm^3. There were 224 opportunistic infections documented in 160 patients, with opportunistic diarrhea (12.22%) and pulmonary tuberculosis (10.83%) being the most common. In our study group, opportunistic infections were documented in two-thirds of the patients (65.87%). The majority of the patients (80.83%) were eligible for the initiation of first-line antiretrovirals at presentation, while all patients from our clinic initiated antiretroviral therapy [7].

In a cohort from Morocco, they treated 525 patients with new HIV diagnoses during the course of 18 months. The sex ratio was 1:1, and the mean age was 36.1 years. While the sex ratio in our study was 3:1, the mean age had similar results (35.35). In 47.8% of instances, the seropositivity was identified based on an evocative symptom. The two primary clinical signs were oral candidiasis (11.2%) and weight loss (16.6%). The majority (23%) of opportunistic infections were tuberculosis. A stage of acquired immunodeficiency syndrome (AIDS) diagnosis was made in 36.1% of cases. In our research, we found that almost half of the patients newly diagnosed were in the AIDS stage. The first CD4 count and viral load tested had median values of $248/mm^3$ and 88.174 copies/mL, respectively, results comparable with our paper (median CD4 count, 300.45 cells/mm^3), but the median viral load was increasingly higher (944,689.55 copies/mL) [8].

Gokengin D et. al. realized a survey about HIV care, which included twenty-four countries (Albania, Armenia, Azerbaijan, Bosnia and Herzegovina, Bulgaria, Croatia, Czech Republic, Estonia, Georgia, Hungary, Kazakhstan, Kosovo, Kyrgyz Republic, FYR of Macedonia, Moldova, Montenegro, Poland, Romania, Russian Federation, Serbia, Slovak Republic, Slovenia, Turkey, and Uzbekistan) out of 31 (77.4%) from Central and Eastern Europe. The major route of transmission was MSM (41.7%, 10/24 countries), followed by heterosexual contact (37.5%, 9/24 countries) and injected drug use (20.8%, 5/24 countries). Men who have sex with men (MSM) (14/24, 58.3%), persons who inject drugs (15/24, 62.5%), and sex workers (12/24, 50.0%) were among the other categories subjected to targeted screening. Pregnant women were only screened in 14 of the 24 countries (58.3%) [9]. The frequency in transmission routes was similar to that in our region.

In a Spanish study, from a total of 1398 HIV-positive individuals, 2.1% of the infections involved injected drugs or slam practices, and 97.9% of the infections were sexually transmitted. The median age was 32.9 years, comparable to our results, and 40.1% of the population was Latin American [10].

In a study from France about comorbidities in people living with HIV in comparison to those in non-HIV people, the researchers showed that PWH had significantly higher rates of alcohol abuse (5.8% vs. 3.1%), chronic renal disease (1.2% vs. 0.3%), cardiovascular disease (7.4% vs. 5.1%), dyslipidemia (22% vs. 15.9%), and hepatitis B (3.8% vs. 0.1%) [11]. Moreover, PWH had higher rates of other comorbidities, including anemia, malnutrition, mental disorders, and tumors [12].

Other researchers observed that the most common non-related HIV-comorbidities were vitamin D deficiency (29.1%), depressive episodes (27.8%), arterial hypertension (16.3%), and hypercholesterolemia (10.8%) in people with HIV in Germany [13]. Another German study found that the prevalence in PWH compared to that in the matched non-HIV cohort of acute renal disease (0.5% vs. 0.2%), bone fractures due to osteoporosis (6.4% vs. 2.1%), chronic renal disease (4.3% vs. 2.4%), cardiovascular disease (12.8% vs. 10.4%), Hepatitis B (5.9% vs. 0.3%), and Hepatitis C infection (8.8% vs. 0.3%) was significantly higher in PWH [14]. Our study showed that the most frequent co-infections/comorbidities were oral candidiasis (34.73%), hepatitis B (17.37%), SARS-CoV-2 infection (8.38%), and hepatitis C (6.39%).

Roomaney et al. found that cardiovascular diseases were more frequent in people with HIV (especially hypertension: 13.3%), and the next prevalent comorbidities were pulmonary diseases (tuberculosis was the main cause: 3.5%), followed by metabolic diseases, such as diabetes (3.0%) and cancer (0.4%). Elderly people were more likely to contract any of the diseases. In general, the prevalence of diseases, such as cancer, diabetes, heart disease, and hypertension, was higher in women [15].

Another recent study observed that HIV infections were seen more in males than in females, a fact that our study showed as well. A significant decrease in the complete blood count was observed in HIV patients when compared to that in healthy individuals. A significant increase in aspartate aminotransferase (AST), alanine aminotransferase (ALT), urea, and creatinine was observed in HIV patients, with results comparable with ours. No significant difference was observed in alkaline phosphatase (ALP), total bilirubin, and albumin levels when compared to those in the healthy controls. Anemia was observed in 59.4% of HIV patients. A total of three (8.1%) patients were found to be co-infected with hepatitis B and one (2.7%) was co-infected with hepatitis C. Our study aimed to correlate hepatitis B or C co-infection in HIV/AIDS patients with comparable results [16,17].

Harklerode et al. found that of the 8664 newly discovered HIV cases throughout the trial period on the territory of Kenia, 3.1% had an HIV retest after the first diagnosis. About half (45.3%) had links to care documented. The median CD4 count at baseline was 332 cells/mm^3. Our study group's mean CD4 count was 300.45 cells/mm^3, and 53.0% of those newly diagnosed with HIV who had received a CD4 test and were 15 years old or older did so at a late stage, with 32.9% already having advanced HIV. Being male and older than 34 years of age were two characteristics linked to a late diagnosis [18].

A clustering of common comorbidities, such as cardiovascular diseases, metabolic disorders, sexually transmitted diseases (STDs), and mental health issues, was identified in two different cohorts of PWH [19,20], further extending our knowledge of comorbidity profiles in HIV. Importantly, it was revealed that these illnesses did not occur together randomly [21,22]. Our evaluation focused on the most common coinfections, although the study group was screened periodically for other possible illnesses. In our cohort of patients, the most frequent co-infections were oral candidiasis (34.73%), hepatitis B (17.37%), SARS-CoV-2 infection (8.38%), and hepatitis C (6.39%).

Among PWH from middle- and low-income countries, it was found that the summary risk for oral candidiasis, tuberculosis, herpes zoster, and bacterial pneumonia was highest (>5%) among ART-naive patients. With the exception of tuberculosis, all opportunistic infections experienced a reduction in incidence over the first year of ART (range: 57–91%). The reductions were greatest for oral candidiasis, *Pneumocystis* pneumonia, and toxoplasmosis [23,24]. To a lesser extent, cases of tuberculosis (TB) (5.39%), syphilis (1.80%), toxoplasmosis (1.80%), *Cryptococcus* (0.60%), *Cytomegalic virus* (CMV) (1.20%), *Herpes virus*, and *varicella-zoster virus* (VZV) (2.40%) infections were recorded. The favorable evolution after ART was described in Romania, which used a single-pill regimen, also adapted to patient's comorbidities according to www.hiv-druginteractions.org [25,26].

Our results can be comparable to those of other studies, but on a smaller scale, given the size of the study group [27,28]. To create the most efficient healthcare programs possible, especially with the aging population, the medical multidisciplinary team must provide the patients with the resources they need to inform themselves about their disease and effectively manage their illness [29,30].

5. Conclusions

Our study found a concerning rise in the incidence of HIV in 2022 compared to that in 2021 in our region, probably because of the rise in post-SARS-COV-2 pandemic addressability.

Advanced immunodeficiency and the burden of opportunistic infections characterize newly diagnosed HIV patients. The physicians should keep in mind that these patients may have more than one clinical condition at presentation.

HIV infection is still detected after a long period in our country, despite decent antiretroviral coverage. The encouragement of voluntary testing, particularly among those at a high risk of infection (medical personnel, men having sex with men, people who inject drugs, youth under 24-years-old, sex workers, and people who are economically disadvantaged), must be the focus.

Additionally, we need to make HIV testing more accessible, with community outreach efforts being especially helpful. These outreach efforts should always be supported by assisted counseling and prompt referral to medical facilities to begin ART.

Author Contributions: Conceptualization, I.I.L. and C.M.D.; Data curation, I.I.L., A.V. and I.F.M.; Formal analysis, I.F.M. and Ș.A.R.; Investigation, I.I.L. and C.M.D.; Methodology, I.I.L. and A.V.; Resources, C.M.L.; Software, G.S. and Ș.A.R.; Supervision, C.M.D.; Validation, I.I.L., C.M.L. and C.M.D.; Visualization, I.I.L. and C.M.D.; Writing—original draft, I.I.L. and G.S.; Writing—review & editing, A.V. All authors have read and agreed to the published version of the manuscript.

Funding: This research received no external funding.

Institutional Review Board Statement: The study was conducted in accordance with the Declaration of Helsinki and approved by the Ethics Committee of the "Sf. Parascheva" Clinical Hospital of Infectious Diseases, Iasi, Romania. (Approval No. 32/5 December 2022).

Informed Consent Statement: This was a retrospective study, and written informed consent had been obtained from the patients when they were admitted to our hospital, according to the hospital policy.

Data Availability Statement: All data generated or analyzed during this study are included in this published article.

Conflicts of Interest: The authors declare no conflict of interest.

References

1. Govender, R.D.; Hashim, M.J.; Khan, M.A.; Mustafa, H.; Khan, G. Global Epidemiology of HIV/AIDS: A Resurgence in North America and Europe. *J. Epidemiol. Glob. Health* **2021**, *11*, 296–301. [CrossRef]
2. HIV/AIDS Surveillance in Europe 2021 Data. Available online: https://www.ecdc.europa.eu/sites/default/files/documents/2022-Annual_HIV_Report_final.pdf (accessed on 28 November 2022).
3. Streinu-Cercel, A.; Săndulescu, O.; Piano, C.; Dorobanțu, M.; Mircescu, G.; Lăzureanu, V.E.; Dumitru, I.M.; Chirilă, O.; Streinu-Cercel, A.; Extended Consensus Group. Consensus statement on the assessment of comorbidities in people living with HIV in Romania. *Germs* **2019**, *9*, 198–210. [CrossRef]
4. UNAIDS. *Global HIV Statistics 2022 Fact Sheet*; UNAIDS: Geneva, Switzerland, 2022.
5. EVOLUȚIA HIV ÎN ROMÂNIA—30 SEPTEMBRIE 2022, Institutul Național de Boli Infecțioase "Prof. Dr. Matei Balș"; Bucuresti. 2022. Available online: https://www.cnlas.ro/images/doc/01122022.pdf (accessed on 17 December 2022).
6. Available online: https://www.cdc.gov/hiv/statistics/surveillance/terms.html (accessed on 20 December 2022).
7. Bishnu, S.; Bandyopadhyay, D.; Samui, S.; Das, I.; Mondal, P.; Ghosh, P.; Roy, D.; Manna, S. Assessment of clinico-immunological profile of newly diagnosed HIV patients presenting to a teaching hospital of eastern India. *Indian J. Med. Res.* **2014**, *139*, 903–912. [PubMed]
8. Lyazidi, S.; Marih, L.; Marhoum El Filai, K.; Hassoune, S.; Nani, S.; Sodqi, M. Clinical and biological profile of newly diagnosed HIV-infected patients in Casablanca. *Eur. J. Public Health* **2021**, *31* (Suppl. 3), ckab165.477. [CrossRef]
9. Gokengin, D.; Oprea, C.; Begovac, J.; Horban, A.; Zeka, A.N.; Sedlacek, D.; Allabergan, B.; Almamedova, E.A.; Balayan, T.; Banhegyi, D.; et al. HIV care in Central and Eastern Europe: How close are we to the target? *Int. J. Infect. Dis.* **2018**, *70*, 121–130. [CrossRef] [PubMed]
10. Ayerdi Aguirrebengoa, O.; Vera Garcia, M.; Puerta López, T.; Clavo Escribano, P.; Ballesteros Martín, J.; Lejarrag Cañas, C.; Fuentes Ferrer, E.; Raposo Utrilla, M.; Estrada Perez, V.; Del Romero Guerrero, J.; et al. Changes in the profile of newly HIV-diagnosed men who have sex with men, Madrid, 2014 to 2019. *Euro Surveill.* **2021**, *26*, 2001501. [CrossRef]
11. McLeod, A.I. Kendall rank correlation and Mann-Kendall trend test. *R Package Kendall* **2005**, *602*, 1–10.
12. d'Arminio Monforte, A.; Bonnet, F.; Bucher, H.C.; Pourcher, V.; Pantazis, N.; Pelchen-Matthews, A.; Touloumi, G.; Wolf, E. What do the changing patterns of comorbidity burden in people living with HIV mean for long-term management? Perspectives from European HIV cohorts. *HIV Med.* **2020**, *21* (Suppl. 2), 3–16. [CrossRef] [PubMed]
13. Funke, B.; Spinner, C.D.; Wolf, E.; Heiken, H.; Christensen, S.; Stellbrink, H.J.; Witte, V. High prevalence of comorbidities and use of concomitant medication in treated people living with HIV in Germany—Results of the BESIDE study. *Int. J. STD AIDS* **2021**, *32*, 152–161. [CrossRef]
14. Christensen, S.; Wolf, E.; Altevers, J.; Diaz-Cuervo, H. Comorbidities and costs in HIV patients: A retrospective claims database analysis in Germany. *PLoS ONE* **2019**, *14*, e0224279. [CrossRef] [PubMed]
15. Roomaney, R.A.; van Wyk, B.; Pillay-van Wyk, V. Aging with HIV: Increased Risk of HIV Comorbidities in Older Adults. *Int. J. Environ. Res. Public Health* **2022**, *19*, 2359. [CrossRef]
16. Anjum, A.; Rehman Au Siddique, H.; Rabaan, A.A.; Alhumaid, S.; Garout, M.; Almuthree, S.A.; Halwani, M.A.; Turkistani, S.A.; Qutob, H.; Albayat, H.; et al. Evaluation of Hematological, Biochemical Profiles and Molecular Detection of Envelope Gene (gp-41) in Human Immunodeficiency Virus (HIV) among Newly Diagnosed Patients. *Medicina* **2023**, *59*, 93. [CrossRef]
17. Palacios-Baena, Z.R.; Martín-Ortega, M.; Ríos-Villegas, M.J. Profile of new HIV diagnoses and risk factors associated with late diagnosis in a specialized outpatient clinic during the 2014–2018 period. *Med. Clin.* **2020**, *155*, 482–487. [CrossRef] [PubMed]

18. Harklerode, R.; Waruiru, W.; Humwa, F.; Waruru, A.; Kellogg, T.; Muthoni, L.; Macharia, J.; Zielinski-Gutierrez, E. Epidemiological profile of individuals diagnosed with HIV: Results from the preliminary phase of case-based surveillance in Kenya. *AIDS Care* **2020**, *32*, 43–49. [CrossRef]
19. De Francesco, D.; Underwood, J.; Post, F.A.; Vera, J.H.; Williams, I.; Boffito, M.; Sachikonye, M.; Anderson, J.; Mallon, P.W.G.; Winston, A.; et al. Defining cognitive impairment in people-living-with-HIV: The POPPY study. *BMC Infect. Dis.* **2016**, *16*, 617. [CrossRef] [PubMed]
20. Schouten, J.; Wit, F.W.; Stolte, I.G.; Kootstra, N.A.; van der Valk, M.; Geerlings, S.E.; Prins, M.; Reiss, P. Cross-sectional comparison of the prevalence of age-associated comorbidities and their risk factors between HIV-infected and uninfected individuals: The AGEhIV cohort study. *Clin. Infect. Dis.* **2014**, *59*, 1787–1797. [CrossRef]
21. Hentzien, M.; Dramé, M.; Delpierre, C.; Allavena, C.; Cabié, A.; Cuzin, L.; Rey, D.; Pugliese, P.; Hédelin, G.; Bani-Sadr, F.; et al. HIV-related excess mortality and age-related comorbidities in patients with HIV aged ≥60: A relative survival analysis in the French Dat'AIDS cohort. *BMJ Open* **2019**, *9*, e024841. [CrossRef]
22. De Francesco, D.; Verboeket, S.O.; Underwood, J.; Bagkeris, E.; Wit, F.W.; Mallon, P.W.G.; Winston, A.; Reiss, P.; Sabin, C.A.; Pharmacokinetic and Clinical Observations in PeoPle Over fiftY (POPPY) Study and the AGEhIV Cohort Study. Patterns of co-occurring comorbidities in people living with HIV. *Open Forum Infect. Dis.* **2018**, *5*, ofy272. [CrossRef] [PubMed]
23. Low, A.; Gavriilidis, G.; Larke, N.; B-Lajoie, M.-R.; Drouin, O.; Stover, J.; Muhe, L.; Easterbrook, P. Incidence of Opportunistic Infections and the Impact of Antiretroviral Therapy Among HIV-Infected Adults in Low- and Middle-Income Countries: A Systematic Review and Meta-analysis. *Clin. Infect. Dis.* **2016**, *62*, 1595–1603. [CrossRef]
24. *European AIDS Clinical Society (EACS) Guidelines*; European AIDS Clinical Society: Brussels, Belgium, 2022; pp. 57–139.
25. Săndulescu, O.; Irimia, M.; Benea, O.E.; Mărdărescu, M.; Preoțescu, L.L.; Dorobăț, C.M.; Loghin, I.I.; Nicolau, I.C.; Jipa, R.E.; Popescu, R.Ș.; et al. Treatment initiation or switch to BIC/FTC/TAF—Real-world safety and efficacy data from two HIV centers in Romania. *Germs* **2021**, *11*, 512–522. [CrossRef]
26. Available online: https://www.hiv-druginteractions.org (accessed on 7 January 2023).
27. Loghin, I.I.; Dorobăț, C.M. *Tabloul Clinic in Infecția cu HIV în Abord Interdisciplinar în Infecția cu HIV, II-a, ed.*; Tehnopress: Iași, Romania, 2019; pp. 68–78.
28. *Management of Opportunistic Infections in HIV/AIDS Clinical Protocol for the WHO European Region*; Denmark, 2007. Available online: https://clinicalinfo.hiv.gov/en/guidelines/hiv-clinical-guidelines-adult-and-adolescent-opportunistic-infections/whats-new (accessed on 14 January 2023).
29. Feinberg, J.; Keeshin, S. Prevention and Initial Management of HIV Infection. *Ann. Intern. Med.* **2022**, *175*, ITC81–ITC96. [CrossRef] [PubMed]
30. Rutstein, S.E.; Ananworanich, J.; Fidler, S.; Johnson, C.; Sanders, E.J.; Sued, O.; Saez-Cirion, A.; Pilcher, C.D.; Fraser, C.; Cohen, M.S.; et al. Clinical and public health implications of acute and early HIV detection and treatment: A scoping review. *J. Int. AIDS Soc.* **2017**, *20*, 21579. [CrossRef] [PubMed]

Disclaimer/Publisher's Note: The statements, opinions and data contained in all publications are solely those of the individual author(s) and contributor(s) and not of MDPI and/or the editor(s). MDPI and/or the editor(s) disclaim responsibility for any injury to people or property resulting from any ideas, methods, instructions or products referred to in the content.

MDPI AG
Grosspeteranlage 5
4052 Basel
Switzerland
Tel.: +41 61 683 77 34

Medicina Editorial Office
E-mail: medicina@mdpi.com
www.mdpi.com/journal/medicina

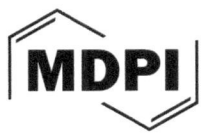

Disclaimer/Publisher's Note: The title and front matter of this reprint are at the discretion of the Guest Editors. The publisher is not responsible for their content or any associated concerns. The statements, opinions and data contained in all individual articles are solely those of the individual Editors and contributors and not of MDPI. MDPI disclaims responsibility for any injury to people or property resulting from any ideas, methods, instructions or products referred to in the content.

www.ingramcontent.com/pod-product-compliance
Lightning Source LLC
LaVergne TN
LVHW072358090526
838202LV00019B/2577